S0-AJV-099

# Progress in Psychobiology and Physiological Psychology

## Volume 9

## Contributors to This Volume

John H. Ashe

Kent Foster

Michael Gabriel

Michael E. Goldberg

Jon H. Kaas

Michael M. Merzenich

Marvin Nachman

Fernando Nottebohm

Edward Orona

Russel J. Reiter

David Lee Robinson

Barbara J. Rolls

Edmund T. Rolls

Steven E. Saltwick

Mark Stanton

Roger J. Wood

Robert H. Wurtz

# Progress in
# PSYCHOBIOLOGY AND
# PHYSIOLOGICAL PSYCHOLOGY

Edited by JAMES M. SPRAGUE

*Institute of Neurological Sciences*
*and Department of Anatomy*
*The School of Medicine*
*University of Pennsylvania*
*Philadelphia, Pennsylvania*

and ALAN N. EPSTEIN

*Institute of Neurological Sciences*
*Department of Biology*
*University of Pennsylvania*
*Philadelphia, Pennsylvania*

Volume 9

1980

**ACADEMIC PRESS**

A Subsidiary of Harcourt Brace Jovanovich, Publishers

New York • London • Toronto • Sydney • San Francisco

COPYRIGHT © 1980, BY ACADEMIC PRESS, INC.
ALL RIGHTS RESERVED.
NO PART OF THIS PUBLICATION MAY BE REPRODUCED OR
TRANSMITTED IN ANY FORM OR BY ANY MEANS, ELECTRONIC
OR MECHANICAL, INCLUDING PHOTOCOPY, RECORDING, OR ANY
INFORMATION STORAGE AND RETRIEVAL SYSTEM, WITHOUT
PERMISSION IN WRITING FROM THE PUBLISHER.

ACADEMIC PRESS, INC.
111 Fifth Avenue, New York, New York 10003

*United Kingdom Edition published by*
ACADEMIC PRESS, INC. (LONDON) LTD.
24/28 Oval Road, London NW1 7DX

LIBRARY OF CONGRESS CATALOG CARD NUMBER: 66–29640

ISBN 0–12–542109–5

PRINTED IN THE UNITED STATES OF AMERICA

80 81 82 83     9 8 7 6 5 4 3 2 1

52.05
943
r.9

# Contents

## Principles of Organization of Sensory–Perceptual Systems in Mammals

*Michael M. Merzenich and Jon H. Kaas*

## Behavioral Modulation of Visual Responses in the Monkey: Stimulus Selection for Attention and Movement

*Robert H. Wurtz, Michael E. Goldberg, and David Lee Robinson*

# Brain Pathways for Vocal Learning in Birds: A Review of the First 10 Years

*Fernando Nottebohm*

# Neuronal Activity of Cingulate Cortex, Anteroventral Thalamus, and Hippocampal Formation in Discriminative Conditioning: Encoding and Extraction of the Significance of Conditional Stimuli

*Michael Gabriel, Kent Foster, Edward Orona, Steven E. Saltwick, and Mark Stanton*

# Neural Mechanisms in Taste Aversion Learning

*John H. Ashe and Marvin Nachman*

# Contents

## Thirst: The Initiation, Maintenance, and Termination of Drinking

*Barbara J. Rolls, Roger J. Wood, and Edmund T. Rolls*

## The Pineal Gland: A Regulator of Regulators

*Russel J. Reiter*

# List of Contributors

Numbers in parentheses indicate the pages on which the authors' contributions begin.

**John H. Ashe,** Department of Physiology, University of California at San Francisco, San Francisco, California 94143 (233)

**Kent Foster,** Department of Psychology, University of Texas, Austin, Texas 78712 (125)

**Michael Gabriel,** Department of Psychology, University of Texas, Austin, Texas 78712 (125)

**Michael E. Goldberg,** Laboratory of Sensorimotor Research, National Eye Institute, National Institutes of Health, Bethesda, Maryland 20205 (43)

**Jon H. Kaas,** Departments of Psychology and Anatomy, Vanderbilt University, Nashville, Tennessee 37240 (1)

**Michael M. Merzenich,** Departments of Otolaryngology and Physiology, University of California at San Francisco, San Francisco, California 94143 (1)

**Marvin Nachman,** Department of Psychology, University of California at Riverside, Riverside, California 92502 (233)

**Fernando Nottebohm,** Department of Behavioral Science, The Rockefeller University, New York, New York 10021 (85)

**Edward Orona,** Department of Psychology, University of Texas, Austin, Texas 78712 (125)

**Russel J. Reiter,** Department of Anatomy, University of Texas Health Science Center at San Antonio, San Antonio, Texas 78284 (323)

**David Lee Robinson,** Laboratory of Sensorimotor Research, National Eye Institute, National Institutes of Health, Bethesda, Maryland 20205 (43)

**Barbara J. Rolls,** Department of Experimental Psychology, University of Oxford, Oxford OX1 3UD, Great Britain (263)

**Edmund T. Rolls,** Department of Experimental Psychology, University of Oxford, Oxford OX1 3UD, Great Britain (263)

**Steven E. Saltwick,** Department of Psychology, University of Texas, Austin, Texas 78712 (125)

**Mark Stanton,** Department of Psychology, University of Texas, Austin, Texas 78712 (125)

**Roger J. Wood,** Department of Experimental Psychology, University of Oxford, Oxford OX1 3UD, Great Britain (263)

**Robert H. Wurtz,** Laboratory of Sensorimotor Research, National Eye Institute, National Institutes of Health, Bethesda, Maryland 20205 (43)

This volume, like its predecessors in this series, attempts to provide contemporary and stimulating reviews and syntheses of selected areas of research relating brain mechanisms and behavior. The selection necessarily reflects the biases and limitations of the Editors, and therefore, is not representative of all major and important developments in this field. We believe, however, that this volume of "Progress in Psychobiology and Physiological Psychology" presents articles of high quality and value to student and expert alike.

The chapter by Merzenich and Kaas gives an insightful account of the evolution of our concepts of cortical organization relevant to perception in mammals. Many of the traditional concepts long regarded as basic to this relationship are now known to be untenable in light of recent research. Wurtz and Goldberg review in detail their studies of single unit activity in awake, behaving monkeys. The enhancement of discharge of visual neurons in different parts of cortex and in superior colliculus depends not only on the physical characteristics of the stimulus but on behavioral factors intrinsic to the animal. Some forms of enhancement may reflect alertness, some may be related to initiation and guidance of specific movements, and some may be participating in mechanisms of attention. Nottebohm has traced his interest and discoveries of the neural control of song in birds from his doctoral dissertation to the present. He stresses the importance of an animal model in the development of a vocal repertoire from auditory input. The brain pathways involved in vocal learning in birds are defined anatomically and physiologically, including the presence of hemispheric dominance and the sensitivity to steroid hormones.

The chapters by Gabriel and his colleagues and by Ashe and Nachman continue the concern of this series for the brain mechanisms of learning. Gabriel et al. describe a research venture that is succeeding in the identification of the response characteristics of the cells in the forebrain that give stimuli their significance for associative learning. Ashe and Nachman review recent work on the neuropsychological mechanisms of taste-aversion learning. They consider both the nature of the effective stimuli (conditioned and unconditioned) and the nature of the brain mechanisms that underly this theoretically important form of learning, and they describe the surprising complexities of both.

Rolls, Wood, and Rolls provide a comprehensive review of their recent work on the psychobiology of thirst. They illustrate the breadth that this problem has now achieved in the variety of mechanisms that underly drinking behavior. Their work is thoroughly comparative, ranging, as it does, from rat to man in search of both similarities and differences.

Lastly, Reiter adds to the many reasons for the renaissance of the pineal gland, that formerly "vestigial" bit of the brain that is now something of a master gland for control of photoperiodic phenomena.

In this, as in our previous volumes, a theme unites the several articles. In all, brain function is discussed but always as the machinery of behavior, and behavior, in turn, is discussed as phenomena that are indispensable for understanding how the brain works. Like the two sides of a coin, each of the two subject matters is inextricable from the other. Each is incomplete without the other. Together they yield fascination and relevance.

James M. Sprague
Alan N. Epstein

# Contents of Previous Volumes

# Progress in
# Psychobiology and
# Physiological Psychology

## Volume 9

# Principles of Organization of Sensory–Perceptual Systems in Mammals

Michael M. Merzenich

*Departments of Otolaryngology and Physiology*
*University of California at San Francisco*
*San Francisco, California*

and

Jon H. Kaas

*Departments of Psychology and Anatomy*
*Vanderbilt University*
*Nashville, Tennessee*

1

Copyright © 1980 by Academic Press, Inc.
All rights of reproduction in any form reserved.
ISBN 0-12-542109-5

# I. Introduction

A common view of the functional organization of the brain, as elaborated from the early proposals by Bolton (1900), Campbell (1905), Brodmann (1909), Elliot-Smith (1906), and others (Mott, 1907; Woolard, 1925), is that sensory input is relayed over a few subcortical stations to a single cortical receiving area, the "primary sensory cortex" with elementary sensory functions, is then sent to an adjacent cortical band of "secondary sensory" or "psychic" cortex with more complex sensory and perceptual functions, and is next relayed to multimodal "association areas" for higher order abilities requiring integration of sensory information. In this view, the "association areas" are the sources of highest level perception, and their resultant outputs can also direct activation of motor cortex to initiate appropriate behaviors. The main point of the present article is that recent electrophysiological, anatomical, and ablation-behavioral studies clearly indicate that a major revision in this traditional viewpoint is required. These studies have revealed that the auditory, somatic, and visual sensory systems all have a number of topographically ordered and complexly interconnected cortical "representations" of sensory surfaces that occupy most of the classical "psychic" and "association" cortex. In addition, interfield connections are too complex to be consistent with a simple hierarchical system of organization. Furthermore, in all three sensory systems, traditional fields have been redefined. Finally, projecting systems delivering information to cortical neurons and to newly defined cortical fields are themselves subdivisible into multiple-component parallel processing systems.

## II. Some Traditional Concepts of Forebrain Organization Relevant to the Genesis of Perception

### A. THERE ARE ONLY A FEW DIVISIONS OF THE FOREBRAIN OF FUNCTIONAL SIGNIFICANCE FOR EACH SENSORY MODALITY, AND THESE DIVISIONS FORM A SERIAL SENSATION-TO-PERCEPTION PROCESSING SEQUENCE, WITH SUCCESSIVE FIELDS PERFORMING SUCCESSIVELY "HIGHER" FUNCTIONS

This concept is most easily related to the visual system. In the traditional view of visual cortex, there are only two or three cortical divisions of functional significance. This view stemmed from early studies of experimental and pathological cases, showing that lesions in caudal occipital cortex resulted in profound disturbances of vision (described as blindness) while more rostral lesions usually produced milder changes (considered to be disruptions of "psychic" or "perceptual" functions; see Bolton, 1900, for review). At about the same time investigators, attempting to subdivide the brain on the basis of differences in histological structure, identified two or three subdivisions of occipital cortex, and, influenced by neurological findings, ascribed either "sensory" or "psychic" functions to different cytoarchitectonically delimited areas. A "sensory" area was regarded as a waystation to a "psychic" area. Thus, Bolton (1900) and Campbell (1905) described a "primary" "visuosensory" area identified by the line of Gennari, and a "secondary" "visuopsychic" area occupying the remaining occipital cortex. Brodmann (1909) and Elliot-Smith (1906) both divided the "visuopsychic" region (somewhat differently) into two bands which they related to increasingly "higher" functions, i.e., the "occipital" and "preoccipital" areas (Areas 18 and 19) of Brodmann and the "parastriate" and "peristriate" areas of Elliot-Smith. Later investigators generally accepted the proposed existence of two hierarchically related "visuopsychic" areas, and the terminology and subdivisions of Brodmann were usually adopted.

With less justification from observations on the consequences of restricted brain damage, early neuroanatomists extended the concept of a few hierarchically related functional divisions of sensory cortex to the auditory and somatosensory systems. Thus, for example, Campbell (1905) spoke of "auditosensory" and "auditopsychic" areas, as well as "somatosensory" and "somatopsychic" areas.

The early viewpoint that each sensory modality was represented by only two or three cortical areas of successively higher levels of function later received strong support from neurophysiological investigators. Most notably, Penfield and colleagues (1952, 1954) interpreted results of extensive human brain stimulation studies as revealing the locations of "sensory," "psychic," and "interpretive" regions. Although the boundaries of these regions did not clearly coincide with the architectonic subdivisions of earlier investigators, the concept of a few hierarchically related regions was strongly reinforced. Similarly, Woolsey (Woolsey and Fairman, 1946; Woolsey, 1958) concluded from evoked potential mapping studies in primates and other mammals that there were two topographic representations in each sensory system, a "primary" and "secondary" area (i.e., AI and AII, SI and SII, V-I and V-II), and, in primates, very large adjoining regions of "association" cortex. Again, these studies reinforced the concept of a tripartite low-to-high level sensory-to-perceptual cortical hierarchy.

Finally, the elegant single unit experiments of Hubel and Wiesel (1965) were interpreted within the framework of a three-level hierarchy of visual areas (V-I, V-II, and V-III). Together with the clear evidence from the studies of Klüver and Bucy (1939) that the temporal lobes of monkeys are important in vision, the view that a three- or four-element hierarchial processing series exists in the visual system became commonly accepted.

B. ORDERLY REPRESENTATIONS OF RECEPTOR
   SURFACES ARE IMPORTANT IN THE EARLY STAGES
   OF SENSORY PROCESSING, BUT ARE NOT
   NECESSARY IN LATER STAGES WHICH DEAL WITH
   ABSTRACTIONS AND HIGHER ORDER FUNCTIONS

A widespread presumption has been that orderly representations of sensory epithelia are limited to a few brain stem structures and to cortical areas "early" in the sensory–perceptual processing chain. Other cortical areas have been presumed to be nonrepresentational or only crudely representational (perhaps as a vestigial trait) since topological organization did not seem to have any bearing on the presumed higher and more abstract functions of these areas. In this vein, an apparent lack of topographic order was and is sometimes interpreted as evidence of higher level processing of information. Thus, an earlier viewpoint was that "at the level of Area 18 and beyond . . . all topological organization in the visual process seems to have disappeared" (Hebb, 1949), and one still commonly finds such opinions as "the topographic map is strictly conserved . . . in 'lower' optic centers" such as the superior colliculus, "but as the coding system becomes more refined, wider departures from strict isomorphism are found" (Young, 1962) and "it would be astonishing if this topological organization were not gradually eroded" (from lower to higher levels) (Zeki, 1971). Recent investigators concluded that there was at best a very "weak" tonotopic organization in even primary auditory cortex (Evans *et al.,* 1965; Goldstein *et al.,* 1970). Tonotopic organization was not considered to be necessarily relevant for the presumed "higher" functions of cortical stations and more complex cortical processing algorithims were sought (e.g., see Swarbrick and Whitfield, 1972; Newman and Wollberg, 1973; Winter and Funkenstein, 1973).

The concept that higher level cortex is nonrepresentational received early support from the electrical stimulation studies of Penfield and colleagues (1952, 1954) which suggested that complex perceptions were in some sense site-specific in "psychic" areas of cortex. The interpretation that a spatially complex perception could arise from activity in one or a few neurons (whose response was specific to that given complex input) was further supported by experiments that sought object-specific or vocalization-specific neurons (e.g., see Gross *et al.,* 1972; Winter and Funkenstein, 1973).

C. ENTRANCE INTO THE "SENSORY" LEVEL OF THIS
   HIERARCHICAL PROCESSING SYSTEM IS FROM A
   LARGE, SINGLE REPRESENTATION OF THE
   SENSORY EPITHELIUM WITHIN THE THALAMUS

Of fundamental importance to the concept of serial hierarchical processing was the view that a single nucleus for each sensory system was the basic source of sensory information "relayed" from the periphery to sensory cortex. Furthermore, the relay was thought to be restricted to the "first" or "primary" cortical sensory representation. Thus, the medial geniculate nucleus was considered the relay nucleus for AI, the ventroposterior nucleus for SI, and the lateral geniculate nucleus for V-I. Minor modifications of this view were necessary to accommodate evidence that (*a*) the medial geniculate nucleus contained subdivisions with different cortical targets; (*b*) the lateral geniculate nucleus projects to extrastriate cortex in cats; and (*c*) there are other thalamic zones or nuclei with sensory input from the periphery. However, these early modifications have had relatively little impact on the basic idea of a single, primary thalamic relay nucleus providing input to primary sensory cortex and to the first stage of the cortical hierarchical processing system.

### D. THERE ARE LARGE REGIONS OF MULTIMODAL "ASSOCIATION CORTEX" IN ADVANCED MAMMALS

It is obvious by comparing the amount of cortex occupied by the "primary" and "secondary" sensory areas in a range of mammals that these sensory representations occupy a greatly varying proportion of cortex. Thus, mammals with little neocortex, such as rats or hedgehogs, have much of the cortex devoted to the primary and secondary sensory representations and little additional sensory cortex, while progressive mammals with greatly expanded neocortex, such as cats, monkeys, and humans, have large regions of cortex outside the primary and secondary representations. Much of this additional cortex has been considered to be nonrepresentational "psychic" or "association" cortex indirectly devoted to more than one modality via cortical connections. It followed that the expansion of "psychic" or "association" cortex was the major advance in the phylogenetic development of mammalian brains.

The idea that large areas of cortex are utilized in associating inputs from two or more sensory systems has a long history. This viewpoint was extensively developed by Flechsig (1896), who concluded that large regions between the visual, auditory, and somatic sensory areas in man received limited or no direct input from the thalamus, and therefore were engaged in the association of information first relayed to the different sensory areas. These very large association regions were three in number and located in the frontal, occipital-temporal, and parietal lobes. Flechsig concluded that association centers were absent in rodents, present in carnivores, well developed in monkeys, and occupied two-thirds of the cortex in humans. Differences in the amount of association cortex were used to account for species differences in "intellectual" ability. The basic theory of Flechsig has been retained (with the exception of early recognition of thalamic input to "association" cortex) in current thinking as well as in standard textbook considerations of neocortex (e.g., see Thompson, 1975). It is also worth noting that the concept of a few "association areas" that expand in phylogeny and relate to a single dimension of increasing intelligence has been subject to a long history of criticism ranging from the early comments of Rámon y Cajal (1911) to a more recent discussion by Diamond and Hall (1969).

### III. Summary of Some Recent Studies of Forebrain Organization

Studies over the past decade provide an understanding of forebrain organization that is inconsistent with many of the classical concepts of the role of the forebrain in the genesis of perception. Several basic features of organization are common to different sensory systems and appear relevant to considerations of the genesis of perception within the brain. These basic features are outlined below and their implications for the classical model of hierarchical processing systems generating sensation-to-perception serial transformations are then discussed.

A. THERE ARE MULTIPLE REPRESENTATIONS OF SENSORY EPITHELIA WITHIN THE CORTEX OF MONKEYS IN ALL SENSORY SYSTEMS

Recent studies have revealed the existence of multiple representations of sensory epithelia within visual, auditory, and somatosensory cortex in primates, carnivores, and at least some other mammals. Some of these studies are reviewed in the following.

*1. Visual Cortical Fields*

There are many topographically ("retinotopically") organized fields within primate cortex. In fact, recent studies have revealed that a strict topography is preserved within fields occupying all or nearly all of cortex that was formerly classified as visual "sensory" and visual "psychic" cortex. In the most completely studied primate species, the owl monkey, topographic representations of the retina have been mapped in detail within six visual fields (Allman and Kaas, 1976; Kaas, 1978; see Fig. 1). The first visual representation, V-I, is coincident with the classical Area 17; the second representation, V-II, corresponds to Area 18 as defined in New World monkeys. The four other fully or partly mapped fields, DM, DL, MT, and M, lie completely or partly within the classical Area 19 (V-III of many formulations) of New World monkeys. Within all six mapped fields, there is a highly ordered and complete representation of the retina. In the unmapped regions between

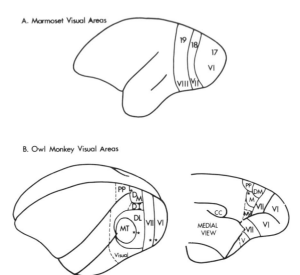

FIG. 1. Traditional (A) and current (B) views on the organization of visual cortex in New World monkeys. Areas 17, 18, and 19 of Brodmann (A) have commonly been considered to be three separate representations of the visual hemifield. In B, the first (V-I) and second (V-II) visual areas are shown, corresponding to Areas 17 and 18 of Brodmann. "Area 19" and adjoining regions of cortex consist of a number of visual areas. Asterisks mark the approximate location of the center of gaze in those visual areas where systematic representations of the visual hemifield have been fully determined. The dorsolateral (DL), dorsointermediate (DI), dorsomedial (DM), medial (M), middle temporal (MT), and posterior parietal (PP) visual areas are from Allman and Kaas (1975). Evidence for a ventral (V) visual area is from unpublished studies of Allman and Kaas. The location of a medial ventral (MV) visual area is suggested by patterns of cortical projections (Wagor et al., 1975). CC, corpus callosum.

and around these fields, the visually responsive cortex also appears to be topographically organized, i.e., in rows of penetrations crossing these regions, successively defined visual fields shift systematically. In particular, a region bordering Area 18 on the ventral surface of the brain has been extensively mapped and a nearly complete representation of the visual hemifield has been revealed (J. M. Allman and J. H. Kaas, unpublished experiments; the Ventral Visual Area, Fig. 1). Other rather extensive mapping data exist for the Dorsal Intermediate Visual Area (Fig. 1). In other words, while the details of internal organization of several fields are not completely defined, evidence suggests that in the owl monkey *all* or nearly all of the caudal visually responsive cortex including all of the classic "visuopsychic area" is occupied by retinotopically organized fields, and that there are, overall, as many as 10 or more topographically organized fields in this species.

While no other primate species has been studied in corresponding detail, evidence in macaque monkeys is consistent with the existence of at least some homologous fields (e.g., see Van Essen, 1979; Weller and Kaas, 1978). In macaques, as in owl monkeys, it would appear that at least most of the "visuopsychic" cortical region is occupied by retinotopically organized fields (e.g., see Van Essen, 1979).

## 2. Somatosensory Cortical Fields

Recent studies of somatosensory cortex have, again, revealed the existence of a number of topographically ("somatotopically") organized fields. Classically, it has been contended that in higher primates, there was a single representation of the body surface in the parietal cortex occupying Brodmann's cytoarchitectonic Areas 3 (3b and 3a), 1 and 2 (Woolsey *et al.,* 1942; Penfield and Boldrey, 1937). This "single" primate representation spanning four distinct cytoarchitectonic fields has long been termed "SI" (Woolsey and Fairman, 1946). A second representation was defined in the dorsal aspect of the Sylvian fissure ("SII") (Woolsey and Fairman, 1946). On the basis of more complete microelectrode mapping studies, the classical view of "SI" organization in primates has been revised (see Fig. 2). "SI" has been found to contain four orderly representations, with Areas 3b and 1 (and in some species Area 2) each containing complete representations of the skin surface (Merzenich *et al.,* 1978; Kaas *et al.,* 1979), and Areas 3a and 2 each containing representations of "deep" receptors in muscles and joints. A narrow strip-like representation of the skin was seen, additionally, between Areas 1 and 2 (Merzenich *et al.,* 1978). Finally, there is the possibility of at least a crude representation of joint and/or muscle receptors caudal to Area 2 within Area 5 (Mountcastle *et al.,* 1975; Sakata *et al.,* 1973; Duffy and Burchfiel, 1971). Similarly, the "SII" region of monkeys has recently been found to be comprised of at least three distinct fields, probably individually topographically organized (Burton and Robinson, 1978). Thus, in a primate like a macaque or owl monkey, there are as many as seven or more somatosensory areas, most of which appear to constitute complete, orderly representations of the body surface or deep body tissues.

## 3. Auditory Cortical Fields

In auditory cortex, classical evoked potential mapping studies provided evidence for only two large fields ("AI" and "AII") in macaque monkeys (Woolsey and Walzl, 1944; Walzl, 1947; see Fig. 3). However,

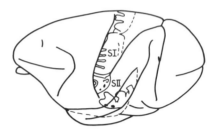

A. Somatic Sensory Cortex

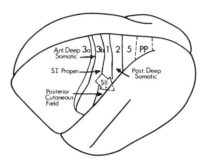

B. Owl Monkey Somatosensory Areas

Fig. 2. Traditional (A) and current (B) views of the subdivisions of parietal somato-sensory cortex in monkeys. Traditionally, somatosensory cortex has been thought of as containing two divisions, the first (SI) and second (SII) somatosensory areas. (A) is redrawn from Woolsey (1958). In (B), the anterior deep somatic field (3a), SI proper (3b), posterior cutaneous field (Area 1), and the posterior deep somatic fields (Area 2) are separate representations of the body as described in Merzenich et al. (1978). The region of "Area 5" and posterior parietal cortex (PP) may also be involved in somatosensory proc-esses, and both may contain subdivisions. The report of Burton and Robinson (1978) sug-gests the existence of additional somatosensory areas on the upper bank of the lateral fissure adjacent to or within the classical "SII."

recent studies have revealed that there are at least six topographically ("cochleotopically" or "tonotopically") organized representations within the auditory cortex of macaque monkeys (Fig. 3B), and at least four topographically organized representations within the auditory cor-tex of owl monkeys (Fig. 4). In both of these primates, a single non-topographically (or weakly topographically) organized field has also been identified.

Domestic cats have been studied in special detail, and four cochleotopically organized fields have been defined (Fig. 3D). In addi-tion, there appear to be at least three other auditory fields without ap-

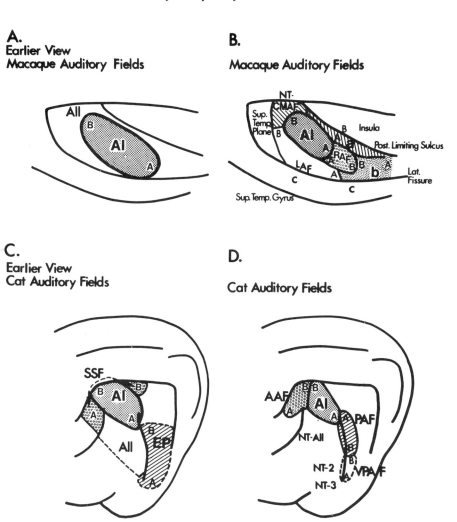

**A.**
Earlier View
Macaque Auditory Fields

**B.**
Macaque Auditory Fields

**C.**
Earlier View
Cat Auditory Fields

**D.**
Cat Auditory Fields

FIG. 3. Traditional (A and C) and current (B and D) views of the organization of auditory cortex in monkeys and carnivores. In all figures, the representation of the cochlear apex (A) and base (B) are indicated in those fields where cochleotopic organization has been described. The traditional view of auditory cortex in the monkey (A) is based on Walzl (1947) and Kennedy (1955). Only primary (AI) and secondary (AII) auditory fields were described. Later, AI was redefined and five additional auditory fields with distinct architectonic and electrophysiological characteristics were described (Merzenich and Brugge, 1973). AI, primary auditory cortex; LAF, lateral auditory field; RAF, rostrolateral auditory field; a, b, and c, other topographically organized fields; NT-CMAF, nontopographic caudomedial auditory field. Fields in A and B are shown on a view of the surface of the superior temporal plane and dorsolateral surface of the superior temporal gyrus. For the location of the auditory fields in owl monkeys, see Imig *et al.*

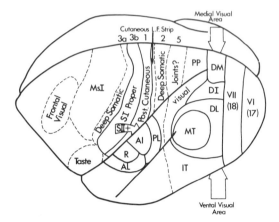

FIG. 4. A summary of the subdivisions of neocortex in a New World monkey as currently understood. Many of these subdivisions are within cortex previously considered "association cortex" (for example, see Thompson, 1975). R, rostral auditory field; AL, anterior lateral auditory field; PL, posterior lateral auditory field; MsI, motor-sensory area I; other abbreviations as in other figures.

parent tonotopic organization. Thus, in the auditory systems of cats and monkeys there is a significant region of sensory cortex that appears to be "nonrepresentational" for the sensory epithelium.

## B. THERE HAVE BEEN IMPORTANT REDEFINITIONS OF SENSORY FIELDS IN ALL THREE SENSORY SYSTEMS

In some instances, the classical terms for sensory representations have been retained, although the areas have been redefined with different boundaries and extents. Unfortunately, these corrected definitions have not yet been widely adopted by neurobiologists, and it is not always clear from the use of a term if the old or new definition is intended. The major changes in definitions are noted in the following.

As illustrated in Fig. 1, the classical Area 19 or V-III of primates has been found to correspond to a number of functionally distinct subdivi-

(1977) and Fig. 4. The traditional auditory fields of the cat have been redrawn from Woolsey (1960). The fields included AI, AII, the suprasylvian fringe (SSF) and the posterior ectosylvian area (EP). The current auditory areas of the cat are based on Merzenich and colleagues (Merzenich et al., 1977; Andersen, 1979, unpublished studies) and on Reale and Imig (1977 and personal communication). Subdivisions redefined with microelectrode mapping methods include a smaller primary field, AI, at least three other cochleotopic fields (the anterior auditory field, AAF; the posterior auditory field, PAF; the ventroposterior field, VPAF), a nontopographic and redefined AII (NT-AII), and at least two other nontopographic fields (NT-2 and NT-3).

sions rather than one. While Area 18 of New World monkeys and prosimians has been found to correspond to a second systematic representation of the visual field, V-II, Area 18 as classically defined in Old World
monkeys (and almost certainly in apes and humans) is far too wide and
includes much more than V-II. Since a V-II appears to exist in most if
not all mammals, and the architectonic zone that is coextensive with V-II
has often been identified as Area 18, we have suggested that Area 18 be
defined as the cortex devoted to V-II in all species (Kaas, 1978). The
classical use of the term Area 18 in advanced primates presently has
uncertain meaning and should be redefined as the cortex that is coextensive with V-II, as Zeki (1969) has done. However, as an added complication, Zeki (1969) has introduced the term V-III for a region of cortex
that is largely within the classical Area 18 of macaque monkeys. The
studies by Zeki helped define the rostral border of V-II (and thereby the
true border of Area 18), but we regard the use of the term V-III or Area
19 for the cortex bordering V-II as unfortunate since there has been no
demonstration that a single visual area forms the rostral border of V-II
with a retinotopic organization mirroring that of V-II as would be required by the traditional concept of Area 19 and V-III. In fact, there is
clear evidence of several visual areas bordering V-II of macaque
monkeys (Van Essen, 1979), as in New World monkeys.

In auditory cortex, a number of distinct fields have been found to be
partly or completely within the classically defined "AI" of primates as
identified by Woolsey and Walzl (1944) and Kennedy (1955). The subdivision "AI" of the auditory cortex in the cat has also been redefined
as occupying only part of its former area (Merzenich *et al.*, 1975, 1977;
Knight, 1977). In both cats and monkeys, the classically defined boundaries of AI were apparently extended by inability of surface recordings
to detect precisely reversals of topographic order. Thus, when Woolsey
and colleagues stimulated the basal end of the cochlea representing
highest frequencies, they must have excited cortex along the lines of
reversal in the representation of highest frequencies both in AI and the
bordering field. Apparently, all of this relatively continuous responsive
zone was included within AI. The same complication arose at low-
frequency field boundaries (e.g., in the cat, the border of AI with the
field posterior to it; or in the monkey, with the field anterior to AI). All
regions in which there were such reversals in representation of frequency
across the boundaries of auditory fields were interpreted to be within
one field. Because AI included parts of adjoining fields, the interpretation of the organization and boundaries of adjoining fields was also
incorrect.

The consequence of recent detailed microelectrode mapping studies of auditory cortex has been a complete redefinition of the organization of the traditional subdivisions (Merzenich and Brugge, 1973; Merzenich *et al.*, 1975, 1977; Knight, 1977; Imig and Reale, 1977). By these new definitions, AI in cats and in monkeys is much smaller than defined by Woolsey and colleagues, large topographically organized fields are found rostral and caudal to AI, and a fourth field is situated ventral to the caudal "posterior auditory field" (Fig. 3). There are reversals (not discontinuities, as defined classically) in the sequence of representation across all of the shared borders of these fields.

In somatosensory cortex, "SI" of monkeys has been redefined with the appreciation that the classical single representation actually contains four or five complete representations. These representations occupy cytoarchitectonically delimitable subdivisions. Area 3b of primates is probably homologous with "SI" of other mammals, and hence has been renamed "SI proper" (Merzenich *et al.*, 1978). The several representations that were previously included in the classical "SI" now have been collectively termed the "parietal somatosensory strip." A similar need for redefining "SII" in primates has recently become apparent with the evidence that the region considered to be a single body surface representation may contain several body surface representations (see Burton and Robinson, 1978).

## C. MOST POSTCENTRAL NEOCORTEX CONTAINS SENSORY REPRESENTATIONS

Contrary to the classical view of somatosensory, visual, and auditory cortical fields occupying narrow core areas separated by large regions of nonrepresentational "association" or "psychic" cortex, most of the cortex caudal to motor cortex and excluding the middle and anterior temporal cortex appears to be occupied by retinotopically, cochleotopically, or somatotopically organized fields. In New World monkeys, many of these representations have been fully defined, and these areas are shown in Fig. 4. In addition, there is incomplete evidence for other sensory representations, and the general conclusion that most of the caudal neocortex responsive to sensory stimuli is occupied by sensory representations appears valid. In some limited regions of cortex, careful investigations have failed to reveal any systematic representations of sensory surfaces. For example, there are at least three cortical fields that are strongly driven by auditory stimuli in cats, but are without any clear cochleotopic organization (Merzenich *et al.*, 1977; Andersen, 1979). At least one such cortical field appears to exist in monkeys (Merzenich and Brugge, 1972; Imig *et al.*, 1977). In addition, there is evidence for a narrow region between auditory, visual, and somatosensory cortex without any clear representation of any of these modalities in the rhesus monkey (Merzenich and Brugge, 1978) and in the owl monkey (Imig *et al.*, 1977). (The possibility of vestibular representation has not been ruled out.) But overall, these "nonrepresentational" cortical regions occupy only a small fraction of the parietal, posterior temporal and occipital cortex, and most of what has long been regarded as the "integrative" or "psychic" cortex is actually occupied by topographically organized fields (Fig. 4).

D. The Number of Cortical Fields (and Overall Cortex Devoted to Topographically Organized Cortex) Has Increased in Several Lines of Mammalian Phylogeny

While modern mapping methods have revealed many sensory representations in advanced mammals with expanded cortex like cats and the various monkeys, fewer representations have been demonstrated in smooth-brained mammals with relatively little neocortex. Perhaps the strongest evidence for the conclusion that the number of sensory representations has increased in phylogeny comes from sensory mapping studies on the hedgehog (Kaas *et al.*, 1970), which is a small insectivore with proportionally less neocortex than almost any extant mammal. While no attempt has been made to subdivide auditory cortex in this species, it appears that there are only two visual representations, and only two somatosensory representations (Fig. 5). Since the visual areas directly adjoin the somatosensory areas, there is no room for "undiscovered" additional representations and the conclusion seems inescapable that, although most of the neocortex of the hedgehog is sensory, there are only a few subdivisions of sensory cortex. Because all present day eutherian mammals evolved from insectivore-like ancestors with little neocortex and an external brain morphology similar to that of the hedgehog (see Kaas *et al.*, 1970), it is reasonable to conclude from studies of the hedgehog that the first mammals had few subdivisions of cortex. Furthermore, this conclusion is supported by similar results on other mammals (such as oposums and rats) with little neocortex. Here too, there seem to be few sensory representations. Thus, small smooth forebrains with few sensory representations is a generalized condition and therefore most likely ancestral, while large forebrains with fissures and many sensory representations has been a product of several parallel lines of evolution.

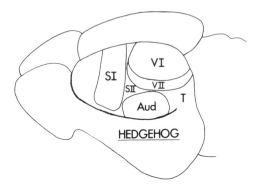

Fig. 5. Subdivisions of neocortex in the hedgehog, an insectivore with little neocortex. Note that there are few subdivisions, and that most of the defined subdivisions are sensory representations. No attempts have been made to divide auditory cortex. After Kaas *et al.* (1970).

If species of mammals differing in amount of neocortical expansion are considered, there is evidence that cortical expansion is related to an increase in the *number* of sensory representations. Thus, two topographic cortical representations of the cochlea have been found in a rodent with a slight expansion of neocortex, the squirrel (Merzenich *et al.,* 1976), at least three auditory representations exist in the tree shrew (Oliver *et al.,* 1976), which has an expanded temporal cortex, while owl monkeys (Imig *et al.,* 1977) have at least four and rhesus monkeys (Merzenich and Brugge, 1973) have at least six auditory representations. All mammals appear to have two somatosensory representations, SI and SII, although opposums do not seem to have a "motor" representation separate from SI (Lende, 1963). However, more somatosensory representations clearly exist in monkeys, although it is not yet certain if New and Old World monkeys vary in numbers of areas, or if prosimians have fewer representations than monkeys, as recent studies suggest (Sur *et al.,* 1979). In the visual system, there is evidence for four or fewer representations in a range of small smooth brained mammals, while cats (Palmer *et al.,* 1978) and monkeys (Kaas, 1978) have 10 or more representations.

E.  INFORMATION IS DELIVERED TO THE THALAMUS
     AND THEN TO THE CORTEX OVER A NUMBER OF
     FUNCTIONALLY DISTINCT PARALLEL PATHWAYS

Classically, descriptions of sensory projection systems have focused on simple, serial "main-line" large-fiber systems complemented in minor ways by "secondary" small-fiber systems (see Rose and Mountcastle, 1959; Bishop, 1959). It is now evident that (*a*) each "mainline" system is actually a composite of several input classes projecting in parallel; (*b*) there are multiple projection systems outside the "main-line" system; and (*c*) most if not all sensory representations have direct thalamic inputs.

The "main-line" projection system in the visual system of primates differs from those of the somatic and auditory systems in that only one sensory representation, V-I, receives the most direct visual information (however, the lateral geniculate nucleus and the medial interlaminar nucleus relay direct retinal projections to several cortical fields in cats). Recently, major advances have been made in the understanding of the functional organization of the "main-line" projection system from the retina. The main-line projection system can be considered to constitute the "X," "Y," and some of the "W" ganglion cell populations projecting to the lateral geniculate nucleus (see Rowe and Stone, 1977, for review). The X cells are considered important in form vision, respond in a sustained manner to static stimuli, are largely color-opponent types in primates, and are concentrated in the central retina. The Y cells are thought to be important in visual attention, respond to stimulus changes, are "broad-band" in response to color, conduct information rapidly to the thalamus over large axons, and are more evenly distributed over the retina. The W cells form a heterogeneous group with a range of response properties, slowly conducting axons, and probably several functional types. It now appears that the X cells project solely or almost solely to the parvocellular layers of the lateral geniculate nucleus of primates, while the Y cells project to the magnocellular layers of the lateral geniculate nucleus and via collaterals to the superior colliculus (Schiller and Malpeli, 1977; Weller *et al.,* 1979). The W cells project to the superior colliculus and possibly to parts of the lateral geniculate nucleus such as the interlaminar zones and the superficial S layers. The segregation of input types in the magnocellular and parvocellular layers is maintained at the next level since these layers project to different layers of cortex. There is also evidence that interlaminar cells project separately to layer I (Carey *et al.,* 1979). Thus, there is evidence for at least three parallel projection systems relaying through the lateral geniculate nucleus and terminating in separate layers of striate cortex.

In addition to the lateral geniculate nucleus as a subdivisible "main-line" structure delivering visual information to cortex, there are at least five separate topographically organized subdivisions of the pulvinar complex, each with its own pattern of projections to cortical visual areas (see Graham *et al.,* 1979; Lin and Kaas, 1979; Symonds and Kaas, 1978). Two of these subdivisions receive topologically ordered projections from the superior colliculus (Fig. 6). Other visual input to the pulvinar complex and other nuclei is from targets of the retina in the pretectum (Benevento *et al.,* 1977).

In the "main-line" somatosensory system (the "lemniscal system"; see Mountcastle, 1974), inputs from populations of neurons innervating different mechanoreceptor types are handled largely in parallel from the skin to the cortex. Thus, in the input layers of somatosensory cortex, response characteristics of neurons can be very much like those of primary afferent fibers (see Mountcastle *et al.,* 1969). Moreover, in the squirrel monkey there is evidence of a segregated processing of information from deep and pacinian, cutaneous quickly adapting, and cutaneous slowly adapting receptor populations within strictly delimited sectors of the ventrobasal thalamus (J. Kaas, M. Sur, R. Nelson, R. Dykes, and M. Merzenich, unpublished results). From the ventroposterior nucleus of the thalamus there is parallel input to both SI proper (Area 3b) and the posterior cutaneous field (Area 1) (see Fig. 7; also Lin *et al.,* 1979; Jones *et al.,* 1979). Some of the input to each area appears to originate in separate sets of thalamic neurons, while some thalamic neurons appear to project to both fields. There is further evidence that a thalamic region dorsal to the ventroposterior nucleus projects to the posterior representation of deep body tissues (Area 2), while sensory information

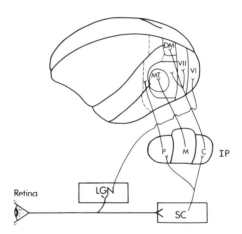

FIG. 6. Some of the thalamocortical connections of the visual system in monkeys. Connections are topographic and reciprocal. Posterior (P), medial (M), and central (C) divisions of the inferior pulvinar complex (IP) are shown. LGN, lateral geniculate nucleus; SC, superior colliculus. Other abbreviations as in Fig. 1. Separate parallel pathways of the X, Y, and W ganglion cell systems through the LGN to V-I, as well as connections with the superior pulvinar complex, are not shown. Based on Lin and Kaas (1979).

Cortex

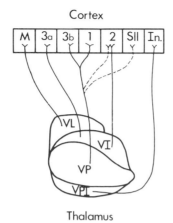

Thalamus

Fig. 7. Some of the thalamocortical connections of the somatosensory system in monkeys. Dashed lines indicate less pronounced connections. Probably all connections are topographic and reciprocal. The approximate spatial relationships of the ventroposterior (VP), the ventroposteroinferior (VPI), ventralis intermedius (VI), and ventralis lateralis (VL) nuclei are indicated. M, motor cortex; In, insular cortex. Other abbreviations as in Fig. 4. Based on Lin *et al.* (1979) and Jones *et al.* (1979, and unpublished studies).

from muscle afferents is relayed from the ventrolateral thalamus to Area 3a (Tanji, 1975; Heath *et al.,* 1976).

Other somatosensory thalamic inputs are to "Area 5" and the SII region. There is evidence for separate anterior and posterior fields within "Area 5" with inputs from the pulvinar and lateral posterior nucleus, respectively (Jones *et al.,* 1979). The ventroposterior nucleus and nuclei of the posterior group project to separate fields in the SII region (Burton and Jones, 1976).

Multiple parallel sensory pathways have been most fully demonstrated for the auditory system of cats (Figs. 8 and 9). While different classes of ganglion cells send distinct types of information centrally in the somatic and visual system, the auditory system has its own way to accomplish the same end. From a relatively homogeneous input from the cochlea, information is distributed to a series of different response-specific neuron populations that, by virtue of different synaptology, extract very different information from this common input. Subsequently, information from the two ears is combined in several binaural "comparator" nuclei apparently abstracting information relevant to the localization of sound sources. Information from the two ears is added in other neuron populations; this adding of information from the two ears results in a two-ear excitatory–excitatory product. Thus, while information from the somatosensory and visual systems at the level of the thalamus is very

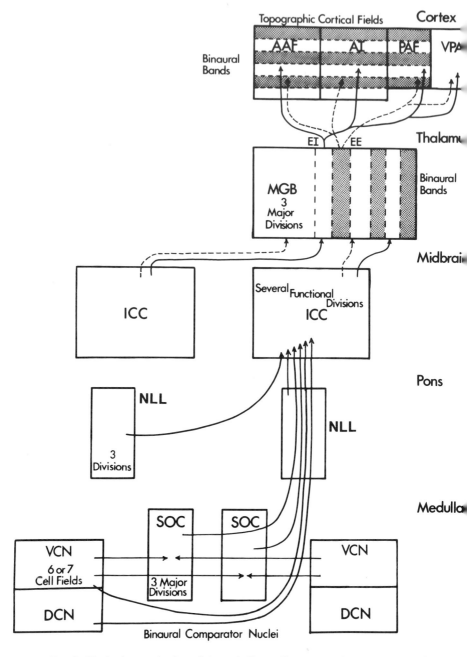

FIG. 8. The basic organization of the main-line auditory system in the cat. Inputs from specific cell fields of the right and left ventral cochlear nulcei (VCN) converge on the binaural comparator nuclei of the superior olivary complex (SOC). Neurons of the ventral and dorsal cochlear nuclei and neurons of subdivisions of the superior olivary complex

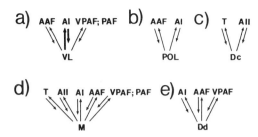

FIG. 9. Some of the thalamocortical connections of the auditory system of the cat. (a) The ventrolateral thalamus (VL) is topographically interconnected with four auditory cortical areas (see Fig. 3 for abbreviations). (b) The lateral "nucleus" of the posterior group (POL) is topographically interconnected with two auditory fields. (c) The caudal part of the dorsal division of the medial geniculate complex (Dc) is interconnected with non-topographic AII and other temporal auditory fields (T). (d) The medial division of the medial geniculate complex (M) is interconnected with all studied auditory fields. (e) The deep dorsal division of the medial geniculate complex (Dd) is topographically interconnected with three auditory fields. Redrawn from Andersen (1979) with reference to Fitzpatrick *et al.* (1977), Winer *et al.* (1977), and Colwell and Merzenich (1980).

like information recorded at the level of the peripheral sensory neurons and the ganglion cells, there is a profound *second-level abstraction of information* in the auditory system. Neuron populations in different subdivisions of the cochlear nuclear complex (there are on the order of six or seven functionally and morphologically distinct classes of projecting neurons), superior olivary complex (three major divisions), and nuclei of the lateral lemnisci (there are three principle projecting nuclei) all have different source-specific response characteristics. Thus, in the sensory system with the most homogeneous input from the sensory epithelium, many response classes of neurons are *created* as a consequence of the second level of abstraction of information in the system. As in the visual and somatosensory systems, once class-specific auditory information is derived, it is delivered forward in parallel over at least largely separate

project to the three nuclei of the lateral lemnisci (NLL). Subdivisions of all these nuclear groups (VCN, DCN, SOC, NLL) project to the principal midbrain auditory center, the central nucleus of the inferior colliculus (ICC). These inputs are segregated into at least four subdivisions of the ICC. The ICC projects bilaterally to the three major thalamic subdivisions of the main-line system, the medial nucleus, the ventral nucleus, and the deep part of the dorsal nucleus of the medial geniculate body (MGB). Details of how information from different midbrain nuclei project are lacking, but it appears that there are alternating slabs of excitatory–excititory and excitatory–inhibitory neurons in at least part of the large ventral nucleus. The main-line thalamic nuclei project to at least four topographically organized cortical fields; abbreviations as in Fig. 3D. Three of these fields (AI, AAF, and PAF, see Fig. 9) are known to contain alternating excitatory-excitity and excitatory-inhibitory binaural bands (see text for further description).

pathways from the midbrain to cortical fields (Roth *et al.,* 1978; Imig and Adrian, 1978; Morest, 1964). That is, inputs from different nuclei in the pons are delivered to different, segregated neuronal populations within the principal midbrain nucleus (the central nucleus of the inferior colliculus), and relayed to subdivisions of the auditory thalamus. Each subdivision of auditory cortex receives input from one or more of the component nuclei or subnuclei of the ventral, dorsal, and medial divisions of the medial geniculate complex (Colwell and Merzenich, 1980; Andersen *et al.,* 1977; Andersen, 1979). Thus, for example, the anterior auditory field receives its principal input from the deep dorsal nucleus of the medial geniculate body and not from the lateral part of the ventral nucleus (which provides the most powerful input to "AI") (Merzenich *et al.,* 1977; Andersen *et al.,* 1977; Andersen, 1979). There are at least seven projecting subdivisions of the medial geniculate body, projecting in a variety of different field-specific combinations to different auditory cortical fields (see Colwell and Merzenich, 1980; Andersen, 1979). Cortical fields that are topographic receive thalamic input from a different group of thalamic nuclei than do the cortical fields without obvious topographic organization.

Thus, rather than the early concept of a simple single thalamic nucleus for each sensory system, it is now apparent that the "main-line" thalamic region for each system is actually a complex of segregated neuron populations with input relayed from different classes of peripheral or second-level neurons. Even the "main-line" systems, then, are multiple-component parallel projection systems, feeding information in different mixes to different cortical representational fields. Rather than a simple serial relay from the thalamus to "primary" sensory cortex, most if not all representations have direct thalamic inputs. This allows each cortical representation to be simultaneously or nearly simultaneously activated by direct thalamic projections as well as by cortical connections.

F. Topographically Organized Cortical
   Fields Are Multiply Interconnected.
   Interconnections Are Often Reciprocal

Our present understanding of the connections of the topographically organized cortical fields is far from complete. Many subdivisions of sensory cortex have been only recently defined, the significance of some previously described architectonic fields has only been recently determined, and all of the subdivisions of sensory cortex are not yet known for any mammalian brain. Yet, enough is known to allow some general statements about connections. First, the ipsilateral connections invariably appear to be homotopic in that they relate similar parts of sensory surfaces in separate representations (although they may spread to include more than the homotopic site in at least some somatosensory fields; see Jones *et al.,* 1978). Second, multiple interconnèctions occur for most (if not all) representations (Fig. 10). Third, reciprocal interconnections between areas are common (Fig. 10). However, "reciprocal" interconnections often differ in the magnitude of the connection and in the laminar termination pattern. Thus, there are anatomical reasons for suggesting that "reciprocal" interconnections are not equivalent in function. Fourth, corpus callosum interhemispheric connections add to the complexity of the system by being of at least three types (Kaas, 1978). One type is homotopic or nearly so and relates the margins of representations in the two hemispheres where they are devoted to adjoining or overlapping parts of the same sensory surface (i.e., along the line of decussation of the retina or along the dorsal midline of the body surface). Another type is homoregional and connects other parts of matched representations of the two hemispheres. A third type is heteroregional and connects a representation on one side of the brain with one or more different representations on the other side of the brain. Fifth, most cortical areas project to other representations within the same sensory domain. Sensory representations of different modalities are not significantly interconnected. When these generalizations about cortical connections are considered, it is obvious that the concept of a hierarchical cortico-cortical sequence of processing is an oversimplification.

G. Sensory Representations Vary in Internal
   Organization. Few Representations Are
   Actually Topologically Equivalent to a
   Sensory Surface

There are a number of significantly different ways in which sensory surfaces are represented in neocortex. These differences are seen in all three sensory systems (Kaas, 1977). They suggest that functional considerations have an important role in determining the organization of sensory representations.

In the visual system, a most obvious difference between representations is in the proportions of tissue devoted to different portions of the hemiretina or hemifield (Fig. 10A). For example, in the owl monkey, the Medial Area devotes little cortex (about 5%) to the central 10° of the visual field while most of the Dorsolateral Area (about 75%) is devoted to the central 10° (Allman and Kaas, 1976). There are also several quite

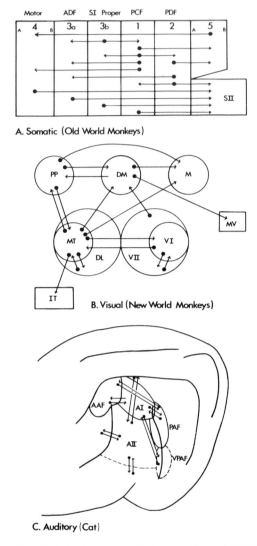

**A. Somatic (Old World Monkeys)**

**B. Visual (New World Monkeys)**

**C. Auditory (Cat)**

Fig. 10. Some of the ipsilateral corticocortical connections of sensory areas of cortex. Connections between topographically organized fields appear to be homotopic. The complex transcallosal interfield connections are not drawn. (A) Connections of somatosensory areas based on Vogt and Pandya (1978) and Jones *et al.* (1978). Connections with the supplementary motor area are not shown. Cortical areas as in Fig. 2. (B) Some of the known connections of visual cortical areas of New World monkeys as summarized by Kaas (1978). The connections of only a few of the visual areas have been fully established and connections with frontal cortex are not shown. The extents and boundaries and possible subdivisions of inferotemporal (IT) and medioventral (MV) cortex are unknown. Other abbreviations as in Fig. 1. (C) Connections of auditory cortex in the cat based on Reale and Imig (1977); Andersen (1979, unpublished observations). Abbreviations as in other figures.

different types of representations or transformations of the hemifield in visual cortical fields. In primates, V-I and MT are basically simple topological transformations of the visual hemifield, or first-order transformations (Allman and Kaas, 1974), if one ignores the complication of rerepresentation of visual space in layer IV of adjoining ocular dominance columns in some primates (see Hubel and Wiesel, 1977). Another type of representation is found in V-II, DL, DM, and M (Fig. 11). In these representations, the hemifield is largely or almost completely split along the zero horizontal meridian. This second-order transformation (Allman and Kaas, 1974) is topological in the representa-

**Retinotopic Transformations in Visual Cortex**

**A.**

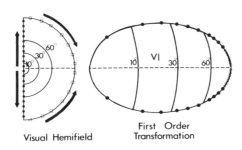

Visual Hemifield

First Order Transformation

**B.**

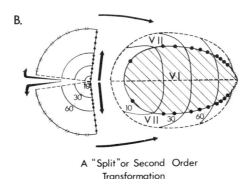

A "Split" or Second Order Transformation

FIG. 11. Two basic types of visual hemifield representation in monkeys. (A) In the first-order transformation, found in V-I and MT, the visual hemifield is distorted but not split in the representation. (B) In the second-order transformation found in V-II, DL, DM, and M, the visual hemifield is distorted and split. Visual areas also differ considerably in the ways they distort the visual hemifield. After definitions of Allman and Kaas (1974).

tion of the upper and lower visual quadrants, but because of the split it is not topological overall. The split in the representation allows a second-order representation (such as V-II or DL) to wrap around a first-order transformation (such as the adjoining V-I or MT) with minimal distortion and matched or congruent borders. This arrangement also permits short interconnections between paired representations. For other areas, the split allows partially matched borders along the horizontal meridian of V-II. Only these two types of representations have so far been found in primates. However, "extended representations" including part of the ipsilateral hemifield have been found in the visual cortex of sheep, and they may occur elsewhere. More complicated "point-to-line" transformations have been described for visual areas of the suprasylvian sulcus of cats (Palmer *et al.,* 1978), but again, this type of representation has not yet been found elsewhere. As more is understood about the organizations of visual areas, less obvious differences in the internal organizations of separate areas no doubt will be revealed. For example, the division of V-I into "ocular dominance" and "orientation" columns or bands (Hubel and Wiesel, 1977) apparently does not occur, at least in the same way, in other visual fields.

In the somatosensory cortex, recent studies have revealed that the separate representations of the skin surface in the parietal somatosensory strip differ in topography in several ways. For example, there are differences in the proportional area of cortex dedicated to specific skin surfaces in the different fields (Merzenich *et al.,* 1978; Kaas *et al.,* 1979; Nelson *et al.,* 1979). Moreover, discontinuities in the representation of the skin surface relate to different skin locations in the separate cortical representations. A striking example is illustrated in Fig. 12, in which the very different schema for representing the dorsal surfaces of the fingers in Areas 3b and 1 of the owl monkey are shown. Another example of an important variation in organization is seen in "SII" in which ipsilateral and contralateral body surface representations are overlying and in register. Important differences in the microorganizations of somatosensory fields can be expected to be revealed by further study. For example, there is evidence that at least part of Area 3b is divided into "columns" or strips devoted to slowly adapting or rapidly adapting receptor inputs (Sur, 1978), much like the ocular dominance "columns" and orientation "columns" divide V-I. A corresponding organization is not yet apparent in Area 1.

The situation is somewhat more complicated in auditory cortex where there are two unique features of organization. First, auditory cortical fields necessarily have a fundamentally different kind of representation of the sensory epithelium (see Merzenich *et al.,* 1977). The auditory sen-

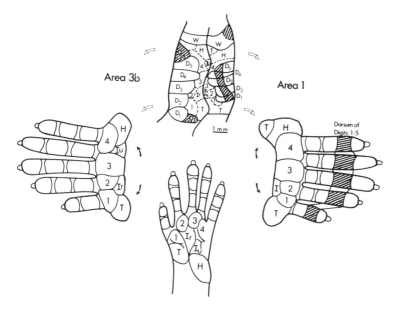

FIG. 12. Differences in the representations of the hand in Area 3b (SI proper) and Area 1 (the posterior cutaneous field) in owl monkeys. Basically, the palmar hand (below) is split (right and left) between the pads of the palm and distorted to form two roughly mirror image representations in Areas 3b and 1 (above). However, major differences in the two representations exist in the proportions of cortex devoted to different parts of the hand and the detailed arrangement of the parts. To point out two clear distinctions, (*a*) there is a greater proportion of representation of the glabrous surfaces of the fingers in Area 3b than in Area 1; and (*b*) the dorsum of the digits (shaded) is centered in the representation of the glabrous digits in Area 1 and split out to dorsal and ventral cortex in Area 3. Many such distinctions are found in the internal topography of these two large representations in this and other primates. Based on Merzenich *et al.* (1978).

sory epithelium, the organ of Corti, is a *line* of cells of insignificant width (3000 or so hair cells long, and one or four hair cells wide). If represented topographically within a cortical field like the point-to-point representations of visual and somatosensory sensory epithelia (which are surfaces), the organ of Corti would occupy a strip of cortex of insignificant width. Of course auditory cortex has an additional dimension, and, in this dimension, the cochlea is rerepresented, i.e., any given short sector of the cochlea is represented across a band of cortex of approximately constant width that extends across AI (or other cortical fields) from edge to edge (Fig. 13) (Tunturi, 1950; Merzenich *et al.*, 1975). Second, recent studies have revealed that there are a series of response-specific bands within AI that are oriented orthogonal to cortical lines of isorepresentation ("isofrequency contour"). Thus, each isofrequency

A. Cochlear Rep. in two Cat
Auditory Fields (AAF and AI)

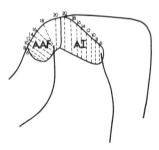

B. Binaural Bands within AI

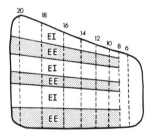

FIG. 13. (A) Cochleotopic representation within two auditory fields (AAF and AI) in the cat. Numbers represent locations along the cochlear sensory epithelium measured from the cochlear apex. When these two fields are unfolded, they are seen to be topographic mirror images of about equal size, with a reversal in the representation of the extreme cochlear base along the border between the two fields. Note that the cochlear sensory epithelium is rerepresented across one axis (the axis of "isofrequency" contours) of cochleotopically organized fields; this axis of rerepresentation is indicated by the broken lines in this schematic drawing. After Merzenich *et al.* (1975); Knight (1977). (B) Highly schematized drawing of the internal organization of AI. This field is marked by a series of alternating functional binaural bands, orthogonal to the isofrequency contours of the field. Within a given binaural band, all neurons are excited by stimulation of both ears (EE bands), or excited by stimulation of the contralateral ear and inhibited by stimulation of the ipsilateral ear (EI bands). The lowest frequency part of AI (at the right) has not been studied in sufficient detail to determine its internal binaural organization. After Middlebrooks *et al.* (1979).

contour crosses five or six major AI subdivisions (Brugge and Imig, 1978; Imig and Adrian, 1977; Imig and Brugge, 1978; Middlebrooks *et al.*, 1978, 1979). In each of these subdivisions, binaural response properties of neurons are similar, and they differ from those of neurons in adjacent bands. At least three (probably four) auditory cortical fields in the cat (the cochleotopically organized fields) appear to have similar subdivisions. However, the several apparently "nontopographic" fields in the cat do not have this organization. These fields not only lack a clearly delineable topographic order, but they also appear to lack the binaural response bands of AI and other topographic fields.

The organization of AI raises a basic question about how to subdivide auditory cortex. Is "AI" the functional unit? Or are the individual bands of AI actually individual representational areas, ultimately processing input from different brainstem sources? Some evidence supports both views (see Middlebrooks *et al.,* 1979; Andersen, 1979). If the individual bands are separate representations, there would actually be on the order of 20 representations of the auditory sensory epithelium within auditory cortex in cats and probably more in primates.

From these examples, it is evident that in all three sensory systems there are different types of sensory representations, and that representations commonly differ from each other in important features of their detailed topography.

H. Neurons in Sensory Representations Have
   Field-Specific Response Properties,
   Presumably Reflecting Different Inputs
   and Processing

While several sensory areas of the same modality may contain neurons that respond similarly to a particular sensory stimulus, there is evidence to support the view that all sensory representations differ in the overall response properties of populations of contained neurons, and, in some cases at least, have clear, field-specific classes of neurons. These differences argue that each sensory representational area is mediating distinct aspects of perception.

In the somatosensory cortex, many field-specific differences in overall response properties have been established. There is evidence, for example, that Area 3b has more neurons activated by slowly adapting peripheral neurons than do Areas 1 or 2 (Paul *et al.,* 1972a). Area 1 has neurons related to quickly adapting Pacinian receptors, while such input is not seen in Area 3b (Paul *et al.,* 1972a; Merzenich *et al.,* 1978; Sur *et al.,* 1978). Furthermore, neurons in Area 3b have a homogeneous receptive field organization, while many cells in Area 1 have a center-surround receptive field organization (Sur, 1978). Area 2 has joint and other "deep" receptor inputs without obvious cutaneous receptor inputs in the anesthetized owl monkey (Merzenich *et al.,* 1978), but in macaque monkeys both deep and cutaneous inputs were apparent in similar recordings (see Nelson *et al.,* 1979). Area 3a is predominantly activated by the stimulation of afferents from muscle (Tanji, 1975; Heath *et al.,*

1976). Finally, neurons in Area 1 have larger receptive fields than do those of Area 3b. There is evidence that these larger receptive fields are a consequence of greater convergence of inputs to Area 1 "columns" (Sur, 1978; Paul et al., 1972b; M. M. Merzenich, J. H. Kaas, Sur and, R. A. Nelson, unpublished).

Differences in response characteristics are less clearly understood in the topographically organized auditory cortical fields, but detailed temporal response characteristics and susceptibility to anesthesia are clearly to some extent field-specific (see Merzenich et al., 1975; Knight, 1977; Andersen, 1979). Of course, response properties are very different in nontopographic and topographic cortical fields (e.g., see Merzenich et al., 1975).

In the visual system, Hubel and Wiesel (1965) noted striking field-specific response characteristics in the visual cortex of cats. They found that a class of neurons, the "simple" cells, were common in V-I but were absent in "V-II" and "V-III." Similarly, "simple" cells and "circularly symmetric" cells appeared to be confined to V-I in monkeys (Hubel and Wiesel, 1968). In further studies of macaque monkeys, Hubel and Wiesel (1970) later described "binocular depth" cells in V-II of a type not found in V-I (also, see Poggio and Fischer, 1977). In more recent investigations, a high proportion of neurons in Area MT of the owl monkey (Newsome et al., 1978) and in the probable homolog in macaque monkeys (Zeki, 1974) have a preference for stimuli moving in a particular direction. Zeki (1977) has also described an area of the superior temporal sulcus of macaque monkeys with a concentration of "color-coded" neurons. Finally, neurons in the various visual areas have different receptive field sizes, again suggesting differing degrees of convergence and/or different sources of inputs.

I. THERE IS SOME DIRECT EVIDENCE THAT
   DIFFERENT TOPOGRAPHIC REPRESENTATIONS
   MAKE SPECIFIC CONTRIBUTIONS TO EVOKED
   PERCEPTIONS

Identification of field-specific contributions to perception constitutes a difficult task because there is very little information about selectively activating or inactivating individual fields. However, one clear demonstration of field-specific contributions to behavior exists in the ablation-behavioral studies of Randolph and Semmes (1974). They demonstrated that removal of the hand representation in Area 1 of somatosensory cortex of monkeys resulted in an impairment on tasks involving discriminations of "texture" while a specific deficit in form discrimination could be attributed to a lesion of the hand representation in Area 2. Thus, distinct changes in perceptual abilities were demonstrated to be field-specific and assignable to these two Areas.

The neurological literature provides numerous examples of highly specific deficits resulting from restricted cortical lesions in humans (see Hines, 1929, for classical review, and Teuber, 1960, and Luria, 1966, for more contemporary reviews). Thus, in classical neurological studies color perception has been lost without loss of form discrimination, or depth perception without pattern discrimination. In the somatosensory system, various limited combinations of losses of vibratory, temperature, pain, tactile pattern, or position sensibility have long been described consequent of different parietal lobe lesions. A wide variety of lesion-specific deficits have been described; in the words of a contemporary neurologist, "for every local lesion functional systems develop specific defects" (Luria, 1966). Unfortunately, information on lesion location and cortical field definition in humans is rarely adequate for unequivocally relating specific sensory deficits to given cortical representations.

## IV. General Conclusions

### A. A Summary of Findings Relevant to the Classical View of Forebrain Organization

Consider again the aforementioned tenets of the classical concept of forebrain organization.

1. There are only a few divisions of the forebrain of functional significance for each sensory modality.

2. These divisions form a system for serial sensation-to-perception processing, i.e., successive fields subserve successively "higher" functions.

3. Orderly representations of receptor surfaces are important in the early stages of sensory processing, but are not necessary in later stages, which deal with abstractions and higher order functions.

4. These higher order functions are the product of large regions of "psychic" or multimodal "association" cortex.

5. Nonrepresentational "psychic" or "association" cortex expands greatly in mammalian phylogeny.

6. Entrance into the sensory level of a cortical hierarchical processing system is primarily from unitary "main-line" projection systems, i.e.,

from a single large representation of the retina, cochlea, or skin surface within the thalamus.

*None of these ideas is now supportable.* To the contrary:

1. There are a number of topographic representations of sensory surfaces in each sensory system. Thus, in the cortex of a macaque monkey, there are six or more representations of the organ of Corti, seven or more representations of the skin surface, and probably 10 or more representations of the retina.

2. Identification of these representations has led to a nearly complete redefinition of cortical field identity and boundaries both in primates and in carnivores.

3. Topographic representations occupy most of cortex caudal to the central sulcus in primates. There is proportionately little non-topographically organized cortex. The existence of an "association cortex" as the site of the generation of the highest level of perceptual information is in doubt.

4. Perhaps nonrepresentational cortex has expanded in primate phylogeny, but not nearly as much as has been proposed. On the other hand, the *numbers* of sensory representations clearly have increased with phylogenetic expansion of the forebrain.

5. The present understanding of cortical connections does not support the traditional concept of a serial cortical sensation-to-perception hierarchy of processing of information. Rather, each cortical field is multiply interconnected with other representations with the inclusion of parallel, serial, and recurrent components. Most connections are within a sensory domain. Parallel thalamocortical projection systems that segregate different classes of information are common.

6. The topography of different fields is field-specific and often dramatic differences are seen.

7. Different cortical fields receive different mixes of input with component-segregated information. Many response characteristics of neurons are consequently field-specific.

8. The response properties of neurons in "secondary" fields in comparison with those of neurons in "primary" fields are not consistently compatible with the concept of higher functions in the "secondary" fields.

9. Finally, some evidence from studies of the effects of lesions or damage of cortical regions indicates that different topographic representations can make field-specific contributions to perceptions.

B. Some Implications for the Genesis of
Perception from the Forebrain

*1. Perception Arises from the Nearly Simultaneous
and Largely Parallel Activation of a Number of
Cortical Fields*

While the responses of cortical neurons are greatly dependent on specific stimulus features, it is also true that rather simple stimuli such as a moving bar of light, onset of a tone, or the depression of the skin will activate neurons in all or nearly all of the cortical representations at about the same time. Thus, a viewed object would generate concurrent topographic patterns of activity in a number of cortical fields. Because cortical areas differ in the source of their inputs, their internal topographics and intrinsic structure, and their overall neural response properties, each area must make a field-specific contribution to the resulting perception of the object. Since a spatially unified perception is generated, the cortical maps must allow the same "peripheral reference" to be established for each cortical site activated by the same stimulus.

*2. There Are Potentially Complex Functional
Interfield Interactions Modifying the Product of
Fields; Cortical Fields Can also Potentially Modify
Their Inputs (and the Inputs to Other Fields)*

While the percept of an observed or felt object must be the product of the nearly simultaneous activation within most or all of the fields of cortex within the appropriate sensory domain, there are many anatomically expressed opportunities for interfield interactions that could modify that percept. Certain clusters of topographic fields are strongly interconnected. This creates tremendous *potential* for interfield interactions, although the functional significance of the complex system of interconnections has not yet been defined. Moreover, most fields have connections that would allow the direct modification of their thalamic input and thalamic input to other fields. Thus, while different cortical fields usually derive their principal inputs from parallel ascending sources, there are complex connections that allow the possibility of both the manipulation of that input and the modification of the cortical field product. As far as is known, at least most interfield and descending connections are homotopic or nearly so. Differences in how an object is perceived could result from such a complexly interconnected system. In other words, under different operational conditions such as in different states of attention or expectancy, complex interactions could produce greatly altered outputs from specific fields, and hence result in quite different perceptions of the same object.

## 3. Implications for Dreaming and Remembering

If perception is generated by the coincident activity of a number of topographic matrices that generate a unified sensation by virtue of their internal topographies, homotopic interconnections, and coincidentally assigned peripheral references, memories and dreams are likely to depend on similar mechanisms. Since memories and dreams have similar spatial referents to ongoing perceptions, it is parsimonious to hypothesize that they all arise as a consequence of the same basic neural representational mechanisms. Thus it seems plausible that a memory or a dream is somehow reintroduced across much of the same representational matrices that are normally activated during perception. Differences in the memory or the dream of an object and the actual perception of the object could be a consequence of a different mix or balance of outputs from different representational areas. In fact, there is recent evidence that regions in topographically organized visual cortex are differentially active during REM (dreaming) sleep. Whether a memory is stored in some way throughout the representational matrices, or whether there is some site-specific memory storage system is an intriguing question. In any case, without knowing how information is stored it is difficult to speculate how stored information could be replayed across representational cortical matrices.

If dreams and memories depend on the activation of a collection of sensory representations, how do we account for the observation that electrical stimulation of single cortical locations in what must be representational cortex in humans sometimes evokes complex memories (see Penfield and Rasmussen, 1952; Penfield and Jasper, 1954). One possibility is that the relatively high levels of stimulation used in such instances are capable of activating complete networks of cortical and subcortical areas, and somehow activating storage and replay mechanisms. Such memories are not commonly activated near the epileptic focus in epileptic patients where presumably cortical depression would reduce the recruitment of other brain structures. In addition, lower levels of cortical stimulation related to the development of a "visual prosthesis" resulted in only simple sensations such as points of light, stars, and small bars (Dr. Daniel Pollen, personal communication). Thus, it appears unlikely that activity restricted to a single sensory representation is capable of inducing complex memories, dreams, or perceptions.

### 4. The Significance of "Association" Cortex: Is It the Highest Level Cortex for Genesis of Perception?

One of the clear implications of recent studies of sensory cortex and thalamus is that there is actually relatively little multimodal processing in sensory systems. Yet, there still may be limited small regions of cortex between the topographic visual, auditory, and somatosensory areas that are reasonably characterized as bimodal or multimodal. Is this the "highest level" cortex from which refined aspects of perception arise, or does multimodal cortex have some other role? Since nontopographic multimodal fields would seem incapable of assigning *topographic* attributes to evoked perceptions, it would seem reasonable to hypothesize that such multimodal nontopographic regions are performing in the perceptual realm what Penfield termed "interpretative" functions. Penfield found that general perceptual attributes ("I've seen (felt, heard) this before," "I like this," "I don't want to do this," "I don't feel (or see or hear) any," etc.) were applied to any ongoing experience of the stimulated patient (see Penfield and Rasmussen, 1952; Penfield and Jasper, 1954). Such interpretative attributes are, in a sense, *lower* level attributes. They are applicable to more than one modality for the very reason that a spatial reference is irrelevant. In terms of its *perceptual* contributions, then, multimodal cortex might possibly subserve interpretative functions.

Of course, as pointed out by Mountcastle and colleagues (1974), multimodal neural integration can probably be expected to have a role in controlling an animal's decision to act. However, the command control of voluntary activity should be separated from considerations of the perception evoked from normal activation of this cortex.

### C. Summary of Principles of a Unified Hypothesis on the Genesis of Perception in the Forebrain Based on Contemporary Results of Studies of Sensory Systems

A hypothesis of the basic mechanism of genesis of spatial aspects of perceptions from the forebrain based on recent studies of sensory systems might contain the following principles:

1. Perception is a product of a nearly simultaneous activation of a number of topographic sensory representations.

2. Inputs to and the response properties of neurons within these topographic representations are in some respects field-specific.

3. The intrafield topographic orders establish a spatial referent for each spatially assignable perceptual attribute generated by these representational areas.

4. Differences in the perception of a given stimulus are to some extent a result of variations in the contributions of individual topographic representations to perception under different conditions of attention, expectancy, or other factors.

5. Contributions to perception are also made by "interpretative" cortical regions that may be multimodal. Perceptual attributes contributed by these cortical fields are not spatially assignable (or are only weakly so). There may be representational cortex between the topographically ordered visual and somatosensory and auditory cortical fields that are of this type.

6. Memories and dreams receive their spatial referents by the same mechanisms as do real-time perceptions. Differences between dreams, memories, and perceptions are a result of differential activations of specific subsets of topographic representations. Remembering must require a mechanism whereby stored information can in some way be replayed across topographic representations so that the memory gains its spatial referents.

7. Complex interfield connections might be involved in (a) the generation of a spatially unified perception, (b) the replaying of memories or dreams across multiple cortical topographic representations, and (c) the production of perceptual variety for given stimuli.

## Acknowledgments

Research by the authors and co-workers included in this review was supported by NIH Grant NS–10414, EY–02686, NSF Grant BNS–81824, Hearing Research, Inc., and the Coleman Fund. Illustrations were drawn by R. J. Nelson. Helpful comments were provided by R. Dykes, A. Epstein, H. Fields, R. Guillery, J. Sprague, M. Stryker, L. Symonds, and J. Wall.

## References

Allman, J. M., and Kaas, J. H. (1974). The organization of the second visual area (VII) in the owl monkey: A second order transformation of the visual hemifield. *Brain Research* **76**, 247–265.

Allman, J. M., and Kaas, J. H. (1975). The dorsomedial cortical visual area: A third tier area in the occipital lobe of the owl monkey (*Aotus trivirgatus*). *Brain research* **100**, 473–487.

Allman, J. M., and Kaas, J. H. (1976). Representation of the visual field in the medial wall of occipital-parietal cortex in the owl monkey. *Science* **191**, 572–575.

Andersen, *R*. A. (1979). Functional Connections of the Central Auditory Nervous System: Thalamocortical, Corticothalamic and Corticotectal Connections of the AI, AII and AAF Auditory Cortical Fields. Thesis, University of California at San Francisco, San Francisco.

Andersen, R. A., Patterson, H., Knight, P. L., Crandall, B., and Merzenich, M. M. (1977). Thalamocortical, corticothalamic and corticotectal projections to and from physiologically identified loci within the auditory cortical fields AAF, AII and AI. *Neuroscience Abstracts* **3**, 3.

Bishop, G. H. (1959). The relation between nerve fiber size and sensory modality: Phylogenetic implications of the afferent innervation of the cortex. *Journal of Nervous and Mental Disorders* **128**, 89–128.

Benevento, L. A., Rezak, M., and Santos-Anderson, R. (1977). An autoradiographic study of the projections of the pretectum in the rhesus monkey (*Macaca mulatta*): Evidence for sensorimotor links to the thalamus and oculomotor nuclei. *Brain Research* **127**, 197–218.

Bolton, J. S. (1900). On the exact histological localisation of the visual area of the human cerebral cortex. *Philosophical Transactions* **193**, 165–222.

Brodmann, K. (1909). "Vergleichende Lokalisationslehre der Grosshirnrinde." Verlag Barth, Leipzig.

Brugge, J. F., and Imig, T. J. (1978). Some relationships of binaural response patterns of single neurons to cortical columns and interhemispheric connections of auditory area AI of cat cerebral cortex. *In* "Evoked Electrical Activity in the Auditory Nervous System" (R. F. Naunton, ed.). Academic Press, New York.

Burton, H., and Jones, E. G. (1976). The posterior thalamic region and its cortical projection in New World and Old World monkeys. *Journal of Comparative Neurology* **168**, 249–302.

Burton, H., and Robinson, C. J. (1978). A single unit study of cortical areas adjacent to the second somatic sensory cortex in the cynomologous monkey. *Neuroscience Abstracts* **5**, 548.

Campbell, A. W. (1905). "Histologic Studies on the Localization of Cerebral Function." University Press, Cambridge.

Carey, R., Fitzpatrick, D., and Diamond, I. T. (1979). Layer I of striate cortex of *Tupaia glis* and *Galago senegalensis:* Projections from thalamus and claustrum revealed by retrograde transport of horseradish peroxidase. *Journal of Comparative Neurology* **186**, 393–430.

Colwell, S. A., and Merzenich, M. M. (1979). Corticothalamic projections from physiologically defined loci in AI in the cat. *Journal of Comparative Neurology,* in press.

Diamond, I. T., and Hall, W. C. (1969). Evolution of neocortex. *Science* **164**, 251–262.

Duffy, F. H., and Burchfiel, J. L. (1971). Somatosensory system: Organizational hierarchy from single units in monkey Area 5. *Science* **172**, 273–275.

Elliot-Smith, G. E. (1906). A new topographical survey of human cerebral cortex, being an account of the distribution of the anatomically distinct cortical areas and their relationship to the cerebral sulci. *Journal of Anatomy and Physiology* **41**, 237–254.

Evans, E. F., Ross, H. F., and Whitfield, I. C. (1965). The spatial distribution of unit characteristic frequency in the primary auditory cortex of the cat. *Journal of Physiology (London)* **179**, 238–247.

Fitzpatrick, K. A., Imig, T. J., and Reale, R. A. (1977). Thalamic projections to the posterior auditory cortical field in cat. *Neuroscience Abstracts* **3**, 8.

Flechsig, P. (1896). "Gehirn und Seele." Veit and Company, Leipzig.

Goldstein, M. H., Abeles, M., Daly, R. L., and McIntosh, J. (1970). Functional organization in cat primary auditory cortex: Tonotopic organization. *Journal of Neurophysiology* **33**, 188–197.

Graham, J., Lin, C.-S., and Kaas, J. H. (1979). Subcortical projections of six visual cortical areas in the owl monkey, *Aotus trivirgatus*. *Journal of Comparative Neurology,* **187,** 557–580.

Gross, C. G., Rocha-Miranda, C. E., and Bender, D. B. (1972). Visual properties of neurons in inferotemporal cortex of the macaque. *Journal of Neurophysiology* **35**, 96–111.

Heath, G. J., Hore, J., and Phillips, C. G. (1976). Inputs from low threshold muscle and cutaneous afferents of hand and forearm to Areas 3a and 3b of baboon's cerebral cortex. *Journal of Physiology (London)* **257**, 199–227.

Hebb, D. O. (1949). "The Organization of Behavior." Wiley, New York.

Hines, M. (1929). On cerebral localization. *Physiological Reviews* **9**, 462–574.

Hubel, D. H., and Wiesel, T. N. (1965). Receptive fields and functional architecture in two non-striate visual areas (18 and 19) of the cat. *Journal of Neurophysiology* **28**, 229–289.

Hubel, D. H., and Wiesel, T. N. (1968). Receptive fields and functional architecture of monkey striate cortex. *Journal of Physiology (London)* **195**, 215–243.

Hubel, D. H., and Wiesel, T. N. (1970). Cells sensitive to binocular depth in Area 18 of the macaque monkey cortex. *Nature (London)* **225**, 41–43.

Hubel, D. H., and Wiesel, T. N. (1977). Functional architecture of macaque visual cortex. *Proceedings of the Royal Society of London B* **198**, 1–59.

Imig, T. J., and Adrian, H. O. (1977). Binaural columns in the primary field (AI) of cat auditory cortex. *Brain Research* **138**, 241–257.

Imig, T. J., and Brugge, T. J. (1978). Sources and terminations of callosal axons related to binaural and frequency maps in primary auditory cortex of the cat. *Journal of Comparative Neurology* **182**, 637–660.

Imig, T. J., and Reale, R. A. (1977). The origins and targets of corticocortical connections related to tonotopic maps of cat auditory cortex. *Neuroscience Abstracts* **3**, 8.

Imig, T. J., Ruggero, M. H., Kitzes, L. M., Javel, E., and Brugge, J. F. (1977). Organization of auditory cortex in the owl monkey (*Aotus trivirgatus*). *Journal of Comparative Neurology* **171**, 111–128.

Jones, E. G., Coulter, J. D., and Hendry, S. H. C. (1978). Intracortical connectivity of architectonic fields in the somatic sensory motor and parietal cortex of monkeys. *Journal of Comparative Neurology* **181**, 291–348.

Jones, E. G., Wise, S. P., and Coulter, J. D. (1979). Differential thalamic relationships of sensory-motor and parietal cortical fields in monkeys. *Journal of Comparative Neurology* **183**, 833–882.

Kaas, J. H. (1977). Sensory representations in mammals. *In* "Function and Formation of Neural Systems" (G. S. Stent, ed.), pp. 65–80. Dahlem Konferenzen, Berlin.

Kaas, J. H. (1978). The organization of visual cortex in primates. *In* "Sensory Systems of Primates" (C. A. Noback, ed.), pp. 151–179. Plenum, New York.

Kaas, J. H., Hall, W. C., and Diamond, I. T. (1970). Cortical visual Areas I and II in the hedgehog: Relation between evoked potential maps and architectonic subdivisions. *Journal of Neurophysiology* **33**, 595–615.

Kaas, J. H., Nelson, R. J., Sur, M., Lin, C.-S., and Merzenich, M. M. (1979). Multiple representations of the body within "SI" of primates: A redefinition of "primary somatosensory cortex." *Science* **204**, 521–523.

Kennedy, T. T. K. (1955). An Electrophysiological Study of the Auditory Projection Areas of the Cortex in Monkey (*Macaca mulatta*). Thesis, University of Chicago, Chicago.

Klüver, H., and Bucy, P. C. (1939). Preliminary analysis of functions of the temporal lobes in monkeys. *Archives of Neurology and Psychiatry* **42**, 979–1000.

Knight, P. L. (1977). Representation of the cochlea within the anterior auditory field (AAF) of the cat. *Brain Research* **130**, 447–467.

Lende, R. A. (1963). Cerebral cortex: A sensorimotor amalgam in the Marsupialia. *Science* **141**, 730–732.

Lin, C.-S., and Kaas, J. H. (1979). The inferior pulvinar complex in owl monkeys: Architectonic subdivisions and patterns of input from the superior colliculus and subdivisions of visual cortex. *Journal of Comparative Neurology* **187**, 655–678.

Lin, C.-S., Merzenich, M. M., Sur, M., and Kaas, J. H. (1979). Connections of Areas 3b and 1 of the parietal somatosensory strip with the ventroposterior nucleus in the owl monkey (*Aotus trivirgatus*). *Journal of Comparative Neurology* **185**, 355–372.

Luria, A. R. (1966). "Higher Cortical Functions in Man." Basic Books, New York.

Merzenich, M. M., and Brugge, J. F. (1973). Representation of the cochlear partition on the superior temporal plane of the macaque monkey. *Brain Research* **50**, 275–296.

Merzenich, M. M., Knight, P. L., and Roth, G. L. (1975). Representation of cochlea within primary auditory cortex in the cat. *Journal of Neurophysiology* **38**, 231–249.

Merzenich, M. M., Kaas, J. H., and Roth, G. L. (1976). Auditory cortex in the grey squirrel: Tonotopic organization and architectonic fields. *Journal of Comparative Neurology* **166**, 387–402.

Merzenich, M. M., Roth, G. L., Anderson, R. A., Knight, P. L., and Colwell, S. A. (1977). Some basic features of organization of the central auditory nervous system. *In* "Psychophysics and Physiology of Hearing" (E. F. Evans and J. P. Wilson, eds.), pp. 1–11. Academic Press, New York.

Merzenich, M. M., Kaas, J. H., Sur, M., and Lin, C.-S. (1978). Double representation of the body surface within cytoarchitectonic Areas 3b and 1 in "SI" in the owl monkey (*Aotus trivirgatus*). *Journal of Comparative Neurology* **181**, 41–74.

Middlebrooks, J. C., Dykes, R. W., and Merzenich, M. M. (1978). Binaural response-specific bands within AI in the cat: Specialization within isofrequency contours. *Neuroscience Abstracts* **4**, 24.

Middlebrooks, J. C., Dykes, R. W., and Merzenich, M. M. (1980). Binaural response-specific bands in primary auditory cortex (AI) of the cat: Topographical organization orthogonal to isofrequency contours. *Brain Research* **181**, 31–48.

Morest, D. K. (1964). The probable significance of synaptic and dendritic patterns of the thalamic and midbrain auditory system. *Anatomical Record* **148**, 390–391.

Mott, F. W. (1907). The progressive evolution of the structure and functions of visual cortex in mammalia. *Archives Neurology (Mott's)* **3**, 1–117.

Mountcastle, V. B. (1974). Neural mechanisms in somesthesia. *In* "Medical Physiology." Mosby, St. Louis.

Mountcastle, V. B., Talbot, W. H., Sakata, H., and Hyvärinen, J. (1969). Cortical neuronal mechanisms in flutter-vibration studied in unanesthetized monkeys. Neuronal peridicity and frequency discrimination. *Journal of Neurophysiology* **32**, 452–484.

Mountcastle, V. B., Lynch, J. C., Georopoulos, A., Sakata, H., and Acuna, C. (1975). Posterior parietal association cortex of the monkey: Command functions for operations within extrapersonal space. *Journal of Neurophysiology* **38**, 871–908.

Nelson, R. A., Sur, M., Felleman, D. J., and Kaas, J. H. (1980). Representations of the body surface in postcentral parietal cortex of *Macaca fascicularis*. *Journal of Comparative Neurology,* in press.

Newman, J. D., and Wollberg, Z. (1973). Multiple coding of species-specific vocalizations in the auditory cortex of squirrel monkeys. *Brain Research* **54,** 287–304.

Newsome, W. T., Baker, J. F., Meizen, F. M. Myerson, J., Petersen, S. E., and Allman, J. M. (1978). Functional localization of neuronal response properties in extrastriate visual cortex of the owl monkey. *ARVO Abstracts* **1,** 174.

Oliver, D. L., Merzenich, M. M., Roth, G. L., Hall, W. C., and Kaas, J. H. (1977). Tonotopic organization and connections of primary auditory cortex in the tree shrew *(Tupaia glis)*. *Anatomical Record* **184,** 491.

Palmer, L. A., Rosenquist, A. C., and Tusa, R. J. (1978). The retinotopic organization of the lateral suprasylvian areas in the cat. *Journal of Comparative Neurology* **177,** 233–256.

Paul, R. L., Goodman, H., and Merzenich, M. M. (1972a). Representation of slowly and rapidly adapting cutaneous mechanoreceptors of the hand in Brodmann's Areas 3 and 1 of *Macaca mulatta*. *Brain Research* **36,** 229–249.

Paul, R. L., Goodman, H., and Merzenich, M. M. (1972b). Alterations in mechanoreceptor input to Brodmann's Areas 1 and 3 of the postcentral hand area of *Macaca mulatta* after nerve section and regeneration. *Brain Research* **39,** 1–19.

Penfield, W., and Boldrey, E. (1937). Somatic motor and sensory representation in the cerebral cortex of man as studied by electrical stimulation. *Brain* **60,** 389–443.

Penfield, W., and Jasper, H. (1954). "Epilepsy and the Functional Anatomy of the Human Brain." Little, Brown, Boston.

Penfield, W., and Rasmussen, T. (1952). "The Cerebral Cortex of Man." Macmillan, New York.

Poggio, G. F., and Fischer, B. (1977). Binocular interaction and depth sensitivity in striate and prestriate cortex of behaving rhesus monkey. *Journal of Neurophysiology* **40,** 1392–1405.

Rámon y Cajal, S. (1911). "Histologie du Systéme Nerveux de L'homme et des Vertébrés," pp. 1909–1911. Maloine, Paris.

Randolph, M., and Semmes, J. (1974). Behavioral consequence of selective subtotal ablation in the post central gyrus of *Macaca mulatta*. *Brain Research* **70,** 55–70.

Reale, R. A., and Imig, T. J. (1977). An orderly representation in the posterior ectosylvian sulcus of the cat. *Neuroscience Abstracts* **3,** 10.

Rose, J. E., and Mountcastle, V. B. (1959). Touch and kinesthesis. *In* "Handbook of Physiology: Neurophysiology I." American Physiological Society, Washington, D.C.

Roth, G. L., Atkin, L. M., Andersen, R. A., and Merzenich, M. M. (1978). Some features of the spatial organization of the central nucleus of the inferior colliculus of the cat. *Journal of Comparative Neurology* **182,** 661–680.

Rowe, M. II., and Stone, J. (1977). Naming of neurons: Classification and naming of cat retinal ganglion cells. *Brain Behavior and Evolution* **14,** 185–216.

Sakata, H., Takaoka, Y., Kawarasaki, A., and Shibutani, H. (1973). Somatosensory properties of neurons in the superior parietal cortex (Area 5) of the rhesus monkey. *Brain Research* **64,** 85–102.

Schiller, P., and Malpeli, J. (1977). Properties and tectal projections of monkey retinal ganglion cells. *Journal of Neurophysiology* **40,** 428–445.

Sur, M. (1978). Some principles of organization of somatosensory cortex. Ph.D. Thesis, Vanderbilt University, Nashville.

Sur, M., Nelson, R. J., and Kaas, J. H. (1980). Representation of the body surface in somatic koniocortex in the prosimian, Galago. *Journal of Comparative Neurology,* in press.

Swarbrick, L., and Whitfield, I. C. (1972). Auditory cortical units selectively responsive to stimulus 'shape.' *Journal of Physiology (London)* **224**, 68–69.

Symonds, L. L., and Kaas, J. H. (1978). Connections of striate cortex in the prosimian, *Galago senegalensis. Journal of Comparative Neurology* **181**, 477–512.

Tanji, J. (1975). Activity of neurons in cortical Area 3a during maintenance of steady postures by the monkey. *Brain Research* **88**, 549–553.

Teuber, H. L. (1960). Perception. *In* "Handbook of Physiology. Vol. 3. Neurophysiology." American Physiological Society, Washington, D.C.

Thompson, R. F. (1975). "Introduction to Physiological Psychology." Harper and Row, New York.

Tunturi, A. R. (1950). Physiological determination of the arrangement of the afferent connections to the middle ectosylvian auditory area in the dog. *American Journal of Physiology* **162**, 489–502.

Van Essen, D. C. (1979). Visual areas of the mammalian cerebral cortex. *Annual Review of Neurobiology,* **2**, 227–263.

Vogt, B. A., and Pandya, D. N. (1978). Cortico-cortical connections of somatic sensory cortex (Areas 3, 1, and 2) in the rhesus monkey. *Journal of Comparative Neurology* **177**, 179–192.

Wagor, E., Lin, C.-S., and Kaas, J. H. (1975). Some cortical projections of the dorsomedial visual area (DM) of association cortex in the owl monkey, *Aotus trivirgatus. Journal of Comparative Neurology* **163**, 227–250.

Walzl, E. M. (1947). Representation of the cochlea in the cerebral cortex. *Laryngoscope* **57**, 778–787.

Weller, R. E., and Kaas, J. H. (1978). Connections of striate cortex with the posterior bank of the superior temporal sulcus in macaque monkeys. *Neuroscience Abstracts* **4**, 650.

Weller, R. E., Kaas, J. H., and Wetzel, A. B. (1979). Evidence for the loss of X-cells of the retina after long-term ablation of visual cortex in monkeys. *Brain Research* **160**, 134–138.

Winer, J. A., Diamond, I. T., and Raczkowski, D. (1977). Subdivisions of the auditory cortex of the cat: The retrograde transport of horseradish peroxidase to the medial geniculate body and posterior thalamic nuclei. *Journal of Comparative Neurology* **176**, 387–418.

Winter, P., and Funkenstein, H. H. (1973). The effect of species specific vocalization on the discharge of auditory cortical cells in the awake squirrel monkey (*Saimiri sciureus*). *Experimental Brain Research* **18**, 489–504.

Woolard, H. H. (1925). The cortical lamination of tarsiers. *Journal of Anatomy* **60**, 86–105.

Woolsey, C. N. (1958). Organization of somatic sensory and motor areas of the cerebral cortex. *In* "Biological and Biochemical Bases of Behavior" (H. F. Harlow and C. N. Woolsey, eds.), pp. 63–81. University of Wisconsin Press, Madison.

Woolsey, C. N. (1960). Organization of cortical auditory system: A review and a synthesis. *In* "Neural Mechanisms of the Auditory and Vestibular Systems" (G. L. Rasmussen and W. Windle, eds.), pp. 165–180. Thomas, Springfield, Illinois.

Woolsey, C. N., and Fairman, D. (1946). Contralateral, ipsilateral, and bilateral representation of cutaneous receptors in somatic Areas I and II of the cerebral cortex of pig, sheep, and other mammals. *Surgery* **19**, 684–702.

Woolsey, C. N., and Walzl, E. M. (1944). Topical projection of the cochlea to the cerebral cortex of the monkey. *American Journal of Medical Science* **207**, 685–686.

Woolsey, C. N., Marshall, W. H., and Bard, P. (1942). Representation of cutaneous tactile sensibility in the cerebral cortex of the monkey as indicated by evoked potentials. *Bulletin Johns Hopkins Hospital* **70**, 399-441.

Young, J. Z. (1962). Why do we have two brains? *In* "Interhemispheric Relations and Cerebral Dominance" (V. B. Mountcastle, ed.), pp. 7-24. Johns Hopkins University Press, Baltimore.

Zeki, S. M. (1969). Representation of central visual fields in prestriate cortex of monkeys. *Brain Research* **14**, 271-291.

Zeki, S. M. (1971). Cortical projections from two prestriate areas in the monkey. *Brain Research* **34**, 19-35.

Zeki, S. M. (1974). Functional organization of a visual area in the posterior bank of the superior temporal sulcus of the rhesus monkey. *Journal of Physiology (London)* **236**, 549-573.

Zeki, S. M. (1977). Color coding in the superior temporal sulcus of rhesus monkey visual cortex. *Proceedings of the Royal Society of London B* **197**, 195-223.

PROGRESS IN PSYCHOBIOLOGY AND PHYSIOLOGICAL PSYCHOLOGY, VOL. 9

# Behavioral Modulation of Visual Responses in the Monkey: Stimulus Selection for Attention and Movement

Robert H. Wurtz

Michael E. Goldberg

and

David Lee Robinson

*Laboratory of Sensorimotor Research*
*National Eye Institute*
*National Institutes of Health*
*Bethesda, Maryland*

ISBN 0-12-542109-5

# I. Introduction

The visual system must be constantly bombarded by a changing pattern of retinal stimulation. An eye movement can occur as often as three times per second, and the pattern of stimulation in the more than a million optic nerve fibers (Ogden and Miller, 1966; Kupfer *et al.*, 1967) can therefore change as often. At some point in the brain there must be a selective reduction of this sensory barrage since only a fraction of it can actually be utilized within a given period of time. Perceptually, this selection seems reasonable since we usually attend to only one thing at a time. This selective attention was described by William James (1890) as "taking possession of the mind, in clear and vivid form, of one out of what seems several simultaneous possible objects or trains of thought. Focalization, concentration of consciousness are of its essence. It implies withdrawal from some things in order to deal effectively with others." The case for selection in preparation for movement is even more powerful. We cannot move our arm or eye in two directions at once; selection of which stimulus to follow is a necessity.

In a series of investigations of the primate visuomotor system we have described a physiological phenomenon that may well be related to selection processes. There are neurons in the visual system that yield enhanced responses to visual stimuli when those stimuli are relevant in some way to the animal's behavior. This article largely summarizes work on this visual enhancement phenomenon done in our respective laboratories. Several experimental strategies underlie our experiments. We concentrated on the visual system because the sensory transformations at successive levels in the brain have been better understood here than in any other sensory system. We have used extracellular recording rather than evoked potentials because issues of control and stimulus specificity are better handled at the level of a single cell, and at least certain ensemble inferences are possible from the study of adequate numbers of single neurons. We have used the rhesus monkey trained in a number of visuomotor tasks because it is easier to infer the bases of human behavior from phenomena studied in a subhuman primate. Finally, we have used a behaving animal because of a conviction that the neurophysiology of the central nervous system is the neurophysiology of behavior. The phenomenon that we have investigated could only have been described in a behaving animal since it represents the union of environmental and internal phenomena.

In outline we will discuss the visual enhancement effect in the brain areas shown in Fig. 1. First we will consider the superior colliculus where the selection effect was initially encountered, where the general methods

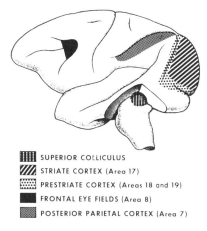

SUPERIOR COLLICULUS
STRIATE CORTEX (Area 17)
PRESTRIATE CORTEX (Areas 18 and 19)
FRONTAL EYE FIELDS (Area 8)
POSTERIOR PARIETAL CORTEX (Area 7)

FIG. 1. Schematic drawing of the lateral surface of the monkey brain showing regions which have been studied for the enhancement effect. The temporal lobe has been drawn as if a large section has been removed in order to expose the superior colliculus lying on the dorsal surface of the brainstem.

were worked out, and where an hypothesis about the source of the effect can be most clearly argued. Then we will go from this midbrain visual pathway to consider the geniculostriate pathway, as well as the prestriate cortex. Two areas of association cortex will then be analyzed: the frontal eye fields of the frontal lobe and the posterior parietal region of the parietal lobe. Finally, we will evaluate the possible functional significance of the enhancement effect.

## II. Superior Colliculus

The superior colliculus has long been identified with both a visual and a movement function (Adamük, 1870; Apter, 1945, 1946) and recent analyses of single cell activity in the colliculus have borne out these earlier suppositions. Single cell analyses in an awake, behaving monkey have indicated that the layers of this structure can be divided into at least two distinct groups as shown in Fig. 2 (Goldberg and Wurtz, 1972a; Wurtz and Goldberg, 1972a). The superficial layers comprise a thin surface layer of fibers, the stratum zonale, a cell layer, the stratum griseum superficiale, and a white layer, the stratum opticum. The input from the retina and striate cortex terminates in these layers (Wilson and Toyne, 1970; Lund, 1972; Hubel *et al.*, 1975). The stratum opticum in part is made up of retinal fibers which terminate near the dorsal surface of the

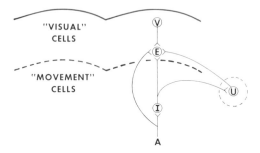

FIG. 2. Schematic drawing of the organization of the superior colliculus and afferents to enhanced cells. The dorsal surface of the colliculus is represented by the solid curved line, and the dashed line parallel to the surface separates the superficial layers from the intermediate layers. Cells in the superficial layers respond to visual stimuli independent of eye movements ("visual cells"); cells in the intermediate layers discharge before eye movements regardless of the stimulus conditions ("movement cells"). Enhanced cells (E) most likely receive their visual inputs from the visual cells (V) in the dorsal parts of the colliculus. The afferent(s) which modulate the visual response to produce the enhancement could arise from: (1) the movement cells deep in the intermediate layers (I), (2) direct projections from or collaterals of those afferents (A) which drive the movement cells, or (3) cells in some unknown (U) nucleus outside of the colliculus which are driven by the movement cells.

stratum griseum superficiale as does a prominent projection from the striate cortex. Cells in these superficial layers respond to visual stimuli (Humphrey, 1968; Cynader and Berman, 1972; Marrocco and Li, 1977) and do not discharge before rapid (saccadic) eye movements (Schiller and Koerner, 1971; Goldberg and Wurtz, 1972a; Schiller et al., 1974; Wurtz and Mohler, 1976a; Robinson and Wurtz, 1976).

The deep layers of the colliculus consist of alternating gray and white layers: the stratum griseum intermediale and stratum album intermediale, the stratum griseum profundum and the stratum album profundum (Kanaseki and Sprague, 1974). Cells in these layers may also have visual responses (Schiller and Koerner, 1971; Goldberg and Wurtz, 1972a; Cynader and Berman, 1972; Updyke, 1975; Mohler and Wurtz, 1976) but their salient feature is that they increase their rate of discharge before rapid or saccadic eye movements (Goldberg and Wurtz, 1970; Wurtz and Goldberg, 1971, 1972a; Schiller and Koerner, 1971; Robinson and Jarvis, 1974; Mohler and Wurtz, 1976; Sparks et al., 1976; Sparks, 1978). The cells discharging before eye movements do so regardless of whether the saccade is made in the light or in the dark.

Goldberg and Wurtz (1972b) in their studies on the superior colliculus were the first to notice the visual enhancement effect. They routinely determined the response of each cell encountered on a microelectrode penetration to both visual stimuli independent of eye movement and to eye movements alone. While they found that cells in the superficial layers did not discharge before eye movements in the dark, they noticed that the *visual* response of such cells to a spot of light that was the target for a saccade was more vigorous when the monkey repeatedly made an eye movement to the spot. They then systematically checked the visual response of cells in the superficial layers as well as how this response was modulated by the monkey's behavior.

## A. Basic Observations and Methods

The behavioral methods used have been applied to other areas of the brain covered in later parts of this article and are worth setting forth clearly. The monkey first learned a task which required him to fixate on a spot of light (the fixation point) for several seconds in order to detect a brief dimming of the spot (Wurtz, 1969). Release of the bar by the monkey during the dimming period was rewarded by a drop of water. If the monkey looked away from the fixation spot, he missed the dimming and missed the reward. The monkey also learned to make a saccadic eye movement from one spot to another if the first fixation spot went out and another spot came on. The training thus provided periods when the eyes were not moving and periods when a particular saccade was repeatedly made to a visual target.

The single unit recording and head restraint techniques used were those developed for monkeys by Evarts (Evarts, 1966, 1968a). During experiments the receptive fields of superior colliculus cells were determined while the monkey fixated on the spot. An outline of such a receptive field is shown in Fig. 3 (top). Collicular fields are easily mapped by spots of light; slits or bars are effective but not required to activate collicular cells in the monkey (Schiller and Koerner, 1971; Goldberg and Wurtz, 1972a; Cynader and Berman, 1972; Schiller *et al.,* 1974; Marrocco and Li, 1977; Robinson and Wurtz, 1976) as they generally are for neurons in monkey striate cortex (Hubel and Wiesel, 1968).

In order to study the visual enhancement effect (Goldberg and Wurtz, 1972b; Wurtz and Goldberg, 1972c), one point within the field was picked and the response of the cell to a spot of light at that point was determined (as illustrated in Fig. 3A). During these trials the monkey need only look at the fixation point to obtain a reward; the receptive field stimulus was not related to the reward. Next, the conditions of the experiment were changed. Now, at the same time that the receptive field stimulus came on, the fixation point went off (Fig. 3B). The monkey knew from previous training that under this condition the spot of light

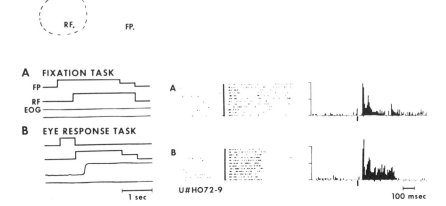

FIG. 3. Schematic illustration of the enhancement paradigm (left) with representative data for a cell in the superior colliculus (right). The diagram on the upper left shows the location of the fixation point (FP), with the dashed circle outlining the extent of the excitatory central area of a visual receptive field (RF). The spot in the receptive field is the stimulus for experiment (A) and the saccade target for experiment (B). (A) (left) illustrates the time of onset of the fixation point in response to the monkey's bar press. After the onset of the fixation point, the monkey fixates it, as indicated by the representative horizontal (top) and vertical (bottom) electro-oculogram traces (EOG). The receptive field stimulus comes on 0.5 seconds later. In the experiment for (B) (left), the fixation point comes on after the monkey presses the bar and then goes off when the light in the receptive field comes on. The monkey makes a saccadic eye movement to fixate the saccade target as indicated by the deflection in the horizontal electro-oculogram trace. The data in (A) (right) show the consistent response of a superior colliculus cell to the spot of light in the receptive field while the monkey fixates. Data in (B) (right) show the enhanced response of this cell to the onset of the same stimulus when the monkey uses it as the target for a saccadic eye movement. Each dot represents an action potential, and each horizontal row of dots represents a single fixation trial for the monkey. The vertical line indicates the time of onset of the visual stimulus. Histograms sum the data in the adjacent dot pattern (raster). The divisions on the vertical scale indicate a discharge rate of 250 spikes/second/trial with 8 msec bin widths. The format and conventions described here will be used throughout this paper unless stated otherwise. After Wurtz and Mohler (1974).

in the receptive field would eventually dim and so he made a saccade to the receptive field stimulus in order to easily detect this dimming. On the first trial the on-response of the cell was not changed by the execution of the saccadic eye movement, but on subsequent trials it was: the response of the cell was more regular and more vigorous—an enhanced visual response. This enhancement in different cells took the form of a more vigorous on-response (an early enhancement), a more prolonged response (a late enhancement), or both effects. About half of the cells studied in the superficial layers showed one of these enhancement effects.

Note that the discharge of the cell is modified at the time that the monkey was presumably preparing to make the saccadic eye movement to the receptive field stimulus but before he actually made the saccade. Thus the retinal stimulation is identical in both fixation and saccade conditions. Since there is a reaction time of about 200 msec for the monkey to make the eye movement and since the visual response occurs with a latency of only 35–60 msec (Wurtz and Mohler, 1976a), the initial visual response of the cell is over well before the eye starts to move. Once this reaction time is over the monkey makes an eye movement and of course moves the stimulus off the receptive field of the cell. This terminates the analysis.

It must be emphasized that the cells showing visual enhancement do not discharge in relation to eye movement per se (Goldberg and Wurtz, 1972b; Wurtz and Mohler, 1976a). They do not discharge before spontaneous eye movements made in the dark; their discharge is synchronous with onset of the visual stimulus, not with onset of saccadic eye movements as is the case with movement related cells in deeper collicular layers. Thus the enhancement effect requires a visual stimulus and is a modulation of the visual response of the cell.

Following a series of saccades to the receptive field stimulus, the conditions of the experiment were returned to the original state as shown for another cell in Fig. 4. Now when the receptive field stimulus came on, the fixation point stayed on, and the monkey no longer made saccades to the receptive field stimulus (Fig. 4C). Over a number of trials, the response of the cell then returned to about the same level as in the original state. If this series of declining responses was examined alone, a reasonable description would be that the response was "habituating"—a point we will consider more extensively in Section V,B.

These experiments show that use of the visual stimulus by the monkey produces an enhancement of the visual response of superior colliculus cells. In these experiments the visual stimulus remained the same when the monkey did and did not saccade to the stimulus. Only the use of the stimulus changed; the physical characteristics did not.

B. SPATIAL SELECTIVITY

The experiments described so far implicitly assume that the enhanced visual response is due to the monkey's saccade to a visual stimulus rather than to some nonspecific modulation. In order to determine how selec-

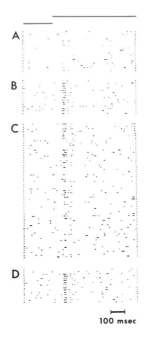

100 msec

FIG. 4. Habituation of the visual response and lack of habituation of the enhanced response. The indicator line at the top represents the time of onset of a spot of light in the receptive field. In (A), the monkey fixates and the spot of light in the receptive field elicits a very weak response. This activity is enhanced in (B) when the animal saccades to the stimulus; when the task is changed, this level of activity habituates over many trials in (C) after the monkey returns to the fixation task. The enhanced response is rapidly dishabituated in (D) and persists as the monkey returns to the saccade task. From Goldberg and Wurtz (1972b).

tive the enhancement effect is, a control experiment for these nonspecific factors was carried out. In this experiment, as the fixation point went off, two spots of light came on and the monkey could saccade to either one of these stimuli (see Fig. 5).[1] One spot of light was in the receptive field as before; the other spot was located outside the receptive field as indicated by the lack of a visual response of the cell when that stimulus was presented alone. The monkey could make a

[1] This control experiment was in fact run in two different ways. Using the first method, both the control point and the receptive field stimulus came on for every trial, and *both* dimmed on every trial when they became the target for a saccade. This method had the advantage that the stimuli were exactly the same throughout on all trials but the disadvantage that the monkey was free to saccade to one or the other at will. Trials on which the monkey made a saccade to the receptive field stimulus were identified from the eye movement records and the raster lines of these trials grouped together. However, since the enhancement effect tends to build up over several successive saccade trials, this method tended to

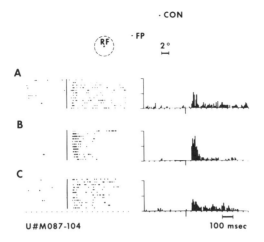

U#M087-104                                      100 msec

Fig. 5. Control experiment for enhancement selectivity. (A) shows the discharge of a collicular neuron to a spot of light in the receptive field (RF) and a control spot (CON) in the ipsilateral visual field while the monkey looks at the fixation point (FP). (B) shows the enhanced response on those trials when the monkey makes a saccadic eye movement to the receptive field stimulus whereas (C) illustrates the lack of enhancement on the trials when the monkey saccades to the control stimulus. Since the stimulus conditions are the same in all three experiments, these data demonstrate that there is a selective facilitation associated with eye movements to the receptive field. From Wurtz and Mohler (1976a).

series of saccades to either stimulus. When the monkey made saccades to the receptive field stimulus, the enhancement effect was clear (Fig. 5b). But when the saccades were made to the control stimulus, no such clear enhancement was seen (Fig. 5C) although a slight nonspecific effect was occasionally present. The enhancement effect was spatially selective; it was related to saccades made to the receptive field stimulus but not to those made to other areas. The enhanced visual response is therefore not related to some general alerting or arousal effect associated with making saccadic eye movements, since the enhancement is not present with all eye movements. For the same reason factors such as pupil dilation during saccades or a visual effect of the fixation light going off as the receptive field stimulus comes on cannot be producing the visual enhancement.

---

minimize the enhancement effect. In the second method both the receptive field stimulus and the control point came on but only *one* dimmed. This made the reward conditions somewhat different between blocks of trials, but required the monkey to make a series of saccades to one target or the other and potentiated the serial effects of enhancement. The enhancement effect is associated with the onset of the stimulus and the dimming occurred seconds later. The first method was used by Goldberg and Wurtz (1972b) and the latter by Wurtz and Mohler (1976a); both methods yielded comparable results.

## C. Hypothesis on Source of the Effect

A specific hypothesis has been developed by Wurtz and Mohler (1976a) to account for this enhancement effect in the superior colliculus. We shall present this hypothesis first and then consider how the characteristics of the enhancement effect fit it. While this discussion is the opposite of the actual sequence of experiments and analysis, it has the advantage of organizing the experimental results to point up both the strengths and weaknesses of the hypothesis.

The hypothesis starts from the fact that the superior colliculus can be divided into two functional parts as outlined in Fig. 2; their separation depends on whether the cells discharge to a visual stimulus or whether they discharge before an eye movement. The simplest explanation of the enhancement effect is that the cells in the intermediate and deep layers of the colliculus, which are the ones which discharge before eye movements, have a projection to those superficial layer cells which show an enhancement. In this hypothesis the enhancement of the visual response of the superficial layer cells results from a facilitation from the movement-related discharge of the deeper cells or a movement-related input to these cells.

Figure 2 shows schematically the organization of the cells showing visual enhancement and connections which might produce the enhancement. The enhanced cells are shown in the deeper part of the superficial layers, since the percentage of the enhanced cells was found to increase as one recorded deeper in the superficial layers (Wurtz and Mohler, 1976a). The visual input to these cells (labeled V in Fig. 2) might well come from superficial layer cells above the enhanced cells; the superficial layer cells in turn receive input from other more dorsal superficial layer cells or directly from retinal afferents. Input to enhanced cells from the visual areas of cortex also cannot be excluded (Schiller *et al.,* 1974). This sequence of visual input is suggested by increased latency for the visual response with increased depth (Wurtz and Mohler, 1976a), but such serial processing is not clearly established. The facilitation acting on these enhanced cells may come from the eye movement-related cells deep in the colliculus (labeled I in Fig. 2), from an external input (labeled A in Fig. 2) which might also project to the movement-related cells, or directly from some other unknown area of the brain (labeled U in Fig. 2). There are several possibilities for the afferents labeled A. One source is the nucleus parabigeminus, which is connected reciprocally with the superior colliculus (Graybiel, 1978b; Baleydier and Magnin, 1979). The intermediate gray layer of the superior colliculus projects to the nucleus parabigeminus, which in turn projects to the superficial layers of the colliculus. The parabigeminal nucleus may also receive eye movement-related information from the nucleus prepositus hypoglossi (Baleydier and Magnin, 1979). A second possible source of this input is the substantial nigra (Graybiel, 1978a), but eye movement-related activity has yet to be described here. Although the ventral lateral geniculate nucleus projects to the superficial layers of the colliculus in the cat (Edwards *et al.,* 1974), the saccade-related activity recorded in the monkey occurs after the saccade onset (Büttner and Fuchs, 1973) and therefore occurs too late to be a plausible candidate for the enhancement afferent. There are no established projections from deep layers to superficial layers within the superior colliculus. The essential point of the hypothesis is that the enhancement comes from a presaccadic discharge which produces facilitation within the superficial layers of the superior colliculus.

The facilitation of the visual input could logically be presynaptic or postsynaptic; no experimental evidence is currently available to distinguish between the two alternatives. For purposes of our analysis this is not a critical point, since the effect of the movement input is simply to change the effectiveness of the visual input.

In the following sections we will consider the relation of this hypothesis to experimental observations on the enhancement effect.

## D. TEMPORAL CHARACTERISTICS

The basic argument that the visual enhancement is a result of eye movement-related activity rests on the temporal properties of the effect: the enhancement varies in relation to the time of onset of the eye movement. This conclusion is based on experiments done by Wurtz and Mohler (1976a). They first showed that the type of enhancement was modified by the time at which the eye movement occurred. Their experiments started from the observation that there are cells showing an early enhancement (the on-response was facilitated), a late enhancement (a prolongation of the on-response), or both (Goldberg and Wurtz, 1972b). By changing the time when the monkey made a saccade to the receptive field stimulus, Wurtz and Mohler (1976a) found that a late enhancement could be converted into an early enhancement and vice versa. Saccades made soon after the onset of the target were associated with early enhancement and later saccades were associated with late enhancement. Conversion of one type of enhancement to the other by changing the monkey's behavior indicates that these variations are due to the monkey's eye movements and do not reveal intrinsic differences among cells. The *type* of enhancement is dependent on the *time* of the eye movement relative to the onset of the stimulus target. This might explain why Goldberg and Wurtz (1972a) were unable to see any orderly relation of early and late enhancement with other characteristics of the cells.[2]

If shifting the onset of the saccade closer in time to the onset of the stimulus produces a potentiated on-response to the visual stimulus, shifting the saccade to a much later time might produce a later enhancement. Goldberg and Wurtz (1972b) tested this by leaving the receptive field stimulus on all the time; there was then no on-response remaining and only the disappearance of the fixation point signaled the monkey to make a saccade. In this situation they found that the on-going response of the cell to the receptive field stimulus was more vigorous just before the onset of the saccade—the ultimate in late enhancement.

Another experiment attempted to determine the time course of the enhancement effect (Wurtz and Mohler, 1976a). In this experiment the monkey made a saccade from the fixation point to a small target within the receptive field area. The experiment tested the response of the cell to a brief light stimulus (50 msec) flashed at various times before and after the signal to initiate the saccade. The goal of the experiment was to use this brief stimulus to test the change in excitability of the cell to stimuli applied progressively closer in time to the onset of the eye movement. If the enhancement effect were a result of input from movement-related activity, the excitability of the cell should change in close temporal relation to the eye movement. This was what happened. A typical result, shown in Fig. 6, indicates that the enhancement effect is present about 200 msec before the onset of the eye movement, becomes larger at the time of the eye movement, and is present even after the eye movement is over. The enhancement effect is therefore transient and synchronous with the eye movement. It is not a tonic process that is set by the monkey's readiness to respond and would be expected to act continu-

[2] The signal to initiate a saccade to a target is actually the fixation point going off. By turning it off before or after the onset of the visual target, the initiation of the saccade could be shifted in time nearer to or farther from the stimulus onset. This paradigm works only within a limited time period. If the fixation light is turned off too long before the stimulus target comes on, the monkey will make a saccade to another point in the visual field of his own choosing before the target point comes on. If the fixation point is turned off too close in time to the onset of the target light, the monkey will not recognize the light as such and will again saccade to a point of his choosing. Why some cells show predominantly earlier enhancement while others show only later enhancement when the monkey controls the timing of his saccades is not entirely resolved by these experiments. One possibility is that the monkey shifts the time at which he initiates saccades at different times during an experimental day and therefore produces early enhancement at some times and late enhancement at others. An alternative explanation might be a differing threshold for the facilitation effect so that the same level of facilitation produces earlier enhancement in some cells than in others.

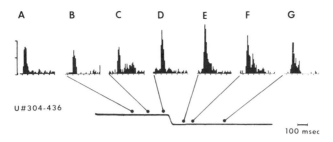

FIG. 6. Transient time course of pre- and posteye movement enhancement. (A) shows the response of a superior colliculus neuron to a spot of light in its receptive field while the monkey fixates. (B) through (G) show the build-up and decay of the facilitated visual response when stimuli are flashed for 50 msec in the receptive field at times close to the time of the saccadic eye movement. From Wurtz and Mohler (1976a).

ously between trials. This phasic development of the enhancement effect is consistent with the phasic discharge of the movement cells before each eye movement; had the enhancement been a tonic effect persisting between trials, it would have been difficult to relate to any other cells in the colliculus since none show such tonic discharge between trials.

That the enhanced visual response occurs several hundred milliseconds before the onset of the eye movement does, however, raise a potential problem. The cells deeper in the colliculus that discharge before eye movements seldom precede a spontaneous eye movement by more than 150 msec. If the response to a visual stimulus occurred in the colliculus 50 msec after stimulus onset, and the reaction time for a saccade to the target were 200 msec, the movement-related activity would barely overlap the visual activity in time. This may not be as much an embarrassment for the hypothesis as it might at first seem, since Mohler and Wurtz (1976) observed that many of the movement cells began to discharge in anticipation of the signal to make an eye movement (Fig. 7B). In cases where the monkey made eye movements to the same visual target on repeated trials, the onset of the eye movement and the discharge of the movement cells came earlier on successive trials. On many trials the movement cells actually started to discharge before the onset of the visual target. In this case the discharge of the movement cells started early enough to act on the visual input of cells in the superficial layer and facilitate the visual response of these cells.

This anticipatory effect in fact fits with a number of other observations on the enhancement effect. First, there is never a demonstrable enhancement of the on-response on the first trial when the monkey is required to make a saccade to the visual stimulus (Goldberg and Wurtz, 1972a; Wurtz and Mohler, 1976a). When Wurtz and Mohler (1976a)

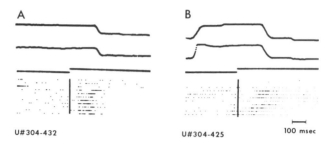

Fig. 7. Sequential build-up of the enhancement effect (A) and progressive anticipation of the discharge of movement cell (B). The monkey fixated on the first three trials in both (A) and (B) and then started making saccades to the visual stimulus on the fourth trial. The vertical line in each dot pattern indicates the onset of the visual target (for the first three trials) and both the onset of the visual target and offset of the fixation point in subsequent trials. The enhanced response of a superficial layer cell in (A) becomes progressively more vigorous on successive trials. Under similar conditions in (B), cells in the intermediate layers of the superior colliculus which discharge before eye movements become active progressively sooner and eventually precede the signal to make an eye movement. From Mohler and Wurtz (1976).

grouped together data from trials in which the monkey first made a saccade to the visual receptive field stimulus no enhancement of the on-response was apparent. Since the monkey cannot anticipate the requirement to make a saccade, there is probably no anticipatory activity by the movement cells, and they would not be expected to facilitate the visual response. However, there are occasional cases of late enhancement on these first trials and this could result from the start of movement cell discharge 150 msec before the onset of the eye movement.

The second observation in relation to anticipation is that visual enhancement of the on-response frequently becomes progressively better on successive trials when the monkey makes saccades to the visual stimulus (Fig. 7A). This could be due to the greater anticipation over a series of trials which is seen in movement cells in similar circumstances.

The final point is that the enhanced response was found to "habituate" over a number of trials after the monkey had stopped making saccades to the visual target (see Fig. 4C). This at first also seemed a problem for our hypothesis, which derived the enhancement effect from eye movement-related activity. This may not be a problem, however, since some movement cells continue to discharge as if the monkey were about to make an eye movement even though the monkey does not in fact make the saccade (Wurtz and Mohler, 1976a). If these cells discharged in such a manner after the end of a series of saccades to a visual stimulus, their continued facilitation of the visual cells would account for the prolongation of the enhancement effect beyond the end of the actual saccade trials. The gradual waning of the enhancement might result from the reduction of the number of movement cells discharging on successive trials.

This independence of discharge of the movement-related cells and the actual occurrence of the saccade has a parallel in the occasional independence of collicular cell discharge and the metrics of a saccade. The discharge of some collicular cells is the same before a 40° saccade as it is when the monkey instead makes two 20° saccades (Mohler and Wurtz, 1976); the cell discharge is the same whether a saccade is 20° or much less due to the modification of the eye movement by simultaneous occurrence of a head movement (Robinson and Jarvis, 1974). These examples probably represent a modification of eye movement control downstream from the superior colliculus, and in the present context serve to indicate that the collicular cells are not locked to the onset of a saccade.

What the temporal properties of the enhancement effect indicate is that it relates not so much to the monkey's eye movement but to the discharge of movement cells in anticipation of such a movement regardless of whether the movement actually occurs or not. The enhancement effect relates to a readiness to respond. The lack of a one-to-one relationship of the enhancement effect to the eye movement originally led Goldberg and Wurtz (1972b) to argue that the enhancement was independent of the saccades. Subsequent investigation of the characteristics of the movement cells deeper in the colliculus (summarized previously) has indicated that some of these cells also can be independent of the actual eye movement. The enhancement effect, as Goldberg and Wurtz (1972b) pointed out, *is* independent of the actual occurrence of eye movement, but we now realize that the discharge of some of the movement-related cells may also be independent.

### E. SPATIAL CHARACTERISTICS

The enhancement effect has been found to have several characteristics related to the spatial organization of the visual receptive field. We shall consider two questions and then see how the answers fit the hypothesis about the source of the enhancement.

To produce the enhancement effect the monkey must saccade to the receptive field stimulus. But need he saccade exactly to it? By having the monkey saccade to a small spot of light at varying distances from the effective receptive field stimulus, Wurtz and Mohler (1976a) answered this question: the enhanced response to the visual stimulus occurred even when the saccade target was outside but close to the receptive field. At target points farther from the receptive field, the enhancement disappeared.[3] In net, saccades near the receptive field produced an enhanced response; saccades remote from the field did not. A convenient description of this observation was that there was an "enhancement field," an area where saccades to any point produced a facilitated response to a stimulus in the center of the receptive field. This enhancement field was sometimes slightly larger than the visual receptive field, the area where spots of light alone produced a visual response.

The next question concerned the effect of the enhancement on receptive field size. Does a stimulus that produces no response from a cell when the monkey fixates produce a response when he makes a saccade to the visual stimulus? The answer to this question is that it does for some cells. But the maximum effect is a slight expansion of the receptive field of several degrees (Goldberg and Wurtz, 1972b; Wurtz and Mohler, 1976a) as indicated in Fig. 8.

The response of most superior colliculus cells to a spot of light falling in the central area of their receptive fields is probably the result of two antagonistic processes: an excitatory effect, concentrated in the central part of the receptive field, and an inhibitory or antagonistic effect spreading throughout the field, including a surrounding area. One possible mechanism underlying the expansion of the receptive field size might be a facilitation of the excitatory inputs to the cell; at the edge of the excitatory area of the field this increases the effectiveness of the stimulus just enough to lift the response above a background noise level and reveal a response to the stimulus. Another possibility might be a decrease in the strength of the suppressive surround which would produce a similar effect. The experiments done so far do not allow an estimate of the relative contribution of these two mechanisms.

The major point, however, is that receptive field size is altered only slightly. The enhancement effect modifies the vigor of the response to a spot of light, but it does not alter significantly the indication by the cell

[3] An important point in this experiment is the control for the effect of the target spot alone. This spot might produce a visual response (even though it was selected to be as ineffective as possible) and this response might be enhanced; what might have been determined in this experiment was simply the addition of the enhanced response to the target spot to the response to the receptive field stimulus. To control for this, other trials were run to determine the response to the target spot alone when the monkey made saccades to the stimulus. Near the edge of the receptive field the response was negligible so that conclusions on "enhancement field" were uncontaminated by any response to the target spot. In the receptive field center it was frequently not possible to distinguish the enhancement response to the saccade target and the visual receptive field stimulus, and no detailed study within the receptive field was therefore attempted. In addition, once the two points were within a few degrees of one another, determination of which stimuli the saccade was directed toward became difficult since eye movements were recorded with an electrooculogram with a resolution limited to about one degree of visual angle.

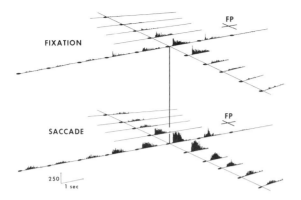

FIXATION

FP

SACCADE

FP

250 | 1 sec

FIG. 8. Expansion of the visual receptive field during the enhancement experiment. Histograms on the top show the response of a collicular neuron to spots of light falling on the tangent screen at the positions illustrated. The histograms on the bottom show the enhanced response to the corresponding spot of light when the monkey uses that stimulus as the target for a saccadic eye movement. FP, fixation point. From Wurtz and Mohler (1976a).

that a point of light lies within the receptive field. In other words, the signal-to-noise ratio of the cell is improved but the meaning of the signal remains the same.

An effect which is similar to the spatial features of the enhancement effect has recently been demonstrated in the cat superior colliculus by Rizzolatti *et al.* (1974). They found that moving a stimulus in the visual field of the paralyzed cat remote from the visual receptive field of a colliculus cell produced a *decrease* in the response to a receptive field stimulus. They suggested that this remote inhibitory effect might be a result of the cat's readiness to respond or to shift its attention to another part of the visual field with a resultant loss of facilitation to the area of the visual field where the receptive field of the cell is located—an inverse of the enhancement effect.

Recent experiments by Richmond and Wurtz (1978) suggest that in the awake monkey, which can move its eyes, this remote inhibitory effect results from visual interactions of the two stimuli rather than from any shift in gaze or attention. During a series of experiments on visual masking, they noticed that a stimulus remote from the central receptive field area, flashed on 50 msec before the onset of a stimulus within the central excitatory area, was effective in reducing the response to that stimulus in the central excitatory area. As in the cat, the effect was a suppressive one: the remote stimulus alone did not alter the discharge rate of the cell; it only reduced the response to a stimulus falling within the central area of the receptive field. The reduction in response persisted when the remote stimulus was turned on several hundred milliseconds before the onset of the stimulus in the central part of the receptive field. The remote stimulus was effective even when it was at least 30° from the edge of the central area but in the same hemifield. However, when the remote stimulus was on the contralateral side of the visual field, it was only slightly effective. No saccades or shift of attention need be invoked in these experiments since the monkey fixated on the small central fixation point throughout the entire experiment. The characteristics of these visual interactions are similar to those observed by Rizzolatti *et al.* (1974) in the cat although other factors, such as the greater effect of a moving rather than a stationary remote stimulus, are not obvious in the monkey. However, the effects in cat and monkey are sufficiently similar to suggest that the effect in the cat, like that in the monkey, is a purely visual sensory interaction, not a shift in attention and not related to the enhancement effect which requires a saccadic eye movement toward the stimulus.

## F. SPECIFIC RELATION TO EYE MOVEMENT

One of the key points in the analysis of the enhancement effect in the colliculus has been that it is related at least loosely to eye movements in both temporal and spatial properties. The temporal relationship between onset of the eye movement or preparation to move the eyes and the enhanced visual response supports this dependence of the enhancement on eye movement-related cells. A supplementary behavioral experiment also supports this view.

In this experiment (Wurtz and Mohler, 1976a), the monkey was trained for one set of trials to respond to a visual stimulus with a saccadic eye movement as in the previously described experiments *or* for another set of trials to indicate use of the stimulus by a hand movement instead of an eye movement. In this latter experiment, the monkey looked at the fixation point but learned that either the fixation point or the receptive field stimulus would dim and that release of the bar was required in either case to obtain a reward. The fixation point was small, the receptive field stimulus large, so that it was possible for the monkey to look at the fixation point and detect a dimming of the receptive field stimulus using peripheral vision. In addition, if the monkey made an eye movement during the fixation period, the trial was automatically terminated. This task forced the monkey not only to fixate but also to respond to a change in the receptive field stimulus with a hand rather than an eye movement. If the enhancement effect were related to use of the stimulus in a general way rather than in a way specifically related to eye movement, the visual cells should show enhancement in this task just as in the eye movement task. This was not the case; the enhancement in this task without eye movement was never as sharp and clear as with the eye movement. Therefore the enhancement seems to be more closely associated with preparation to make eye movements than to either make limb movements or possibly general use of the stimulus. Further details on the variations of the experiment and the limitations on interpretation are considered by Wurtz and Mohler (1976a).

If the enhancement effect, and indeed the function of the superior colliculus as a whole, is related to the initiation of eye movements, damage to the structure should produce a deficit at least in visually initiated and guided eye movements. This appears to be the case: following lesions placed in the superior colliculus, Wurtz and Goldberg (1972b) found an increased latency to make saccades, and Mohler and Wurtz (1977) found an additional tendency to make saccades somewhat shorter than required to reach a visual target.

## III. Striate and Prestriate Cortices

Striate (area 17) and prestriate cortices (roughly areas 18 and 19 for the present discussion) have traditionally been thought to be involved in the detailed analysis of visual input. Area 17 receives a massive projection from the retina via the lateral geniculate nucleus (Wilson and Cragg, 1967; Hendrickson et al., 1970; Garey and Powell, 1971; Hubel and Wiesel, 1972; Bunt et al., 1975) and damage along this pathway leads to devastating visual deficits in primates (see Doty, 1973, for review; Weiskrantz, 1972; Mohler and Wurtz, 1977). Furthermore, neurons in striate and prestriate cortices are selective for the types of visual stimuli which excite them (Hubel and Wiesel, 1968; Wurtz, 1969; Dow and Gouras, 1973; Schiller et al., 1976; Poggio and Fischer, 1977; Baizer et al., 1977; Michael, 1978).

It was of interest to determine whether the visual enhancement effect seen in the superior colliculus is a general phenomenon found throughout the visual system or whether it might be restricted to the midbrain visual areas. Wurtz and Mohler (1976b) found that there is occasionally a facilitation of the visual response when monkeys made saccadic eye movements to a stimulus in the receptive field of a striate cortical neuron. However, this enhancement occurs in a smaller proportion of striate neurons than collicular cells and is never as intense as that found in the colliculus. In contrast to the rather homogeneous receptive field properties found in the colliculus, there are several different types of receptive fields for neurons in striate cortex; all types in striate cortex have this behavioral modulation of their visual response (Wurtz and Mohler, 1976b).

The facilitation in striate cortex is seen in association with many directions of eye movements: those into the receptive field as well as those to points distant from the receptive field (Wurtz and Mohler, 1976b) (Fig. 9). The effect is therefore spatially nonselective. In addition, this modulation in striate cortex does not require an eye movement as does the collicular effect (Wurtz and Mohler, 1976a,b). If, while recording from a cell in striate cortex that shows this enhancement, the monkey is required to detect the dimming of a stimulus in the receptive field but not make an eye movement to it, the enhancement effect can still be demonstrated. Thus the enhancement in striate cortex is qualitatively different from that in the colliculus, being spatially nonselective and dissociable from the eye movement. It is also quantitatively different, occurring less frequently and less intensely than the selective enhancement in the superior colliculus.

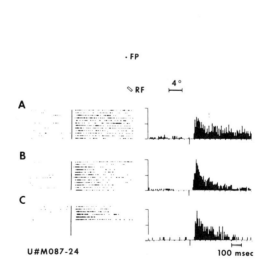

FIG. 9. Nonselective enhancement for a cell in striate cortex. The drawing at the top shows the location of the receptive field (RF) and control (CON) stimuli which fell on the screen while the monkey fixated. (A) illustrates the response of a cell to these stimuli. (B) and (C) demonstrate the enhanced responses in the saccade condition whether the monkey saccades to the stimulus in the receptive field (B) or to the control stimulus (C). FP, fixation point. From Wurtz and Mohler (1976b).

One of the efferent pathways from the superficial layers of the colliculus in primates is to the inferior pulvinar (Myers, 1963; Harting *et al.*, 1973; Mathers, 1971; Benevento and Fallon, 1975; Partlow *et al.*, 1977; Raczkowski and Diamond, 1978) and then to areas 18 and 19 (Glendenning *et al.*, 1975; Benevento and Rezak, 1976; Raczkowski and Diamond, 1978). Thus prestriate cortex may have inputs indirectly from the colliculus as well as directly from striate cortex (Kuypers *et al.*, 1965; Cragg, 1969; Zeki, 1975, 1978a,b), and it is of interest to know which of the types of enhancement, if any, occurs here. The visual properties of cells in areas 18 and 19 resemble those in striate cortex in most ways except for their increased size of the receptive fields (Baizer, 1976; Baizer *et al.*, 1977; Zeki, 1978a,b; Poggio and Fischer, 1977), and these visual properties are dependent on striate afferents (Schiller and Malpeli, 1977). For prestriate cells in the posterior bank of the lunate sulcus, enhancement is present and resembles that in striate cortex in that it is spatially nonselective, occurring with a wide variety of eye movements, and is seen with all cell types tested (Robinson *et al.*, in preparation). However, it occurs with greater frequency in prestriate cortex than in striate cortex.

Since the enhancement effects seen in areas 17, 18, and 19 are qualitatively and quantitatively different from that seen in the superior colliculus, it is unlikely that this cortical enhancement is derived from that seen in the superior colliculus. More likely it directly enters the geniculostriate system and may then be transmitted to areas 18 and 19.

We conclude that those parts of striate cortex and the prestriate cortex studied to date are well organized for the fine-grained analysis of the visual scene but poorly endowed for the evaluation of the behavioral context in which visual stimulation takes place. The only modulation observed in these areas appears to be a nonspecific one possibly related to alertness.

Initial experiments in the pulvinar nuclei of the thalamus have shown that the enhancement effect is present; here it is spatially nonselective but specific for eye movements (Keys and Robinson, 1979).

A major efferent of layer V of the striate cortex projects to the superficial layers of the superior colliculus (Hayaishi, 1969; Toyama *et al.*, 1969; Wilson and Toyne, 1970; Lund, 1972; Holländer, 1974; Palmer and Rosenquist, 1974; Lund *et al.*, 1975; Finlay *et al.*, 1976). Because the enhancement in striate cortex is so different from that seen in the colliculus, it seems unlikely that collicular enhancement is mediated through this corticotectal pathway, and this is in fact the case. Monkeys that have recovered from focal striate lesions have cells in the colliculus which show enhancement in the visual field representation corresponding to the damaged region of striate cortex (Wurtz and Mohler, 1976a). In fact, cells showing visual enhancement are slightly more frequent in the portions of the colliculus deprived of input from the ipsilateral striate cortex than in those areas with intact corticotectal afferents; such tectal cells contralateral to the striate lesion appear to be less frequent.

## IV. Parietal and Frontal Association Cortices

Stimulation experiments in the nineteenth century implicated two areas of association cortex as being important in the generation of eye movements (see Wagman, 1964). These areas, the frontal eye fields (Brodmann's area 8) and the posterior parietal eye fields (Brodmann's area 7) have also been considered important in the neural processes underlying visual attention (Welch and Stuteville, 1958; Critchley, 1953; Mountcastle *et al.,* 1975; Lynch *et al.,* 1977; Robinson *et al.,* 1978). Recent work has shown that cells in both of these areas are visually responsive and that these responses are behaviorally modifiable (Mohler *et al.,* 1973; Wurtz and Mohler, 1976b; Goldberg and Robinson, 1977a,b; Yin and Mountcastle, 1977; Robinson *et al.,* 1978). However, there are striking differences between the kinds of behavioral modifiability found in these two association cortices.

### A. FRONTAL EYE FIELDS

More recent stimulation experiments (Robinson and Fuchs, 1969) have indeed shown that electrical excitation of area 8 reliably induces saccadic eye movements in the unanesthetized monkey. Nonetheless, single cell recording studies did not confirm a role of frontal neurons in the generation of spontaneous eye movements. This is in contrast to primary motor cortex, area 4, where cells discharge reliably before limb movements (Evarts, 1968b). Bizzi (1968) showed that there was a small percentage of neurons in the frontal eye fields of the monkey that discharged in relation to saccades, but these cells discharged during and after the eye movements. Bizzi and Schiller (1970) described neurons discharging before head movement. Neither of these cell types could account for eye movements induced by stimulation.

Mohler *et al.* (1973) showed that roughly half of the cells they sampled in the frontal eye fields had visual responses with well-defined receptive fields. The receptive fields of the cells were large and were generally contralateral to the cerebral hemisphere containing the cells. The cells did not respond selectively to orientation or direction of movement. Like

neurons in the superior colliculus, cells in the frontal eye fields were easily driven by small spots of light, but unlike collicular neurons they
responded better to small spots within their excitatory regions than they
did to larger spots which lay entirely within their excitatory regions. A
major difference between these visual responses in the frontal eye fields
and in superior colliculus was the latency of the visual response, 40–60
msec for the superior colliculus and 80–120 msec for frontal eye fields.
Any serial relationship between these two areas must therefore be from
superior colliculus to frontal cortex. Figure 10,I shows the visual response and receptive field outline of a neuron in the frontal eye fields
of the monkey.

Half of these visually responsive neurons show enhancement when the
stimulus in the receptive field is the target for an eye movement (Wurtz
and Mohler, 1976b) (Fig. 10,II). The enhancement of the frontal eye
fields is present only when the animal makes a saccade to the stimulus in
the field and not when the animal makes a saccade to a stimulus outside
the field. The enhancement is therefore spatially selective, like that
found in the superior colliculus but unlike that found in the striate and
prestriate cortices.

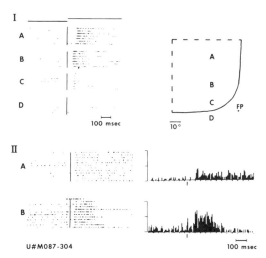

FIG. 10. Visual receptive field (I) and enhanced response (II) for a cell in the frontal eye
fields. The dot patterns in (I) show the discharge of a frontal eye field cell in response to a
spot of light flashed on the tangent screen at the locations illustrated on the right. The solid
line indicates the boundary determined for the receptive field; dashed lines are for indeter-
minant edges of the field. The lettered rasters (A–D) illustrate the cell's response to a spot
of light in the correspondingly lettered location in the receptive field. FP, fixation point.
Part (II) shows the response of another cell in area 8 to a spot of light in the fixation (A)
and saccade (B) conditions. From Mohler *et al.* (1973) and Wurtz and Mohler (1976b).

Since visually responsive frontal eye field neurons do not discharge before eye movements made spontaneously in the dark, any increased activity before visually guided eye movements must result from a modulation of a visual response. For the same reason, the enhancement cannot be the addition of a gaze-related discharge to a visual discharge. This is in contrast to those cells in the intermediate layers of the superior colliculus that do have such a dual visual- and movement-related discharge (Wurtz and Goldberg, 1972a).

Bushnell *et al.* (1978) have recently shown that neurons in area 8 display enhancement only when the monkey actually makes a saccadic eye movement to the stimulus. There is no enhancement when the monkey uses the stimulus as data for some other movement, such as the signal for a bar release or the target for a hand movement unassociated with an eye movement. These enhanced visual responses, occurring only when the animal intends to make a saccadic eye movement, may provide a retinal error signal for the generation of visually guided saccades. This retinal error signal may be the activity mimicked by the electrical stimulation which induces saccades from the frontal eye fields.

In summary, the frontal eye fields show a clear visual enhancement effect similar to that observed in the superior colliculus (spatially selective and specifically related to saccadic eye movements) but very different from that seen in striate and prestriate cortices (spatially nonselective and independent of saccadic eye movements). In addition, the type of visual stimulus required to activate cells is similar in frontal eye fields and superior colliculus but different from stimuli required to activate striate and prestriate cortical cells.

B. POSTERIOR PARIETAL CORTEX

Area 7 of the posterior parietal cortex is another visual area which may be linked to the eye movement process through the phenomenon of enhancement. Hyvärinen and Poranen (1974) described cells in area 7 of the awake rhesus monkey that discharged in association with eye movements. Using monkeys trained in an eye movement task, Mountcastle and his colleagues (Mountcastle *et al.*, 1975; Lynch *et al.*, 1977) described neurons that discharged in association with visually guided eye movements. Yin and Mountcastle (1977, 1978) described a small population of neurons in area 7 that responded to the onset of small light-emitting diodes, the response of some of which was enhanced when the animal made a saccade to the diode. Robinson *et al.* (1978) showed that every neuron they isolated in area 7 that discharged in association with some form of visually guided behavior could be driven by some visual stimulus independent of behavior. They proposed that all of the eye movement-related activity in area 7 could be explained as either passive visual responses or as behaviorally enhanced visual responses to stimuli falling in the receptive fields of the parietal cells, rather than as a movement signal independent of the sensory properties of the neurons. Figure 11 shows a neuron discharging before an eye movement, its time relationship to the eye movement, and its response to the stimulus in the absence of the eye movement (Fig. 11C). The response of the neuron is significantly enhanced when the animal makes a saccade to fixate the stimulus (Fig. 11B and C).

Parietal neurons also require the presence of the stimulus: if the animal makes the equivalent eye movement in total darkness, there is no change of the rate of discharge of the cell in relation to the eye movement (Mountcastle *et al.*, 1975; Lynch *et al.*, 1977; Robinson *et al.*, 1978). Therefore in area 7, too, the eye movement-related activity is a modulation of the visual response rather than an independent movement-related response.

Like the superior colliculus and the frontal eye fields, the enhancement in parietal cortex is spatially selective. A neuron that gives an

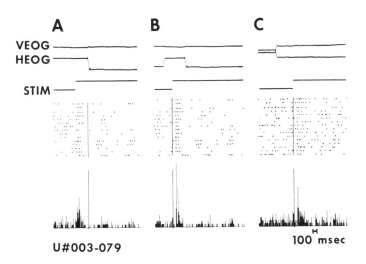

Fig. 11. Enhanced response and synchrony of activity with target onset for a cell in posterior parietal cortex. Data in (A) show the activity of the cell aligned with the onset of the saccadic eye movement, whereas (B) illustrates the same activity aligned with the onset of the target to which the eye movement was made. (C) demonstrates the visual response of the same cell to the same stimulus while the monkey fixates throughout the trial. VEOG, vertical electrooculogram; HEOG, horizontal electrooculogram; STIM, stimulus or target onset. From Robinson *et al.* (1978).

enhanced response when a stimulus in its receptive field is a target for a saccade will not give an enhanced response when the animal makes a saccade to a target outside the receptive field (Robinson *et al.,* 1978).

Enhancement in posterior parietal cortex is very different from that in the colliculus and frontal eye fields in its independence of the motor aspects of the response to the stimulus. Bushnell *et al.* (1978) trained monkeys to respond to a peripheral stimulus but not to fixate it. As in experiments previously described, in each trial the animal was presented with two stimuli, a small central fixation point and a larger peripheral stimulus. Either one might dim in a given trial, and the animal learned to release the bar at the dimming of either. If the animal made an eye movement to fixate the peripheral stimulus, the trial was aborted. At the onset of the peripheral stimulus the animal did not know which stimulus might dim, and his response was the same regardless of which actually did dim. Since the animal released the bar whenever either stimulus dimmed, the investigators concluded that on each trial he was attending to the peripheral stimulus as well as to the fixation point. Those area 7 neurons that display presaccadic enhancement also show enhancement during a series of trials when the animal attends to but does not fixate the stimulus in the receptive field. Figure 12 compares the response of a neuron in area 7 in this no-saccade attention task to the response of the same neuron to the same stimulus during a series of trials in which the stimulus was irrelevant to the animal. There is a marked enhancement when the animal attends to the stimulus.

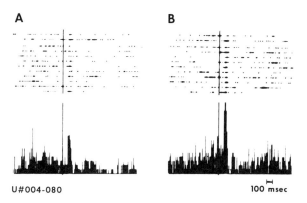

FIG. 12. Enhancement elicited by attention without movement. Responses in (A) were produced by the onset of a visual stimulus presented while the monkey fixated. The enhanced discharge in (B) was present when the monkey was required to attend to the same stimulus but did not make an eye movement to fixate the light. From Bushnell, Goldberg, and Robinson (unpublished data).

## V. Functional Implications

In the monkey brain the intensity of the response of a neuron to a visual stimulus may depend not only on the physical characteristics of the stimulus but frequently on behavioral factors intrinsic to the animal. We have found that we can best understand the significance of this sensory modulation, the visual enhancement, by defining the set of behavioral circumstances under which it takes place. By correlating behavioral circumstances with neuronal responses we have shown that there are at least three different kinds of enhancement in the monkey visual system as summarized in Table I. The enhancement seen in the striate and prestriate cortices is spatially nonselective and response nonspecific. That seen in the superior colliculus and frontal eye fields is spatially selective and response specific. That seen in the posterior parietal cortex is spatially selective but response independent. We will argue that each of these types of enhancement might well have a different role to play in the sensory processes underlying behavior. The enhancement that is both spatially and response nonspecific may well be related to alertness; that which is spatially selective and response specific may be more related to the initiation and guidance of specific movements; that which is spatially selective and independent of the specific motor response may well be participating in the neuronal mechanisms underlying attention.

### A. AROUSAL AND ALERTING

The role of arousal in modifying behavior was stimulated by the work of Moruzzi and Magoun (1949) on the reticular formation of the brainstem (see Lindsley, 1961; Magoun, 1958). These physiological studies in turn produced a surge of interest on the effects of activation or vigilance on a number of psychological factors including sensory processing (Duffy, 1962; Hebb, 1955). The nonselective enhancement effects seen

TABLE I
VARIETIES OF ENHANCEMENT

| Type | Brain location | Possible function |
|------|----------------|-------------------|
| Spatially nonselective | Striate cortex, prestriate cortex, pulvinar | Arousal or alertness |
| Spatially selective response specific | Superior colliculus frontal eye fields | Initiation of movement |
| Spatially selective response independent | Parietal cortex | Selective attention |

in areas 17 and 18 have the characteristics one would expect of a general arousal process: the enhancement modifies the response to all adequate stimuli and is independent of the behavioral response made to the stimuli. It is therefore tempting to correlate spatially nonselective enhancement with arousal, but there is one problem: behavioral state extends over a large spectrum from deep sleep to the performance of a difficult task. We have studied the responses of these neurons only over a limited portion of this range—while the animal was performing intricate visuomotor tasks of varying degrees of difficulty. If the enhancement that we have seen is related to arousal then we have seen only a small fraction of its total range of modulation; had we studied the neurons when the animals were less alert we might have seen a more pronounced modulation of sensitivity.

The responsiveness of the monkey's visual pathway has been shown to change following stimulation of the midbrain reticular formation (Singer, 1977). Bartlett and Doty (1974a,b) showed that the responses of neurons in the striate cortex of the squirrel monkey are augmented by electrical stimulation of the mesencephalic reticular formation. This group had previously shown that stimulation of the same area can also facilitate the transmission of impulses through the lateral geniculate of the monkey (Doty *et al.*, 1974) and that the efficacy of the stimulation is related to the animal's level of alertness (Bartlett *et al.*, 1973): reticular stimulation when the monkey was already alert had much less effect than when the animal was drowsy.

Posner has described a possible psychophysical counterpart of these physiological effects in his human performance experiments (Posner, 1975). He described alertness as the measure of receptivity of the organism to all external signals. Human subjects, for example, decrease their reaction time to a visual stimulus when the stimulus is preceded by a warning signal, and this more efficient processing is independent of the nature of the material to be processed. In the striate and prestriate cortices of the monkey, where the nonselective enhancement was the only effect seen, such enhancement could easily be a physiological representation of an alertness change: the brain becomes more receptive to all visual stimuli, not only those directly relevant to the task. When the animal is alert, it is more receptive to all stimuli, and its striate cortex is similarly more receptive throughout its entire retinotopic map.

B. HABITUATION

Enhancement also may be related to the phenomenon of habituation. If a stimulus is given repeatedly, the behavioral and physiological response to that stimulus wanes or habituates (see Humphrey, 1933, and Sokolov, 1960). This habituation occurs in most sensory systems when the stimuli are of no more than moderate strength and when the stimuli are given at regular intervals. There are remarkable similarities across species and experimental conditions in the habituation process (Thompson and Spencer, 1966).

In the visual system of mammals such habituation has been repeatedly observed, particularly in the superior colliculus (Horn and Hill, 1966; Horn, 1970), but we have seldom seen it in our analysis of the visual system of awake monkeys. One possible reason is that the responses that we study have already habituated to a stable state. This would not be surprising because the monkey has seen the same type of visual stimulus tens and frequently hundreds of times in the course of determining the receptive field of the neuron. Over the experimental lifetime of the animal he may well see similar stimuli hundreds of thousands of times, and although a neuron may respond to that stimulus a few times when the electrode is near, one can assume that the neuron has responded similarly when the electrode was in another group of cells. This situation in an awake animal may be profoundly different from an acute physiological experiment where the animal sees the experimental environment as a novel event, and the visual stimuli used to explore the responses on the neurons are truly new.

A habituated response recovers to original levels if no additional stimulation is given, or the habituated response may be dishabituated by presentation of a different stimulus (Thompson and Spencer, 1966). The dishabituation process and its relation to habituation have been studied intensively over the last 15 years, particularly in the flexor reflex of the cat (Spencer et al., 1966) and frog (Groves and Thompson, 1970; Thompson and Glanzman, 1976) and in the gill withdrawal reflex of the aplysia (Castellucci and Kandel, 1974; Kandel, 1978). A salient point that has emerged from these lines of investigation is that dishabituation is a separate process superimposed upon habituation rather than a reversal of habituation. The dishabituation studied in the cat and frog spinal cord and the aplysia abdominal ganglion is a sensitization effect: a general change in responsiveness which could result from a number of different stimulus changes in the environment or motivational changes in the animal. If the factor producing the sensitization is removed, the response returns to its habituated level. It is the dishabituation process that might have a clear parallel in our experiments on the visual enhancement effects. The response of visual cells we study might ordinarily be habituated, and the enhancement effect might be a dishabituation of this habituated response (Goldberg and Wurtz, 1972b). The visual enhancement effect could be regarded as an example of this separate process which is superimposed upon an habituated response and increases the response of the cell to a stimulus.

In the places where the enhancement effect is nonselective (as in striate and prestriate cortices) the enhancement is similar to the sensitization effect, and this is in turn very similar to arousal. However, we have not studied enough of the aspects of nonspecific enhancement to make a detailed comparison between it and sensitization.

When the enhancement effect is specifically related to a particular movement (as in the superior colliculus and frontal eye fields), it is clearly different from sensitization. Our findings emphasize that in the central nervous system of the primate the dishabituation can be the result of a selective facilitation which acts on just one aspect of visual processing without modifying all of sensory processing as does sensitization.

This reversal of habituation may indicate one of the basic functions of the enhancement effect in those areas where it is selective. The brain cannot respond to all sensory stimuli in the same way all the time, and a mechanism must exist to select novel and important stimuli from the sensory environment. Habituation is one mechanism; it assumes that all novel stimuli are important. When a stimulus ceases to be novel it ceases to have a significant effect, and the response wanes, or habituates. The dishabituation produced by selective enhancement prevents an important stimulus from being lost and enables it to continue to have an effect on behavior.


C. SELECTIVE ATTENTION

Along with initial reports of the visual enhancement effect in the superior colliculus, Goldberg and Wurtz (1972a,b) suggested that the effect might be related to a shift in visual attention. Denny-Brown (1962) and Sprague and Meikle (1965) had suggested earlier, on the basis of lesion experiments, that the superior colliculus might be related to attentional processes. Attention is a concept as old as psychology, and like most classical concepts in psychology has been defined nearly as frequently as it has been discussed. In order to discuss how physiological experiments might relate to this important concept, it is necessary to define what we mean by the term.

Attention has been frequently regarded as having at least two components. The first is an intensive (Berlyne, 1969) or alerting (Posner and Boies, 1971; Kahneman, 1973; Moray, 1969) component. This is essentially what we have considered as arousal or alerting and have compared to nonselective visual enhancement. The intensive effect is general and is probably a necessary condition for the second factor of attention to operate; selection of one stimulus from among many (James, 1890; Broadbent, 1958; Berlyne, 1969; Treisman, 1969; Berlyne, 1969; Kahneman, 1973; Moray, 1969; Posner and Boies, 1971). Selection can operate across sensory modalities or within modalities on the basis of the significance of a stimulus or its characteristics.[4] We have dealt with the visual modality and with selection of spatial location within that modality. Enhancement of sensory response provides a possible mechanism for stimulus selection; neuronal activity induced by the important stimulus has more effect than neuronal activity induced by a less important stimulus. The enhancement is spatially specific in the superior colliculus, frontal eye fields, and parietal cortex, and these areas could therefore be logically involved in focusing attention on certain areas of the visual field.

In both the behavioral experiments of others and our own physiological experiments, selective attention is always indicated by the occurrence of a response to a stimulus, and this presents a difficulty with the measurement of attention. Man can contemplate an object in the environment or in his memory, select that object for analysis, and yet make no externally observable response related to the object. We know that we attend, but an observer need not know. The investigator performing behavioral or physiological experiments cannot rely on the "ineffable, effable, effanineffable"[5] process of attention, but rather on the occurrence of a response to the attended stimuli, from which he must reason backward that attention was there. In fact, some discussions of attention regard it as being closely related to response—Woodworth (1929) refers to an attentional response as in the case of a cat waiting by

---

[4] An additional type of attention related to limited channel capacity is listed by Posner and Boies (1971). This type of attention is derived largely from reaction time interference studies which have indicated that the brain has a limited capacity to process sensory signals, and concentration on one set of tasks will increase the reaction time to a sporadically presented task using different sensory cues. In our physiological experiments, this channel capacity limitation probably is not distinguishable from a selection process, and for the purposes of our discussion this can be regarded as a type of selection. Other authors have identified as many as six types of attention (Moray, 1969), but for purposes of physiological comparison most of these can be subsumed under the rubric of selection.

[5] T. S. Eliot (1952) dealt with this issue in his marsupial analysis of carnivores:

The name that no human research can discover—
But THE CAT HIMSELF KNOWS, and will never confess.
When you notice a cat in profound meditation,
The reason, I tell you, is always the same:
His mind is engaged in a rapt contemplation
Of the thought, of the thought, of the thought of his name:
His ineffable effable
Effanineffable
Deep and inscrutable singular Name.

a mouse hole. This, in turn, is similar to the orienting response of Pavlovian conditioning (Pavlov, 1928). A problem arises when one confounds the response with the act of attention itself. Thus attention in man is well studied by measuring eye movement patterns (Yarbus, 1967) since it is the human style to look at what we attend.

Although visual attention is most often associated with movement, it can be dissociated from eye movement. For example, young monkeys never look at a dominant male, since eye contact is a threatening gesture, yet clearly they attend to the male (Perachio and Alexander, 1975). We therefore propose that although attention can be studied by looking at movements, particularly eye movements, true selective attention must be considered independent of the type of movement response.

In the posterior parietal cortex (area 7), Bushnell et al. (1978) found that visual responses are enhanced whenever the animal uses the stimulus in the receptive field for some behavior, regardless of the nature of the response. Thus the enhanced response will be seen if the animal makes an eye movement to the stimulus, reaches out to touch it, or merely knows that he may have to respond to it. We propose that these neurons have the properties one would expect to underly selective attention; they must be spatially selective and they must be independent of the movement the animal uses to respond to the stimulus. Posterior parietal cortex may well contain the neuronal substrate of visual attention in the form of its enhancement effect.

While we have postulated that the enhancement process in posterior parietal cortex participates in the mechanisms of selective attention, the enhancement effect in this area might in fact be derived from activity in other areas. The enhancement effect which is independent of particular movement might be summed from enhancements related to various movements. For example, the eye movement-related enhancement might come from enhanced visual input directly from the frontal eye fields or indirectly from the superior colliculus via the lateral posterior nucleus of the thalamus. Other enhancements may arise from the rich limbic connections of area 7 (Divac et al., 1977; Stanton et al., 1977; Mesulam et al., 1977; Kasdon and Jacobson, 1978). This caution emphasizes that the sources of enhancement remain unexplored.

It is interesting that all of the areas studied where cells show spatially selective enhancement share the property of having visual responses that do not require very specific stimuli. The requirements for visual orientation and directional selectivity which are the hallmarks of striate (Hubel and Wiesel, 1968, 1977) and prestriate cortices (Zeki, 1975, 1978a,b; Baizer et al., 1977) are not found in the superior colliculus and the frontal and parietal association cortices. This may indicate that pattern analysis is a function separate from the behavioral processes found out-side of the geniculostriate system. These nongeniculostriate areas may only need to analyze the location of an object in space and its functional relevance but not the specific details of its visual properties.

An important practical point that emerges from this analysis is that in an awake animal it may not be possible to look at passive input alone and describe the function of a cell. For example, Robinson *et al.* (1978) showed that cells in area 7 respond more briskly to passively presented large, bright stimuli. However, it is difficult to argue that these cells, which also respond to small spots of light used as targets for eye movements, are in fact bigness and brightness detectors. Rather, it is likely that the animals cannot escape attending to distracting stimuli of this magnitude; therefore, in this seemingly passive situation, the animals are indeed attending to the stimulus. The behavioral modulation of the response may be unavoidable here and must be considered at each step in sensory processing to determine the extent of its effect. The awake, behaving animal offers the only opportunity to study this effect, but it also presents the hazard of being misled by it.

D. INITIATION OF MOVEMENT

The enhancement in the superior colliculus and the frontal cortex does not fit our requirement for selective attention because the selection oc-curs only when the stimulus is intimately linked to a specific motor act, an eye movement, and not when the stimulus is linked to other re-sponses. If a stimulus is to be the target for an eye movement, it is con-venient for that stimulus to have a greater effect on the motor system than equivalent stimuli that are not to be targets of eye movements. This has been well studied in the pyramidal motor system. For example, Evarts and Fromm (1977) demonstrated that brisk load perturbations are accurately represented in motor cortex only when the load perturba-tion is relevant to the movement. A similar situation may obtain in the visual system, where in both the superior colliculus and the frontal eye fields, neurons have markedly enhanced responses only when the visual stimulus is the target for a saccadic eye movement.

One of the persisting problems in analyzing sensorimotor behavior is the transition from stimulus input to movement output. The machinery for the generation of a saccadic eye movement of a given amplitude has been analyzed and modeled (Robinson, 1975), but where in the brain the visual to motor transition lies for the generation of visually guided sac-cades remains unknown. One possible transition might occur through the phenomenon of enhancement, where a premovement signal acts on a visual signal. Stimulation in the frontal eye fields and superior colliculus evokes eye movements; the effect of this stimulation may be to mimic an enhanced visual response and send such a compelling message to the gaze system that the stimulus of interest is placed on the fovea. Thus these enhancements might represent intermediate stages between visual input and oculomotor output. The anatomical connections of both the frontal eye fields and the superficial layers of the superior colliculus make this an excellent possibility. The former projects to regions in the intermediate layers of the superior colliculus including those layers that have cells discharging before eye movements (Kuypers and Lawrence, 1967; Astruc, 1971; Künzle et al., 1976). The subtlety of the transition between an enhanced visual response and a visually triggered movement response in the superior colliculus (Wurtz and Mohler, 1976a) makes it likely that cells of the two sorts could share local circuit communications. The enhancement could then be the first stage in the definition of which object in the environment will be the target for the next saccadic eye movement.

## VI. Conclusion

The apparent necessity for selection among the myriad stimulus inputs of the visual system at the behavioral level seems to have been confirmed by findings at the physiological level; there is, in fact, a selection operating at many different levels of the visual system, ranging from a primary afferent area, the superficial layers of the superior colliculus, to several "association" areas of cerebral cortex, areas 7 and 8. Selective enhancement may also be present in the auditory (Beaton and Miller, 1975; Hocherman et al., 1976) and somatosensory systems (Hayes et al., 1979) although these systems are just beginning to be investigated in detail for these nonsensory modulations.

We have suggested that enhancement may be a mechanism by which sensory association areas combine data from the external world and data from the internal organism to generate a signal for the organization of behavior. While we have suggested a number of functions for the various types of enhancement in different parts of the brain, experiments have not been done which show that an absence of this visual enhancement leads to a pronounced deficit at the behavioral level. However, recent psychophysical experiments in man (Singer et al., 1977) have shown that a saccadic eye movement to a spot of light lowers the detection threshold for that spot of light. These authors suggest that this threshold change is a correlate of the enhancement effect; since it occurs in the absence of occipital cortex, it might be related to activity of the superior colliculus. Demonstration of the behavioral importance of enhancement is probably the most important experimental issue to be resolved.

### References

Adamük, E. (1870). Ueber die innervation der augenbewegungen. *Zeitschrift für Medizinische Wissenschaft* **8**, 65.

Apter, J. T. (1945). Projection of the retina on superior colliculus of cats. *Journal of Neurophysiology* **8**, 123–134.

Apter, J. T. (1946). Eye movements following strychninization of the superior colliculus of cats. *Journal of Neurophysiology* **9**, 73–86.

Astruc, J. (1971). Cortifugal connections of area 8 (frontal eye field) in *Macaca mulatta*. *Brain Research* **33**, 241–256.

Baizer, J. S. (1976). Receptive fields in areas 18 and 19 of the awake, behaving monkey. *Neuroscience Abstracts* **2**, 1101.

Baizer, J. S., Robinson, D. L., and Dow, B. M. (1977). Visual responses of area 18 neurons in awake, behaving monkey. *Journal of Neurophysiology* **40**, 1024–1037.

Baleydier, C., and Magnin, M. (1979). Afferent and efferent connections of the parabigeminal nucleus in cat revealed by retrograde axonal transport of horseradish peroxidase. *Brain Research* **161**, 187–198.

Bartlett, J. R., and Doty, R. W., Sr. (1974a). Response of units in striate cortex of squirrel monkeys to visual and electrical stimuli. *Journal of Neurophysiology* **37**, 621–641.

Bartlett, J. R., and Doty, R. W., Sr. (1974b). Influence of mesencephalic stimulation on unit activity in striate cortex of squirrel monkeys. *Journal of Neurophysiology* **37**, 642–652.

Bartlett, J. R., Doty, R. W., Pecci-Saavedra, J., and Wilson, P. D. (1973). Mesencephalic control of lateral geniculate nucleus in primates. III. Modifications with state of alertness. *Experimental Brain Research* **18**, 214–224.

Beaton, R., and Miller, J. M. (1975). Single cell activity in the auditory cortex of the unanesthetized, behaving monkey: Correlation with stimulus controlled behavior. *Brain Research* **100**, 543–562.

Benevento, L. A., and Fallon, J. H. (1975). The ascending projections of the superior colliculus in the rhesus monkey (*Macaca mulatta*). *Journal of Comparative Neurology* **160**, 339–362.

Benevento, L. A., and Rezak, M. (1976). The cortical projections of the inferior pulvinar and adjacent lateral pulvinar in the rhesus monkey (*Macaca mulatta*): An autoradiographic study. *Brain Research* **108**, 1–24.

Berlyne, D. E. (1969). The development of the concept of attention in psychology. *In* "Attention in Neurophysiology" (C. R. Evans and T. B. Mulholland, eds.), pp. 1–26. Appleton-Century-Crofts, New York.

Bizzi, E. (1968). Discharge of frontal eye field neurons during saccadic and following eye movements in unanesthetized monkeys. *Experimental Brain Research* **6**, 69–80.

Bizzi, E., and Schiller, P. H. (1970). Single unit activity in the frontal eye fields of unanesthetized monkeys during eye and head movement. *Experimental Brain Research* **10**, 151–158.

Broadbent, D. E. (1958). "Perception and Communication." Pergamon, London.

Bunt, A. H., Hendrickson, A. E., Lund, J. S., Lund, R. D., and Fuchs, A. F. (1975). Monkey retinal ganglion cells: Morphometric analysis and tracing of axonal projections, with a consideration of the peroxidase technique. *Journal of Comparative Neurology* **164**, 265-285.

Bushnell, M. C., Robinson, D. L., and Goldberg, M. E. (1978). Dissociation of movement and attention: Neuronal correlates in posterior parietal cortex. *Neuroscience Abstract* **4**, 621.

Büttner, M., and Fuchs, A. F. (1973). Influence of saccadic eye movements and unit activity in Simian lateral geniculate and pregeniculate nuclei. *Journal of Neurophysiology* **36**, 127-141.

Castellucci, V., and Kandel, E. (1974). An invertebrate system for cellular study of habituation and sensitization. *In* "Habituation" (T. J. Tighe and R. N. Leaton, eds.), pp. 1-47. Erlbaum, Hillsdale, New Jersey.

Cragg, B. G. (1969). The topography of the afferent projections in the circumstriate visual cortex of the monkey studied by the Nauta method. *Vision Research* **9**, 733-747.

Critchley, M. (1953). "The Parietal Lobes." Arnold, London.

Cynader, M., and Berman, N. (1972). Receptive-field organization of monkey superior colliculus. *Journal of Neurophysiology* **35**, 187-201.

Denny-Brown, D. (1962). The midbrain and motor integration. *Proceedings Royal Society Medicine* **55**, 527-538.

Divac, I., LaVail, J. H., Rakic, P., and Winston, K. R. (1977). Heterogeneous afferents to the inferior parietal lobule of the rhesus monkey revealed by the retrograde transport method. *Brain Research* **123**, 197-207.

Doty, R. W. (1973). Ablation of visual areas in the central nervous system. *In* "Handbook of Sensory Physiology" (R. Jung, ed.), Vol VII/3B, pp. 483-541. Springer, Berlin.

Doty, R. W., Wilson, P. D., Bartlett, J. R., and Pecci-Saavedra, J. (1973). Mesencephalic control of lateral geniculate nucleus in primates. I. Electrophysiology. *Experimental Brain Research* **18**, 189-203.

Dow, B. M., and Gouras, P. (1973). Color and spatial specificity of single units in rhesus monkey foveal striate cortex. *Journal of Neurophysiology* **36**, 79-100.

Duffy, E. (1962). "Activation and Behavior." Wiley, New York.

Edwards, S. B., Rosenquist, A. C., and Palmer, L. A. (1974). An autoradiographic study of ventral lateral geniculate projections in the cat. *Brain Research* **72**, 282-287.

Eliot, T. S. (1952). The Naming of Cats. "The Complete Poems and Plays," p. 149. Harcourt Brace, New York.

Evarts, E. V. (1966). Methods for recording activity of individual neurons in moving animals. *In* "Methods in Medical Research" (R. F. Rushmer, ed.), Vol. II, pp. 241-250. Year Book, Chicago.

Evarts, E. V. (1968a). A technique for recording activity of subcortical neurons in moving animals. *Electroencephalography and Clinical Neurophysiology* **24**, 83-86.

Evarts, E. V. (1968b). Relation of pyramidal tract activity to force exerted during voluntary movement. *Journal of Neurophysiology* **31**, 14-27.

Evarts, E. V., and Fromm, C. (1977). Sensory responses in motor cortex neurons during precise motor control. *Neuroscience Letters* **5**, 267-272.

Finlay, B. L., Schiller, P. H., and Volman, S. F. (1976). Quantitative studies of single-cell properties in monkey striate cortex. IV. Corticotectal cells. *Journal of Neurophysiology* **39**, 1352-1361.

Garey, L. J., and Powell, T. P. S. (1971). An experimental study of the termination of the lateral geniculo-cortical pathway in the cat and monkey. *Proceedings of the Royal Society of London* **179**, 41-63.

Glendenning, K. K., Hall, J. A., Diamond, I. T., and Hall, W. C. (1975). The pulvinar nucleus of *Galago senegalensis*. *Journal of Comparative Neurology*, **161**, 419-457.

Goldberg, M. E., and Robinson, D. L. (1977a). Visual responses of neurons in monkey inferior parietal lobule: The physiologic substrate of attention and neglect. *Neurology* **27**, 350.

Goldberg, M. E., and Robinson, D. L. (1977b). Visual mechanisms underlying gaze: Function of the cerebral cortex. *In* "Control of Gaze by Brainstem Neurons. Developments in Neuroscience" (R. Baker and A. Berthoz, eds.). Elsevier North Holland, Amsterdam.

Goldberg, M. E., and Robinson, D. L. (1978). The superior colliculus. *In* "Handbook of Behavioral Neurobiology. Vol. 1. Sensory Integration" (R. B. Masterton, ed.), pp. 119–164. Plenum, New York.

Goldberg, M. E., and Wurtz, R. H. (1970). Effects of eye movement and stimulus on units in monkey superior colliculus. *Federation Proceedings* **29**, 453.

Goldberg, M. E., and Wurtz, R. H. (1972a). Activity of superior colliculus in behaving monkey. I. Visual receptive fields of single neurons. *Journal of Neurophysiology* **35**, 542–559.

Goldberg, M. E., and Wurtz, R. H. (1972b). Activity of superior colliculus in behaving monkey. II. Effect of attention on neuronal responses. *Journal of Neurophysiology* **35**, 560–574.

Graybiel, A. M. (1978a). Organization of the nigrotectal connection: An experimental tracer study in the cat. *Brain Research* **143**, 339–348.

Graybiel, A. M. (1978b). A satellite system of the superior colliculus: The parabigeminal nucleus and its projections to the superficial collicular layers. *Brain Research* **145**, 365–374.

Groves, P. M., and Thompson, R. F. (1970). Habituation: A dual process theory. *Psychological Review* **77**, 419–450.

Harting, J. K., Glendenning, K. K., Diamond, I. T., and Hall, W. C. (1973). Evolution of the primate visual system: Anterograde degeneration studies of the tecto pulvinar system. *American Journal of Physical Anthropology* **38**, 383–392.

Hayaishi, Y. (1969). Recurrent collateral inhibition of visual cortical cells projecting to superior colliculus in cats. *Vision Research* **9**, 1367–1380.

Hayes, R. L., Price, D. D., and Dubner, R. (1979). Behavioral and physiological studies of sensory coding and modulation of trigeminal nociceptive input. *Advances in Pain Research and Therapy* **3**, 219–243.

Hebb, D. O. (1955). Drives and the CNS. *Psychological Review* **62**, 243–254.

Hendrickson, A., Wilson, M. E., and Toyne, M. J. (1970). The distribution of optic nerve fibers in *Macaca mulatta*. *Brain Research* **23**, 425–427.

Hocherman, S., Benson, D. A., Goldstein, M. H., Jr., Heffner, H. E., and Heinz, R. D. (1976). Evoked activity in auditory cortex of monkeys performing a selective attention task. *Brain Research* **117**, 51–68.

Holländer, H. (1974). On the origin of the corticotectal projections in the cat. *Experimental Brain Research* **21**, 433–439.

Horn, G. (1970). Changes in neuronal activity and their relationship to behaviour. *In* "Short Term Changes in Neural Activity and Behavior" (G. Horn and R. A. Hinde, eds.), pp. 567–606. Cambridge University Press, Cambridge.

Horn, G., and Hill, R. M. (1966). Responsiveness to sensory stimulation of units in the superior colliculus and subjacent tectotegmental regions of the rabbit. *Experimental Neurology* **14**, 199–223.

Hubel, D. H., and Wiesel, T. N. (1968). Receptive fields and functional architecture of monkey striate cortex. *Journal of Physiology* **195**, 215–243.

Hubel, D. H., and Wiesel, T. N. (1972). Laminar and columnar distribution of geniculo cortical fibers in the macaque monkey. *Journal of Comparative Neurology* **146**, 421–450.

Hubel, D. H., and Wiesel, T. N. (1977). Functional architecture of macaque monkey visual cortex. *Proceedings of the Royal Society of London* **B 198**, 159.

Hubel, D. H., LeVay, S., and Wiesel, T. N. (1975). Mode of termination of retinotectal fibers in the macaque monkey: An autoradiography study. *Brain Research* **96**, 25–40.

Humphrey, G. (1933). "The Nature of Learning." Harcourt, New York.

Humphrey, N. K. (1968). Responses to visual stimuli of units in the superior colliculus of rats and monkeys. *Experimental Neurology* **20**, 312–340.

Hyvärinen, J., and Poranen, A. (1974). Function of the parietal associative area 7 as revealed from cellular discharges in alert monkeys. *Brain* **97**, 673–692.

James, W. (1890). "The Principles of Psychology." Holt, New York (reprinted, Dover, New York, 1950).

Kahneman, D. (1973). "Attention and Effort." Prentice Hall, New York.

Kanaseki, T., and Sprague, J. M. (1974). Anatomical organization of pretectal and tectal laminae in the cat. *Journal of Comparative Neurology* **158**, 319–337.

Kandel, E. R. (1978). "A Cell Biological Approach to Learning," Grass Lecture Monograph 1, Society for Neuroscience, Bethesda, Maryland.

Kasdon, D. L., and Jacobson, S. (1978). The thalamic afferents to the inferior parietal lobule of the rhesus monkey. *Journal of Comparative Neurology* **177**, 685–706.

Keys, W., and Robinson, D. L. (1979). Eye movement-dependent enhancement of visual responses in the pulvinar nucleus of the monkey. *Neuroscience Abstracts* **5**, 791.

Künzle, H., Akert, K., and Wurtz, R. H. (1976). Projection of area 8 (frontal eye field) to superior colliculus in the monkey. An autoradiographic study. *Brain Research* **117**, 487–492.

Kupfer, C., Chumbley, L., and Downer, J. de C. (1967). Quantitative histology of optic nerve, optic tract and lateral geniculate nucleus of man. *Journal of Anatomy* **101**, 393–401.

Kuypers, H. G. J. M., and Lawrence, D. G. (1967). Cortical projections to the red nucleus and the brain stem in the rhesus monkey. *Brain Research* **4**, 151–188.

Kuypers, H. G. J. M., Szwarcbart, M. K., Mishkin, M., and Rosvold, H. E. (1965). Occipitotemporal corticocortical connections in the rhesus monkey. *Experimental Neurology* **11**, 245–262.

Lindsley, D. B. (1961). The reticular activating system and perceptual integration. *In* "Electrical Stimulation of the Brain" (D. E. Sheer, ed.), pp. 331–349. University of Texas Press, Austin.

Lund, R. D. (1972). Synaptic patterns in the superficial layers of the superior colliculus of the monkey, *Macaca mulatta*. *Experimental Brain Research* **15**, 194–211.

Lund, J. S., Lund, R. D., Hendrickson, A. E., Bunt, A. H., and Fuchs, A. F. (1975). The origin of efferent pathways from the primary visual cortex, area 17, of the macaque monkey as shown by retrograde transport of horseradish peroxidase. *Journal of Comparative Neurology* **164**, 287–304.

Lynch, J. C., Mountcastle, V. B., Talbot, W. H., and Yin, T. C. T. (1977). Parietal lobe mechanisms for directed visual attention. *Journal of Neurophysiology* **40**, 362–389.

Magoun, H. W. (1958). "The Waking Brain." Thomas, Springfield, Illinois.

Marrocco, R. T., and Li, R. H. (1977). Monkey superior colliculus: Properties of single cells and their afferent inputs. *Journal of Neurophysiology* **40**, 844–860.

Mathers, L. H. (1971). Tectal projection to the posterior thalamus of the squirrel monkey. *Brain Research* **35**, 295–298.

Mesulam, M.-M., Van Hoesen, G. W., Pandya, D. N., and Geschwind, N. (1977). Limbic and sensory connections of the inferior parietal lobule (area PG) in the rhesus monkey: A study with a new method for horseradish peroxidase histochemistry. *Brain Research* **136**, 393–414.

Michael, C. R. (1978). Color vision mechanisms in monkey striate cortex: Dual opponent cells with concentric receptive fields. *Journal of Neurophysiology* **41**, 572–588.

Mohler, C. W., and Wurtz, R. H. (1976). Organization of monkey superior colliculus: Intermediate layer cells discharging before eye movements. *Journal of Neurophysiology* **39**, 722–744.

Mohler, C. W., and Wurtz, R. H. (1977). Role of striate cortex and superior colliculus in visual guidance of saccadic eye movements in monkeys. *Journal of Neurophysiology* **40**, 74–94.

Mohler, C. W., Goldberg, M. E., and Wurtz, R. H. (1973). Visual receptive fields of frontal eye field neurons. *Brain Research* **61**, 385–389.

Moray, N. (1969). "Attention. Selective Processes in Vision and Hearing." Hutchinson, London.

Moruzzi, G., and Magoun, H. W. (1949). Brain stem reticular formation and activation of the EEG. *Electroencephalography and Clinical Neurophysiology* **1**, 455–473.

Mountcastle, V. B., Lynch, J. C., Georgopoulos, A., Sakata, H., and Acuna, C. (1975). Posterior parietal association cortex of the monkey: Command functions for operations within extrapersonal space. *Journal of Neurophysiology* **38**, 871–908.

Myers, R. E. (1963). Projections of superior colliculus in monkey. *Anatomical Record* **145**, 264.

Ogden, T. E., and Miller, R. F. (1966). Studies of the optic nerve of the rhesus monkey: Nerve fiber spectrum and physiological properties. *Vision Research* **6**, 485–506.

Palmer, L. A., and Rosenquist, A. C. (1974). Visual receptive fields of single striate cortical units projecting to the superior colliculus in the cat. *Brain Research* **67**, 27–42.

Partlow, G. D., Colonnier, M., and Szabo, J. (1977). Thalamic projections of the superior colliculus in the rhesus monkey, *Macaca mulatta*. A light and electron microscopic study. *Journal of Comparative Neurology* **171**, 285–317.

Pavlov, I. P. (1928). "Lectures on Conditioned Reflexes." International Publishers, New York.

Perachio, A. A., and Alexander, M. (1975). The neural basis of aggression and sexual behavior in the rhesus monkey. *In* "The Rhesus Monkey. Vol. I. Anatomy and Physiology" (G. H. Bourne, ed.), pp. 381–409. Academic, New York.

Poggio, G. F., and Fischer, B. (1977). Binocular interaction and depth sensitivity in striate and prestriate cortex of behaving rhesus monkey. *Journal of Neurophysiology* **40**, 1392–1405.

Posner, M. I. (1975). Psychobiology of attention. *In* "Handbook of Psychobiology" (M. S. Gazzaniga and C. Blakemore, eds.), chap. 15, pp. 441–480. Academic Press, New York.

Posner, M. I., and Boies, S. J. (1971). Components of attention. *Psychological Review* **78**, 391–408.

Raczkowski, D., and Diamond, I. T. (1978). Cells of origin of several efferent pathways from the superior colliculus in *Galago senegalensis*. *Brain Research* **146**, 351–357.

Richmond, B. J., and Wurtz, R. H. (1978). Visual masking by remote stimuli in monkey superior colliculus. *Neuroscience Abstracts* **4**, 642.

Rizzolatti, G., Camarda, R., Grupp, L. A., and Pisa, M. (1974). Inhibitory effect of remote visual stimuli on visual responses of cat superior colliculus: spatial and temporal factors. *Journal of Neurophysiology* **37**, 1262–1275.

Robinson, D. A. (1975). Oculomotor control signals. *In* "Basic Mechanisms of Ocular Motility and Their Clinical Implications" (G. Lennerstrand and P. Bach-Y-Rita, eds.), pp. 337–374. Pergamon Press, Oxford.

Robinson, D. A. and Fuchs, A. F. (1969). Eye movements evoked by stimulation of frontal eye fields. *Journal of Neurophysiology* **32**, 637–648.

Robinson, D. L., and Goldberg, M. E. (1977). Visual properties of neurons in the parietal cortex of the awake monkey. *Investigative Ophthalmology and Visual Science* **16**, Supplement, 156.

Robinson, D. L., and Jarvis, C. D. (1974). Superior colliculus neurons studied during head and eye movements of the behaving monkey. *Journal of Neurophysiology* **37**, 533–540.

Robinson, D. L., and Wurtz, R. H. (1976). Use of an extraretinal signal by monkey superior colliculus neurons to distinguish real from self-induced stimulus movements. *Journal of Neurophysiology* **39**, 852–870.

Robinson, D. L., Goldberg, M. E., and Stanton, G. B. (1978). Parietal association cortex in the primate: Sensory mechanisms and behavioral modulations. *Journal of Neurophysiology* **41**, 910–932.

Robinson, D. L., Baizer, J. S., and Dow, B. M. Visual response enhancement in prestriate cortex (in preparation).

Schiller, P. H., and Koerner, F. (1971). Discharge characteristics of single units in superior colliculus of the alert rhesus monkey. *Journal of Neurophysiology* **34**, 920–936.

Schiller, P. H., and Malpeli, J. G. (1977). The effect of striate cortex cooling on area 18 cells in the monkey. *Brain Research* **126**, 366–375.

Schiller, P. H., Stryker, M., Cynader, M., and Berman, N. (1974). Response characteristics of single cells in the monkey superior colliculus following ablation or cooling of visual cortex. *Journal of Neurophysiology* **37**, 181–194.

Schiller, P. H., Finlay, B. L., and Volman, S. F. (1976). Quantitative studies of single cell properties in monkey striate cortex. I. Spatiotemporal organization of receptive fields. *Journal of Neurophysiology* **39**, 1288–1319.

Singer, W. (1977). Control of thalamic transmission by corticofugal and ascending reticular pathways in the visual system. *Physiological Review* **57**, 386–420.

Singer, W., Zihl, J., and Pöppel, E. (1977). Subcortical control of visual thresholds in humans: Evidence for modality specific and retinotopically organized mechanisms of selective attention. *Experimental Brain Research* **29**, 173–190.

Sokolov, E. N. (1960). Neuronal models and the orienting reflex. *In* "The Central Nervous System and Behavior" (M. A. B. Brazier, ed.), pp. 187–276. Josiah Macy, Jr. Foundation, New York.

Sparks, D. L. (1978). Functional properties of neurons in the monkey superior colliculus: coupling of neuronal activity and saccade onset. *Brain Research* **156**, 1–16.

Sparks, D. L., Holland, R., and Guthrie, B. L. (1976). Size and distribution of movement fields in the monkey superior colliculus. *Brain Research* **113**, 21–34.

Spencer, W. A. Thompson, R. F., and Neilson, D. R., Jr. (1966). Response decrement of the flexion reflex in the acute spinal cat and transient restoration by strong stimuli. *Journal of Neurophysiology* **29**, 221–239.

Sprague, J. M., and Meikle, T. H., Jr. (1965). The role of the superior colliculus in visually guided behavior. *Experimental Neurology* **11**, 115–146.

Stanton, G. B., Cruce, W. L. R., Goldberg, M. E., and Robinson, D. L. (1977). Some ipsilateral projections to areas PF and PG of the inferior parietal lobule in monkeys. *Neuroscience Letters* **6**, 243–250.

Thompson, R. F., and Glanzman, D. L. (1976). Neural and behavioral mechanisms of habituation and sensitization. *In* "Habituation" (T. J. Tighe and P. H. Leaton, eds.), pp. 49–93. Erlbaum, Hillsdale, N.J.

Thompson, R. F., and Spencer, W. A. (1966). Habituation: A model phenomenon for the study of neuronal substrates of behavior. *Psychological Review* **73**, 16–43.

Toyama, K., Matsunami, K., and Ohno, T. (1969). Antidromic identification of association, commissural and corticofugal efferent cells in cat visual cortex. *Brain Research* **14**, 513–517.

Treisman, A. M. (1969). Strategies and models of selective attention. *Psychological Review* **76**, 282–299.

Updyke, B. V. (1975). Characteristics of unit responses in superior colliculus of the Cebus monkey. *Journal of Neurophysiology* **37**, 896–909.

Wagman, I. H. (1964). Eye movements induced by electric stimulation of cerebrum in monkeys and their relationship to bodily movement. *In* "The Oculomotor System" (M. B. Bender, ed.), pp. 18–39. Harper and Row, New York.

Weiskrantz, L. (1972). Behavioral analysis of the monkey's visual system. *Proceedings of the Royal Society of London, Ser B*. **182**, 427–455.

Welch, K., and Stuteville, P. (1958). Experimental production of unilateral neglect in monkeys. *Brain* **81**, 341–347.

Wilson, M. E., and Cragg, B. G. (1967). Projections from the lateral geniculate nucleus in the cat and monkey. *Journal of Anatomy* **101**, 677–692.

Wilson, M. E., and Toyne, M. J. (1970). Retinotectal and corticotectal projections in *Macaca mulatta. Brain Research* **24**, 395–406.

Woodworth, R. S. (1929). "Psychology." Holt, New York.

Wurtz, R. H. (1969). Visual receptive fields of striate cortex neurons in awake monkeys. *Journal of Neurophysiology* **32**, 727–742.

Wurtz, R. H., and Albano, J. E. (1980). The primate superior colliculus. *Annual Review of Neuroscience* **3**, 189–226.

Wurtz, R. H., and Goldberg, M. E. (1971). Superior colliculus cell responses related to eye movements in awake monkeys. *Science* **171**, 82–84.

Wurtz, R. H., and Goldberg, M. E. (1972a). Activity of superior colliculus in behaving monkey. III. Cells discharging before eye movements. *Journal of Neurophysiology* **35**, 575–586.

Wurtz, R. H., and Goldberg, M. E. (1972b). Activity of superior colliculus in behaving monkey. IV. Effects of lesions on eye movements. *Journal of Neurophysiology* **35**, 587–596.

Wurtz, R. H., and Goldberg, M. E. (1972c). The primate superior colliculus and the shift of visual attention. *Investigative Ophthalmology* **11**, 441–449.

Wurtz, R. H., and Mohler, C. W. (1974). Selection of visual targets for the initiation of saccadic eye movements. *Brain Research* **71**, 209–214.

Wurtz, R. H., and Mohler, C. W. (1976a). Organization of monkey superior colliculus: Enhanced visual response of superficial layer cells. *Journal of Neurophysiology* **39**, 745–762.

Wurtz, R. H., and Mohler, C. W. (1976b). Enhancement of visual responses in monkey striate cortex and frontal eye fields. *Journal of Neurophysiology* **39**, 766–772.

Yarbus, A. L. (1967). "Eye Movements and Vision" (L. A. Riggs, trans.). Plenum, New York.

Yin, T. C. T., and Mountcastle, V. B. (1977). Visual input to the visuomotor mechanisms of the monkey's parietal lobe. *Science* **197**, 1381–1383.

Yin, T. C. T., and Mountcastle, V. B. (1978). Mechanisms of neural integration in the parietal lobe for visual attention. *Federation Proceedings* **37**, 2251–2257.

Zeki, S. M. (1975). The functional organization of projections from striate to prestriate visual cortex in the rhesus monkey. *Cold Spring Harbor Symposium on Quantitative Biology* **40**, 591–600.

Zeki, S. M. (1978a). The cortical projections of foveal striate cortex in the rhesus monkey. *Journal of Physiology* **277**, 227–244.

Zeki, S. M. (1978b). Uniformity and diversity of structure and function in rhesus monkey prestriate visual cortex. *Journal of Physiology* **277**, 273–290.

PROGRESS IN PSYCHOBIOLOGY AND PHYSIOLOGICAL PSYCHOLOGY, VOL. 9

# Brain Pathways for Vocal Learning in Birds: A Review of the First 10 Years

### Fernando Nottebohm

*Department of Behavioral Science*
*The Rockefeller University*
*New York, New York*

Copyright © 1980 by Academic Press, Inc.
All rights of reproduction in any form reserved.
ISBN 0–12–542109–5

# I. Introduction

I have been fortunate to collaborate in research with a talented group of colleagues.[1] Together we have, over the years, stumbled onto a series of unexpected observations having to do with how the brain of songbirds approaches the task of vocal learning. Most of these observations were done on canaries, *Serinus canarius*. In canaries, we noticed brain pathways for vocal learning include discrete stations, hemispheric dominance, gross sexual dimorphism, a brisk response to hormones, and remarkable neural plasticity that extends well into adulthood. The following is an account of this work, most of which was conducted between 1969 and 1979. I have tried to preserve the original order of events because in this manner, I feel, the story tells itself well. Observations on canaries are supplemented with others on chaffinches, *Fringilla coelebs*, and zebra finches, *Poephila guttata*. All three species belong to the suborder Passeres of the avian order Passeriformes. I will also have something to say about two Psittaciformes, the orange-winged Amazon parrot, *Amazona amazonica*, and the budgerigar, *Melopsittacus undulatus*. All these species learn their vocal repertoire by reference to auditory information.

This is a comparative approach to the question of how brain pathways are organized to cope with the learning of a complex motor task. We do not know how learning is coded, nor do we know where in the brain it occurs. But if there is something special about networks evolved to maximize the learning of complex motor skills, we expect to find this "something" well represented in the vocal control pathways of songbirds and parrots.

## II. Hypoglossal Dominance

A. A SERENDIPITOUS FINDING

My interest in efferent and afferent aspects of song control in birds started with my doctoral dissertation (Nottebohm, 1966, 1968). Earlier Thorpe (1958) had reported that male chaffinches learn their song by copying that of other adult male chaffinches. Working with this same species I noticed that if both cochleas were removed before the onset of song learning, the song pattern that developed was virtually lacking in

---

[1] Arthur P. Arnold, William V. Bleisch, Cheryl Harding, Darcy B. Kelley, Christiana M. Leonard, Ivan Lieburg, Victoria Luine, Bruce McEwen, Donald W. Pfaff, Tegner M. Stokes, and Richard E. Zigmond.

structure. If the same operation was done after song had been learned, the learned pattern remained unaltered even 3 years later. Konishi (1965), reporting on similar findings in white-crowned sparrows, *Zonotrichia leucophrys*, had speculated that during song learning young birds modified their motor output until the auditory feedback it generated matched a learned auditory memory or "template." Once this match was achieved, he suggested, control shifted from auditory template to proprioceptive template, so that the learned pattern persisted in a stereotyped manner even after loss of hearing. Songs developed by chaffinches and white-crowned sparrows deafened before they learned their song were abnormal in their structure as well as in their lack of stereotypy. Presumably completion of a match between an auditory model or expectation and auditory feedback generated during song learning was necessary to achieve normal stereotypy (Konishi and Nottebohm, 1969). One way to test the role of proprioceptive feedback in the maintenance of the acquired pattern was to interfere peripherally with song control, after song had been learned.

It is necessary here to remind the reader about the anatomy of sound production in songbirds (Figs. 1 and 2). Sounds are produced by the syrinx during expiration. The expiratory muscles contract the abdominal air sacs which then function as bellows, and so provide a preliminary gross control over the patterning of song. In oscine (suborder Passeres of order Passeriformes) songbirds the syrinx consists of two functionally equivalent halves. Sounds are produced by the periodic oscillations of the internal tympaniform membranes (i.t.m.). There is one i.t.m. in each right and left syringeal half, forming the medial wall of the upper reaches of each bronchus. Each i.t.m. is drawn into the bronchus as a result of the Bernoulli effect, periodically interrupting air flow. As each i.t.m. occludes the lumen of the corresponding bronchus, the pressure head of expired air rises, pushing the membrane outward. This pattern of oscillation is presumably in phase with turbulence generated as air flows through the narrow opening connecting bronchus and trachea. The syringeal muscles modulate the frequency and amplitude of the sounds produced by setting membrane tension and controlling airflow past them. By acting in this manner the syrinx also works as a valve, setting the resistance against which the expiratory muscles work during sound production. The anatomy and physiology of the syrinx are reviewed in greater detail in Greenewalt (1968) and Nottebohm (1975). Each syringeal half is innervated by the tracheosyrineal (ts) branch of the ipsilateral hypoglossus nerve.

Two approaches were considered when seeking to interfere with proprioceptive feedback accompanying song. The first of these, deafferen-

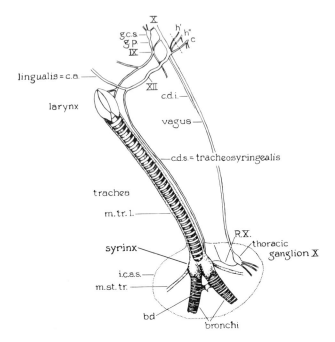

FIG. 1. Ventral view of the syrinx of an adult male canary, surrounded by the interclavicular air sac (i.c.a.s.). The sternotrachealis muscle (m.st.tr.) anchors the syrinx to
the anterior process of the sternum (not shown). Innervation to the syringeal musculature
is provided by the tracheosyringealis branch (ts) of the hypoglossus (XII) nerve. The recur-
rens branch of the vagus (R.X.) innervates the crop (not shown) which lies dorsal to the
syrinx. The bronchidesmal membrane (bd) anchors the syrinx to the dorsal wall of the
i.c.a.s. h′, h″, and c, hypoglossal and cervical roots of XII nerve; g.c.s. and g.p., cervical
superior and petrosum ganglia of IX; c.a. and c.d.i., cervicalis ascendens and descendens
inferior branches of XII; m.tr.l., tracheolateralis muscle.

tation of the expiratory musculature, seemed impractical. The second
one, deafferentation of the syrinx, was somewhat hypothetical since no
sensory innervation to the syrinx had been described. Motor innervation
to the syrinx is provided by the ts branch of the hypoglossus. It was
argued that denervation of the syrinx would disrupt not only the
modulation of song frequency and amplitude, but would also alter song-
related proprioception from all parts of the vocal tract and expiratory
system. However, the bird would not be muted since the expiratory
pulses normally generating song would still set the internal tympaniform
membranes into oscillation, though this oscillation would now be poorly
controlled. If the new pattern of pulsed sounds representing song retained a relation to preoperative song and remained stereotyped, this
would be evidence for the independence of vocal patterning from
learned proprioceptive feedback.

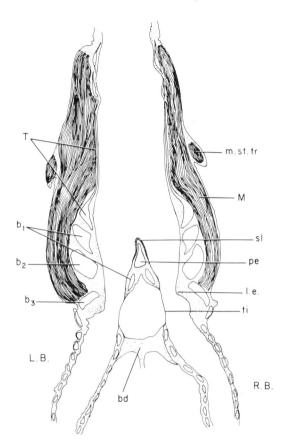

Fig. 2. Longitudinal section of the syrinx of an adult male canary. Abbreviations: R.B. and L.B., right and left bronchi; M, section through lateral mass of intrinsic syringeal muscles; T, tympanum; b₁, b₂, and b₃, bronchial half-rings; bd, bronchidesmus; pe, pessulus; sl, semilunar membrane; l.e., labium externum; ti, *internal tympaniform membrane;* m.st.tr., sternotrachealis muscle. Notice that the muscle mass serving the left syringeal half is heavier than its right counterpart. From Nottebohm and Nottebohm (1976) reproduced with permission from *Journal of Comparative Physiology, A.*

The outcome of this experiment was as follows (Nottebohm, 1967). In hearing chaffinches or in chaffinchs deafened after they learned their song, section of syringeal innervation led to abnormal but stereotyped sounds. Initially these sounds were very faint, but they became louder, though still abnormal, over a period of 1–2 months, as the syringeal muscles regained some of their innervation. This outcome showed that a *complete* match between a learned auditory or proprioceptive template and feedback resulting from song was not necessary to maintain *vocal sterotypy*. These results suggested that even though audition played a crucial role in song learning in chaffinches, once song was learned it became a "motor" tape, that is to say it became a motor program no longer requiring patterned or phasic feedback. At about the same time as our work, Wilson and Wyman (1965) had demonstrated the occurrence of "motor tapes" in insect flight. The possibility of a motor tape for song made some intuitive sense if one considers that the syrinx is surrounded by a stable internal milieu, the interclavicular air sac. A learned motor program for singing does not have to remain "open" since there is no need to include unpredictable peripheral feedback. However, though our research suggested the possibility of a motor tape, it did not demonstrate it. Perhaps for song stereotypy to persist it was sufficient for only part of proprioceptive feedback to remain unaltered. Because of the complexity of the system it was virtually impossible to test this possibility.

## 1. The Role of the Syrinx in Respiration

The preceding research encountered an unexpected difficulty. Many of the operated birds had respiratory trouble. A bird stressed by fright or by heat hyperventilates. Following bilateral syringeal denervation stressed chaffinches hypoventilated. Respiration became noticeably more laborious and was accompanied by a wheezing sound. The interpretation of this was that normally during respiration the syringeal muscles tense or otherwise keep the internal tympaniform membranes from protruding into the bronchial lumen. Following syringeal denervation the two internal tympaniform membranes were sucked into the bronchial lumen during inspiration and possibly to some extent during expiration, producing the wheezing sound and restricting airflow. This handicap was so severe, that some of the birds affected would fall off their perch and die. The reason why this occurred during stress, supposedly, was that during hyperventilation the distension and contraction of the air sacs is faster than during normal breathing, and as a result inflow and outflow of air is also faster. It is this increased speed of airflow, particularly during inspiration, that leads to a collapse of the internal tympaniform membranes into the bronchial lumen (Bernoulli effect).

## 2. The Vocal Left

In order to continue studying the role of altered proprioception without grave effects on respiration, only *one* side of the syrinx was denervated. The expectation was that this operation would interfere significantly with the production of song, modifying proprioception and auditory feedback, yet would produce tolerable respiratory inconvenience. Arbitrarily, it was decided to cut only the left ts. As expected song was much affected and respiration much less. Several months after having done the first group of unilateral nerve sections, a new group was started. The first bird in this second group had its right ts cut. Surprisingly, this chaffinch continued to sing in a completely undisturbed manner. A second operation was attempted on this same bird, now cutting the entire right hypoglossus, with the same result. It was then decided that this difference between right and left syringeal denervation was in itself worthy of study, and of course this led to the discovery of left hypoglossal dominance for song control (Nottebohm, 1970, 1971, 1972b). It was the first report of a consistent right–left asymmetry of neural function in a vertebrate other than man. The research that followed during the next 10 years stemmed from this very simple and accidental observation.

## B. SCORING LEFT HYPOGLOSSAL DOMINANCE

The song of adult chaffinches and canaries consists of more or less complex units called "syllables," which are repeated several times to form a "phrase." A song consists of a number of phrases. Syllables, in turn, consist of one or more "elements"; an element is a continuous trace in a sound-spectrograph. This terminology is illustrated in Fig. 3.

In canaries and chaffinches elements or syllables that are affected by section of either hypoglossus are replaced by silent gaps or grossly distorted sounds (Fig. 4). The affected portion of the song is presumed

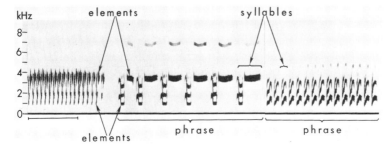

FIG. 3. Fragment of song of an intact adult male canary. This example includes three different phrases; each of the syllables in the first and second phrase is composed of two elements; syllables in the third phrase consist of a single element. Vertical and horizontal axes correspond, respectively, to frequency in kHz and time in seconds; horizontal bar indicates 0.5 sec. Second and third harmonics occur at twice and three times the frequency of the fundamental and should not be counted as different elements. From Nottebohm and Nottebohm (1976), reproduced with permission from *Journal of Comparative Physiology, A.*

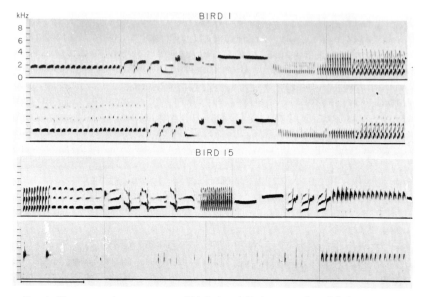

FIG. 4. Upper soundspectrograms of birds 1 and 15 show samples of their preop songs. The lower soundspectrograms show, in each case, the effects of cutting the right (bird 1) or left (bird 15) tracheosyringealis nerve. From Nottebohm and Nottebohm (1976), reproduced with permission from *Journal of Comparative Physiology, A.*

to be controlled by the cut hypoglossus and the unchanged portion by the other, intact, hypoglossus. It is only rarely that one encounters evidence of an element of song being controlled by the interaction of both hypoglossus nerves.

In chaffinches 75% or more of all elements are contributed by the left hypoglossus (Nottebohm, 1971). In canaries 90% or more of all syllables are contributed by the left hypoglossus (Nottebohm and Nottebohm, 1976). These scores are objective and reproducible. Female canaries do not normally sing; when brought into song by testosterone treatment (Section V, A) they show left hypoglossal dominance similar to that of males (F. Nottebohm, unpublished observations).

C. ONTOGENY OF LEFT HYPOGLOSSAL DOMINANCE

Left hypoglossal dominance occurs when the left syringeal innervation contributes a majority or all of song components. This could result from peripheral asymmetries in syringeal innervation or from asymmetries in the anatomy of the sound-generating membranes. Neither is the case. In chaffinches and in canaries each ts innervates only the ipsilateral syringeal half. The anatomy of the syrinx reveals two virtually identical right and left halves. The musculature on the left side is somewhat heavier, as one might expect from greater use of the left than of the right syringeal half. In chaffinches early section of the left ts leads to normal song development under right ts control (Nottebohm, 1971). Similarly, in canaries, when the left ts is cut during the first 2 weeks after hatching the normally subordinate right ts assumes a dominant role in song control. If the left ts is cut 14–28 days after hatching it regrows and both right and left ts contribute comparable numbers of song syllables (Nottebohm *et al.,* 1979). Thus, either syringeal half and its corresponding innervation can develop normal wild-type song, and copy a song model, or the two sides can collaborate in this task. In this respect the two sides are equipotential. It is not known why during ontogeny, and to what evolutionary purpose, the left syringeal innervation normally assumes a dominant role in song control, though this dominance may be related to an asymmetry in airflow during song. The left bronchus seems to handle a greater fraction of the air expired during song (Nottebohm, 1971; Nottebohm *et al.,* 1979).

## D. HYPOGLOSSAL DOMINANCE AND MOTOR TAPES

In some chaffinches and canaries section of the right ts has no effect on song. Though the muscles on that side undergo full atrophy, not a single song element is lost or altered. More commonly, though, a few elements are replaced by silent gaps or distorted sounds. When this happens, the remainder of sounds, presumably contributed by the intact side, stays unaltered. Similarly, when the left ts is cut elements contributed by the right side stay unaltered (Fig. 5). This would not be expected if output of the syringeal halves was integrated by reference to proprioceptive or auditory feedback. Evidence against auditory integration of right–left syringeal output also comes from the observation that such integration persists in deaf birds. Presumably integration of the performance of the right and left syringeal halves is central, and song, once learned, persists as a motor tape. This interpretation, of course, does not exclude a possible role for reafferent circuits.

The notion of a learned motor tape is useful since it focuses attention on possible long-term changes in the relations between neurons of motor control stations. It serves to reduce the number of putative centers where one might expect to find changes attributable to the learning of new motor patterns. As we shall see later, the stability of the putative motor tapes differs dramatically between chaffinches and canaries.

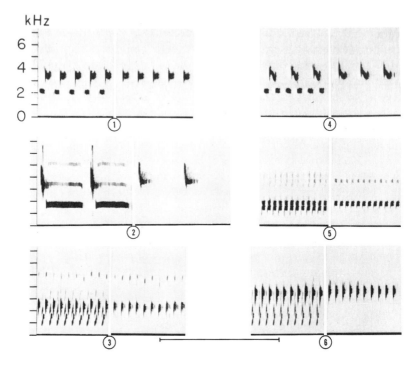

FIG. 5. Preop (left) and postop (right) versions of six complex syllables, numbered (1) to (6) produced by an adult male canary. In each case the lower frequency element disappears after section of the left tracheosyringealis, as shown by the postop condition. Notice that in syllable number (5) the intact bird delivered simultaneously the contributions of both syringeal halves. From Nottebohm and Nottebohm (1976), reproduced with permission from *Journal of Comparative Physiology, A.*

## E. HOW WIDESPREAD IS HYPOGLOSSAL DOMINANCE?

Left hypoglossal dominance has been described in 16 chaffinches (Nottebohm, 1971), 49 canaries (Nottebohm and Nottebohm, 1976; Nottebohm *et al.*, 1979), 2 white-crowned sparrows (Nottebohm and Nottebohm, 1976), and 14 white-throated sparrows (Lemon, 1973). A fifteenth white-throated sparrow included in the latter study reportedly had right hypoglossal dominance. However, this bird was wild-caught, operated, released, and recorded again several days later. It could have been a young bird that was able to redevelop song with its right syringeal half. It is impressive that out of a total of 82 individuals tested, covering four different species, all but one had a dominant left hypoglossus. This phenomenon is more homogeneous and reliable than handedness or hemispheric dominance in man.

Left hypoglossal dominance is probably common among oscine songbirds, but we do not know how widespread it is. One oscine songbird, the zebra-finch, requires participation of both syringeal halves to generate the overlapping fundamentals that give the song of this bird its typical nasal quality. Price (1977) has shown that within this bilateral involvement the right ts has the greater participation in song control, though the right-left differences are nowhere as marked as in chaffinches or canaries. In the orange-winged Amazon parrot, *Amazona amazonica* (order Psittaciformes), each ts innervates both syringeal halves and neither ts is dominant; section of the left or right ts is followed by a temporary reduction in the amplitude of the sounds produced, with no change in patterning (Nottebohm, 1976). All the species previously mentioned learn their song by reference to auditory information. Clearly left or right hypoglossal dominance has not been an inevitable consequence of the evolution of vocal learning!

F. OTHER INSTANCES OF NEURAL
   ASYMMETRY IN NONHUMAN VERTEBRATES

Since the discovery of left hypoglossal dominance, consistent right-left differences in neural function have been reported in other nonhuman vertebrate systems. The left hemisphere of macaques is thought to play a dominant role in some auditory tasks (Dewson, 1977), including perception of conspecific sounds (Peterson *et al.*, 1978). There have been claims of consistent differences in the roles assumed by the right and left hemispheres of chicks of domestic fowl in tasks of visual discrimination, visual and auditory habituation, and inhibition of sexual behavior (Rogers and Anson, 1979). Recent evidence shows that occlusion of the *right* middle cerebral artery dramatically increases wheel-running in rats. Occlusion of the left middle cerebral artery has no such effect (Robinson, 1978). This flurry of recent reports of functional asymmetry in a variety of vertebrate neural systems is quite extraordinary if one considers that it comes after a century during which humans seemed to enjoy the sole monopoly of this phenomenon (Broca, 1865; Wernicke, 1874; review in Geschwind, 1970; Sperry, 1974; Gazzaniga, 1970). Lengthy reviews about the known facts and significance of neural asymmetries appear elsewhere and will not be repeated here (e.g., Levy, 1973, 1977; Corballis and Morgan, 1978; Gazzaniga and LeDoux, 1978; Nottebohm, 1979).

## III. Brain Pathways for Vocal Control

### A. An Atlas of the Songbird Brain

The discovery of hypoglossal dominance opened the possibility of studying in an animal model questions that until then had been addressed solely in human material and with very limited success. These questions had to do with the developmental and evolutionary significance of neural asymmetry of function in the vertebrate brain. But first, of course, it was important to establish whether hypoglossal dominance, as described in the chaffinch and canary, was linked to hemispheric dominance for vocal control. Only then would it be possible to start drawing meaningful comparisons between hemispheric dominance for vocal tasks in humans and birds. Before this could be done, it was necessary to identify the vocal control pathways of the songbird brain. In 1970, when the program for these studies was laid down, there was no atlas of the songbird brain. Fortunately Karten and Hodos (1967) had recently published a quite detailed atlas of the pigeon brain. As an indispensable first step in charting the vocal control pathways in songbirds, and with the generous advice of Dr. Harvey Karten, we produced a stereotaxic atlas of the telencephalon, diencephalon, and mesencephalon of the canary brain (Stokes *et al.,* 1974).

### B. Efferent Pathways for Vocal Control

The next step was to identify efferent pathways controlling song. First the motor neurons innervating syringeal muscles had to be found. It was possible to show that after unilateral section of the ts nerve the relatively large cells ($\sim$ 20–30 $\mu$m diameter) in the caudal half of the ipsilateral nucleus intermedius became chromatolytic, and if the nerve was cut in very young canaries these cells disappeared. Nucleus intermedius (Karten and Hodos, 1967) was then a misnomer; this was the hypoglossal nucleus, nXII. The rostral half of nXII innervates muscles of the tongue, the caudal half (nXII, pars tracheosyringealis, or nXIIts) innervates muscles of trachea and syrinx. Clearly, brain pathways for vocal control would have to project to nXIIts.

Since canaries develop their song with reference to auditory information, we expected to find the highest vocal control station in the caudal telencephalon, close to the highest auditory projection, field L. This was so. Unilateral electrolytic lesions centered on a large cytoarchitectonically discreet nucleus, Hyperstriatum ventrale, pars caudale (HVc), had marked effects on the patterning of song. Using the Fink–Heimer silver stain for degenerating nerve fibers it was possible to show that HVc projected to a second, also discreet region of the telencephalon, the robust nucleus of the archistriatum (RA). RA in turn sent a direct pathway to the caudal half of the hypoglossal nucleus (nXIIts) (Nottebohm *et al.,* 1976). HVc also sent a very strong projection to area X of the lobus parolfactorius. However, whereas unilateral lesions of HVc and RA disrupted song, no such effects followed lesions of area X, which therefore did not seem to play a direct role in the efferent control of song. RA sends a strong projection to the nucleus intercollicularis of the midbrain (ICo). The anatomical relations between HVc, X, RA, ICo, and nXIIts are shown schematically in Fig. 6.

Until then, ICo had been highlighted as the main brain station controlling vocal behavior in birds. This conclusion had been drawn from the fact that electrical stimulation of ICo elicits calls in a number of species (Brown, 1965, 1971; Potash, 1970; Delius, 1971). However unilateral lesions of ICo in canaries failed to have a marked effect on song patterning. Thus ICo may be responsible for motivational correlates leading to vocalization, but does not seem to be part of a direct pathway responsible for song patterning in adult canaries. This interpretation is in line with the observation that bilateral destruction of ICo dampens response of domestic fowl chicks to novel stimuli (deLanerolle and Andrew, 1974; Andrew and deLanerolle, 1974; Andrew, 1974). The

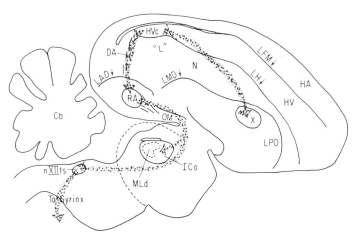

FIG. 6. Saggital section of the brain of an adult canary male showing efferent projections from the main vocal control stations. All projections shown here are ipsilateral. Cb, cerebellum; nXIIts; tracheosyringeal part of hypoglossal nucleus; MLd, nucleus mesencephalicus lateralis, pars dorsalis; ICo, nucleus intercollicularis; OM, occipitomesencephalic tract; RA, robust nucleus of archistriatum; LAD, lamina archistriatalis dorsalis; DA, tractus archistriatalis dorsalis; HVc, hyperstriatum ventrale, pars caudale; "L", field L; N, neostriatum; LMD, lamina medullaris dorsalis; LFM, lamina frontalis suprema; LH, lamina hyperstriatica; X, area X; LPO, lobus parolfactorius; HV, hyperstriatum ventrale; HA, hyperstriatum accessorium. From Nottebohm *et al.* (1976), reproduced with permission from *Journal for Comparative Neurology.*

role of ICo in vocal control in songbirds deserves further attention. Similarly, there should be connections between vocal control pathways and pathways controlling respiration, but they have not yet been described.

## C. AUDITORY PATHWAYS AND THEIR
## RELATION TO MOTOR PATHWAYS FOR
## VOCAL CONTROL

The central auditory pathways of birds resemble those of other vertebrates (reviewed in Boord, 1969). The major ascending pathway consists of the cochlear nuclei, nucleus mesencephalicus lateralis pars dorsalis (MLD) of the torus (presumed homolog to the inferior colliculus), and the nucleus ovoidalis (OV) of the thalamus (homolog to the medial geniculate). The nucleus ovoidalis projects to a discreet area of the telencephalon in the neostriatum caudale, field L. The anatomy of this pathway (Fig. 7) was characterized in pigeons by Boord and Rasmussen (1963), Boord (1968), and Karten (1967, 1968), using degeneration techniques. This summary is not complete: there are additional auditory nuclei such as nucleus laminaris (thought to be the homolog of the medial superior olive) and descending as well as ascending pathways. Further, the major nuclei are probably composed of

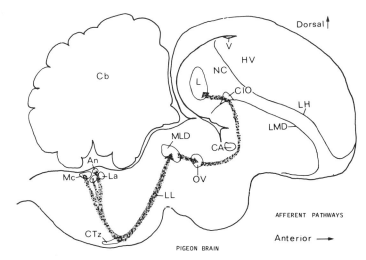

FIG. 7. Auditory pathways in the pigeon brain. After Karten (1967) and Boord (1969). This saggital reconstruction was drawn by Darcy B. Kelley and is reproduced with her permission. Mc, An, and La, magnocellularis, angularis, and laminaris nuclei of the cochlear complex; CTz, trapezoid body; LL, lateral lemniscus; OV, nucleus ovoidalis; CA, anterior commissure; CIO, capsula interna occipitalis; NC, neostriatum caudale; V, ventricle; other abbreviations as in Fig. 6.

closely associated but architectonically different regions (see Boord, 1969, for a more complete description).

A bird imitating the song of another bird must first acquire a memory of what the model sounds like. To match this model efferent pathways for song control must have access to auditory feedback. Efferent commands must be altered until vocal output matches the model. At this time the efferent stations can be presumed to receive an input which states "match completed—retain that efferent program." Thus, it is of importance to be able to demonstrate the relation between auditory stations and efferent pathways involved in vocal control. Such relations must exist in species that show vocal learning.

Using autoradiography to demonstrate the anterograde transport of tritiated proline and leucine injected into field L it was possible to show a projection from L to a "shelf" of tissue outlining the medial and ventral borders of ipsilateral nucleus HVc. Injection of labeled amino acid into an area of neostriatum immediately posteroventral to field L demonstrates an ipsilateral projection to the anteroventral borders of nucleus RA (Kelley and Nottebohm, 1979). The relations between field L and HVc and RA are represented in Fig. 8. Since HVc and RA are the two highest efferent stations controlling song, it seems likely that their close apposition to projections from field L and surroundings provides the expected opportunity for auditory information to reach motor centers, and thus vocal learning to occur. It will be of interest to find out whether this kind of auditory-motor interface exists in species that lack vocal learning.

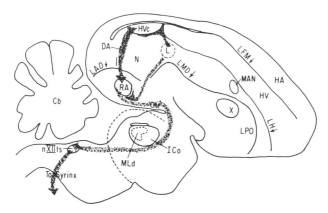

FIG. 8. Saggital section of the brain of an adult male canary. Shown here is the relation between the telencephalic auditory projection, *field L,* and stations of the efferent vocal control system. Abbreviations as in Figs. 6 and 7; MAN, nucleus maguscellularis of the anterior neostriatum. From Kelley and Nottebohm (1979), reproduced with permission from *Journal for Comparative Neurology.*

D. OTHER AFFERENT PROJECTIONS
TO VOCAL CONTROL STATIONS

Afferent projections *into* HVc and RA were investigated by means of
the retrograde tracer horseradish peroxidase (HRP) and tritiated adenosine. Nucleus HVc receives input from the magnocellular nucleus of
the anterior neostriatum (MAN) and from nucleus interface (NIF), to be
found in the neostriatum anterolateral to field L. Nucleus RA receives
projections from HVc and from MAN. HVc also receives a projection
from nucleus Uva of the thalamus. NIF and Uva had not been described
before. All these projections are ipsilateral and are demonstrated in Fig.
9 (Nottebohm and Kelley, 1978 and in preperation). Their significance
remains unclear.

E. SEXUAL DIMORPHISM IN VOCAL CONTROL PATHWAYS

Canary males and the males of a majority of songbird species sing
profusely. Their song, as described earlier, is learned by reference to
auditory information. Females sing little if at all. The amount of brain
volume devoted to song control seems to be proportional to this
behavioral dimorphism (Fig. 10). HVc, RA, and area X are several times

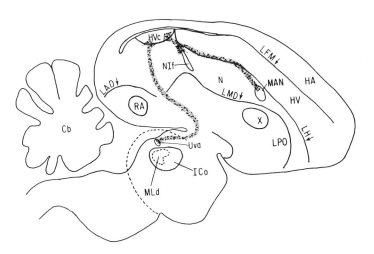

FIG. 9. Afferent projections to nucleus HVc include nucleus Uva of the thalamus,
nucleus interface (NIF) of the neostriatum, and nucleus magnocellularis of the anterior
neostriatum (MAN). MAN also projects to RA. All projections are ipsilateral. Abbreviations as in Figs. 6, 7, and 8; NIf, nucleus interface. From Nottebohm and Kelley (1978, and
in preparation).

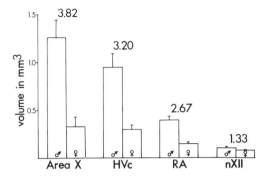

FIG. 10. Volume in mm³ (right plus left) and ratio of male to female volumes for four canary brain nuclei related to vocal control. The numbers on top of the histogram bars for each brain station correspond to this male/female volume ratio. From Nottebohm and Arnold (1976), reproduced with permission from AAAS.

larger in male than in female canaries. This dimorphism is even more marked in zebra finches in which area X is not cytoarchitectonically discreet in females (Nottebohm and Arnold, 1976). Though earlier reports had described microanatomical differences between brains of male and female mammals, ours was the first description of gross sexual differences in volume affecting regions controlling a specific sexually dimorphic task.

F. HEMISPEHRIC DOMINANCE

The description of left hypoglossal dominance raised the possibility that songbirds such as the canary would show hemispheric dominance for song control. This has proven to be the case. Destruction of the left HVc or RA has a much greater disruptive effect on song than comparable lesions of right HVc and RA (Nottebohm, 1977). Whereas destruction of the left HVc results in a virtually total loss of preoperative syllables and phrase structure, destruction of the right HVc is followed by loss of some syllables and phrase structure remains intact. The difference between these two outcomes, demonstrated in Fig. 11, has been recorded in five canaries lesioned on the left side and five on the right side. Despite this greater involvement of the left hemisphere in song control, there is no noticeable difference in volume between the right and left HVc, or between the right and left RA (F. Nottebohm, in preparation).

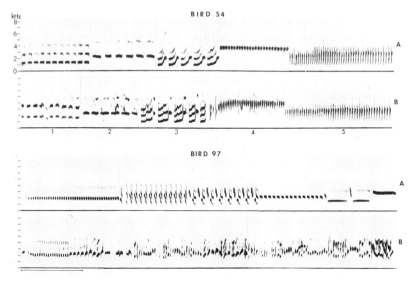

FIG. 11. (A) Soundspectrographs of the song of two intact adult male canaries, bird 54 and bird 97. (B) Same birds after lesion of right HVc (bird 54) or left HVc (bird 97). From Nottebohm *et al.* (1976), reproduced with permission from *Journal for Comparative Neurology*.

## G. REVERSAL OF HEMISPHERIC DOMINANCE

When hemispheric dominance in canaries was first described, it was tempting to think of left HVc dominance in terms of parallels with left hemisphere networks dominant for speech and language. In this sense, song deficits following left HVc damage were seen as possibly reminiscent of some kinds of aphasia which follow left hemisphere insult in humans (Broca, 1865; Penfield and Roberts, 1959; Sperry, 1974). When such insult occurs in adult humans, prognosis for recovery is poor. By analogy, we expected that whereas song deficits following left HVc lesion would be long lasting, those following right HVc lesion would show prompt recovery. The outcome has been different. Seven months after destruction of *either* right or left HVc of adult canaries that had developed stable song, a new repertoire occurs, and this song repertoire is much like that of an intact adult canary (Nottebohm, 1977). An example of such recovery is shown in Fig. 12. Thus, not only are the right and left syringeal halves and their corresponding hypoglossal innervation equipotential for song control, as described earlier, but either HVc can, by itself, assume full song control and develop normal song. What is

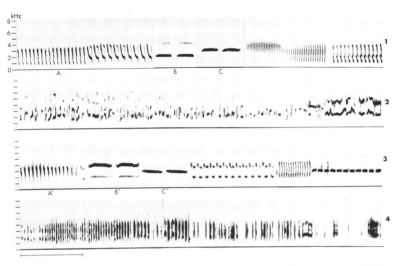

FIG. 12. (1) Fragment of preoperative song of an intact adult male canary. (2) Same bird recorded 7 days after destruction of left HVc; only one preoperative syllable, not shown here, survived this operation. (3) Same bird recorded 7 months later, after it developed a new song repertoire. (4) Still same bird, now recorded 4 days after section of right tracheosyringealis. Letters A, B, and C identify preoperative syllables; A', B', and C' identify the somewhat altered relearned version of these same syllables. No syllable survived section of the right ts, which now has become dominant. From Nottebohm (1977), reproduced with permission from Academic Press.

surprising is that reversal of hypoglossal and hemispheric dominance can occur in adulthood.

In canaries that had the left ts cut soon after hatching, lesion of the left HVc in adulthood has effects similar to those following destruction of the right HVc in otherwise intact birds. In birds that had the left HVc sectioned at 1 year of age and developed a new repertoire, section of the right ts at 2 years of age affected song drastically (Fig. 12), that is to say, the right ts was now behaving as the left ts of otherwise intact birds. A plausible interpretation is that following destruction of the left HVc or section of the left ts, the right HVc and its efferent pathways take over and redevelop normal song. Thus it is possible to induce a reversal of hemispheric dominance for song control either by cutting the left ts or by destroying the left HVc (Nottebohm, 1977 and in preparation).

These observations demonstrate a considerable plasticity of canary vocal control pathways even in adulthood. It should be possible to ask the question, how do the connectivity or properties of left HVc neurons differ from those in right HVc, and how do properties of the latter change as they go from a subordinate to a dominant role? Reversal of hypoglossal and hemispheric dominance should offer good material with which to study the changes in the adult brain that may occur as previously subordinate pathways assume a leading role in song learning and production.

## H. RELATIONS BETWEEN IPSILATERAL AND CONTRALATERAL PATHWAYS FOR CANARY SONG CONTROL

As was described earlier, the efferent pathways from HVc to RA and from RA to nXIIts are ipsilateral in canaries and this is also the case for the projection from HVc to area X. The projections from field L and surrounding neostriatum to tissue adjacent to HVc and RA are also ipsilateral. Similarly, the projections from MAN to HVc and RA, and from NIF and Uva to HVc are all ipsilateral. This is puzzling since we know that *both* left and right efferent pathways participate in song control. Indeed, even lesions to the subordinate right HVc normally result in the loss of anywhere from one-fifth to two-thirds of the preoperative syllable types (Nottebohm, 1977). Also the contribution of the right ts of intact canaries, though quantitatively minor, is closely integrated with the output of the left ts. Such integration suggests communication between the right and left ipsilateral pathways.

Sone of the stations linked to vocal control have crossed projections. The nucleus intercollicularis (ICo) of the midbrain, which receives a strong ipsilateral projection from RA, projects to the contralateral ICo. However, it is possible to eliminate either left or right ICo with only minor effects on song (Nottebohm *et al.,* 1976), and this suggests that ICo is not important in integrating the right and left song control pathways.

The auditory pathway (see Fig. 7) abounds more in crossed projections than the efferent pathways for vocal control. So, for example, Boord (1969) and Karten (1967) describe how in pigeons each cochlea sends information to the cochlear nuclei on both sides of the medulla and to left and right nucleus mesencephalicus lateralis, pars dorsalis (MLD), and from there to ovoidalis and field L. The bihemispheric representation of inputs to either cochlea is emphasized by the fact that in canaries early removal of either cochlea is followed by normal song development under left hypoglossal dominance (Nottebohm and Nottebohm, 1976).

## 1. A Role for the Commissura Infima?

One possible site for R–L hypoglossal integration are the right and left nXIIts. A well-developed commissura infima joins the right and left halves of the medulla at the level of the anterior reaches of nXIIts (Fig. 13). Motor neurons in each nXIIts may send collateral fibers across this commissure, or interneurons may be in charge of linking the right and left nXIIts, distributing excitatory and inhibitory influences so as to assure a harmonious vocal output of both tracheosyringeal nerves. This possibility has yet to be tested.

Auditory feedback from song can be regarded as one way whereby the output of the right and left syringeal halves could be centrally integrated. However, it was pointed out earlier that in chaffinches and canaries right–left integration persists for long periods of time after both cochleas are removed from an *adult* bird that had already learned to

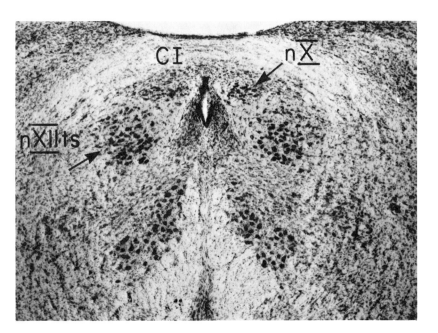

FIG. 13. Cross-section of the medulla of an adult male canary at the level of nXIIts (tracheosyringealis part of hypoglossal nucleus) which can be seen as a ball of large motor neurons ventrolateral to the motor nucleus of the vagus, nX. The commissura infima, CI, can be seen to bridge the right and left sides of the medulla. Dorsal is up. Cresyl violet stain. From Nottebohm *et al.* (1976), reproduced with permission from *Journal of Comparative Neurology.*

sing. It was also noted that proprioception is not likely to be used in the coordination of right–left syringeal output. We must conclude that *maintenance* of right–left syringeal integration does not require sensory feedback. Because of this observation and the absence of evidence for connections between right and left telencephalic stations for song control, it seems justified to suggest that such integration may occur at the level of the hypoglossal nucleus.

## 2. Effects on Song of Combining Left HVc Lesion and Left ts Section

A series of still unpublished experiments test the extent to which ipsilateral and contralateral efferent pathways contribute to song control. The nature of the experiments was to destroy the right or left HVc, cut the left ts, or combine these operations in 1-year-old canaries that had already developed stable adult song. These same birds were recorded again 1 year later, and the number of different syllable types counted and compared with those of 2-year-old intact canaries. Results are presented in Table I.

Interpretation of the results presented in Table I is as follows. Destruction of either right or left HVc is followed by the development of a new syllable repertoire, which yields a syllable count intermediate between that of 1- and 2-year-old intact birds. This repertoire is significantly larger than that developed by the birds who suffered only section of left ts. Two alternative hypotheses could explain this observation. (*a*) The meager syllable count of birds with left ts section in

TABLE I

Syllable Counts for 2-Year-Old Male Canaries That
Underwent Various Operations at 1 Year of Age [a]

| Group number | $n$ | Nature of operation | Mean number of different syllable types (SD in parentheses) |
|:---:|:---:|:---|:---:|
| 1 | 12 | Intact, 1-year-old | 23.2 (4.7) |
| 2 | 6 | Intact, 2-year-old | 30.0 (2.7) |
| 3 | 6 | Cut L ts | 16.8 (1.9) |
| 4 | 3 | Destroyed L HVc | 25.3 (4.9) |
| 5 | 3 | Destroyed R HVc | 28.0 (3.5) |
| 6 | 6 | Cut L ts and destroyed L HVc | 11.5 (4.6) |

[a] Comparing group 3 vs group 4: $t = 3.48$; $p = 0.01$, two-tailed; comparing group 3 vs group 6, $t = 2.61$; $0.05 > p > 0.02$, two-tailed.

adulthood results from the fact that an intact left HVc continues to vie for hegemony, hindering the right HVc in its attempts to use its ipsilateral pathways to develop a new repertoire. (b) Following left ts section, motor neurons on the left nXIIts atrophy and disappear. The size of the syllable repertoire is somehow dependent on the interaction of a right and left nXIIts. If hypothesis (a) is correct, then section of the left ts combined with lesion of the left HVc would free the right HVc from any possible inhibition from its left counterpart: the right HVc and its ipsilateral pathways would develop a normal repertoire no different from that developed by birds with just a left HVc lesion. But this was not the outcome. The double operation of Lts and LHVc leads to a repertoire even smaller than that of Lts alone. This suggests that following lesion of just the left HVc, as the right HVc takes over it relies on an intact right and an intact left nXIIts, thus lending support to hypothesis (b). It should be noted, however, that hypothesis (b) applies only to section of the left ts in adulthood. The same operation done soon after hatching does not hinder the development of a normal syllable count.

I. VOCAL CONTROL PATHWAYS
   IN THE PARAKEET BRAIN

The syrinx of Psittaciformes (parrots and their allies) differs from that of songbirds in that sounds are produced as air rushes by a narrowing at the bottom of the trachea, at the confluence of bronchi and trachea (Fig. 14). The parrot syrinx does not have two independent sound sources, as in oscines, and to that extent performs more like the human larynx. Earlier studies have indicated that in the orange-winged Amazon parrot, *Amazona amazonica*, the ts branch of each hypoglossus innervates both syringeal halves, and normal syringeal performance can be sustained by either hypoglossus. Left hypoglossal dominance in canaries and other oscines can be likened to handedness. It will be of interest to know whether hemispheric dominance for vocal control in birds also occurs in the absence of hypoglossal dominance. The latter situation would resemble more closely the left hemispheric dominance for speech tasks in humans. As a first step, Darcy B. Kelley and I have started mapping the vocal control pathways in the brain of another Psittaciform, the budgerigar, *Melopsittacus undulatus*. Preliminary observations have identified what probably is the budgerigar homolog of RA in oscine songbirds. It is of great interest that lesions to this putative left RA homolog followed by a survival of 7 days and use of the Fink–Heimer silver stain for degenerating axons revealed a strong projection to the *ip-*

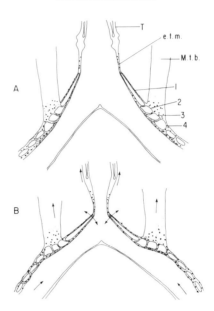

FIG. 14. Schematic longitudinal section of the syrinx of the parrot *Amazona amazonica* (A) at rest, and (B) during phonation. T, tympanum; e.t.m., external tympaniform membrane; M.t.b., musculus tracheobronchialis. Arrows inside bronchi indicate air movement during phonation; two-headed arrows through tip of first bronchial half-ring indicate its oscillatory movements as it pivots on its articulation with second bronchial half-ring. Whereas the cephalad pull by M.t.b. will tip the first bronchial half-ring inward, pull by M. syringeus (not shown, but indicated by arrows) will draw the tip of the first bronchial half-ring cephalad and outward. Unlike the oscine syrinx, the parrot syrinx has no internal tympaniform membrane. Phonation presumably occurs at the confluence of the right and left bronchial air streams and the syrinx acts as a single sound source. From Nottebohm (1976), reproduced with permission from *Journal of Comparative Physiology, A.*

*silateral* as well as to the *contralateral* nXIIts (F. Nottebohm and D. B. Kelley, unpublished observations). We do not know yet whether there are anatomical or behavioral differences between lesions to the right or left RA of budgerigars, or whether budgerigars have a homolog to the songbird's HVc. This work continues.

## IV. Relations between Song Ontogeny and the Ontogeny of Song Control Pathways

Song in canaries develops gradually during the first year. Starting at approximately 40 days after hatching canaries produce variable, low-amplitude patterns of frequency modulation called "subsong." Subsong persists during the next 2 or 3 weeks, at which time it begins to be transformed into "plastic song." As a canary sings, the units of repetition or "syllables" are rendered in quick succession, forming a "phrase." During plastic song syllables and phrases are delivered in a variable manner, and this stage of song development lasts several months. A canary hatched in April or May sings the loud stereotyped song typical of adults by the following January, when 8 to 9 months old. The song of such a bird, reared in a colony room where it can hear many other canaries, typically includes a mean of 24.5 different syllable types (Nottebohm and Nottebohm, 1978).

The development of vocal control stations HVc and RA in male canaries shows an interesting relation to song ontogeny. By day 15 after hatching the brain of a young male canary has achieved full adult weight. At that time HVc is not recognizable in cresyl violet-stained material, but RA is already manifest. In a sample of birds sacrificed at 15-day intervals HVc can be first recognized in cresyl-stained sections 30 days after hatching. Its volume, at that time, is 20% of that of an adult 1-year-old male. RA at that time has 30% of the adult volume. Both HVc and RA show a very marked spurt of growth from the thirtieth to the sixtieth day after hatching. At 60 days the volume of HVc is close to 50% that of an adult 1-year-old male. After then the rate of growth slows down (Nottebohm, in preparation).

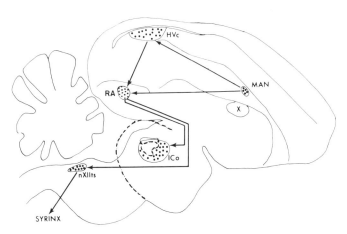

Fig. 15. Sagittal section of adult male canary brain. Arrows indicate connections between components of the vocal control pathways. Dots indicate label concentration following systemic injections of [³H]testosterone. The pattern of uptake shown here is similar in male canaries and male zebra finches. From Arnold et al. (1976), Arnold (1979), and Nottebohm and Kelley (1978 and in preparation).

One can think of song learning in canaries as falling into two stages, each of which may achieve a different purpose. Subsong is essentially a noncommunicatory stage. It is delivered at very low amplitude, it does not require the presence of conspecifics, and often occurs as the bird, eyes closed, seems to doze. It is my guess that during subsong the young bird is learning how to use its vocal tract, learning the auditory consequences of particular efferent commands. In a similar vein Thorpe and Pilcher (1958, p. 512) speculated that "subsong is in the nature of practice for the true song." In all these respects subsong is very reminiscent of the cooing and babbling stages of vocal development in infants. These similarities were not lost to Charles Darwin who in the "Descent of Man" (as quoted by Thorpe and Pilcher, 1958, p. 509) notes: "The first attempts to sing may be compared to the imperfect endeavour in a child to babble."

The temporal overlap young canaries show between occurrence of subsong and a period of fast growth of HVc and RA may be coincidental; or it may mean that subsong does not commence earlier because brain pathways for its production are not available. An interesting possibility is that subsong experience may be made available at a time when it can be incorporated into the growth of vocal control pathways: HVc and RA connectivity being established at that time may correspond, in some manner, to the auditory mapping of vocal tract function. Once this developmental stage is complete, then the bird is ready to imitate external models.

During their second year of life male canaries develop a new song repertoire, which normally includes a significantly larger number of syllables than that of the previous year (Nottebohm and Nottebohm, 1978). It will be interesting to see whether this new episode of song learning is accompanied by further anatomical changes in HVc and RA.

## V. Relation of Testosterone to Vocal Behavior

A. Effects of Testosterone on Song

The vocal behavior of birds plays an important role in reproduction. Song is an important component of territorial defense and courtship (e.g., Howard, 1920; Marler, 1956, 1960; Catchpole, 1973; Krebs, 1976; Kroodsma, 1976). Perhaps it is not surprising that androgens, whose levels rise and fall in a seasonal manner and particularly in response to photoperiod (Rowan, 1926; Brisson and Vaugien, 1957; Follett and Farner, 1966; Menaker and Keatts, 1968; Lofts et al., 1970) and change with the various stages of the reproductive cycle (Feder et al., 1977; Silver, 1978), should also be involved in song control. In adult zebra finch males, the amount of singing is linearly correlated with the naturally occurring amounts of testosterone in the blood plasma (Pröve, 1978).

In adult chaffinches castration eliminates song (Collard and Grevendal, 1946). Testosterone administered to chaffinches in November, when they normally do not sing, induces song (Thorpe, 1958). Female chaffinches normally do not sing, but will do so when treated with testosterone (Nottebohm, 1966; Hooker, 1968). Chaffinches learn to sing during the first 10 months after hatching. This is the "critical period" for song learning. If a chaffinch is castrated at 6 months of age, before the onset of spring song development, it will not sing. When such a bird is treated with testosterone at 2 years of age, well after the normal end of the "critical period," it will learn to sing and imitate chaffinch song played on tape. Thus the end of the critical period is influenced by the availability of testosterone (Nottebohm, 1969).

Male canaries castrated soon after hatching go through the early stages of song development. However, during that first year they fail to develop the loud, stable song typical of adults. Whereas intact first year canaries sing profusely from January to June, which coincides with the breeding season, early castrates of the same age remain silent (Nottebohm, 1980). Female canaries, which normally do not sing, can be induced to do so by testosterone administration (Shoemaker, 1939; Baldwin *et al.,* 1940).

Zebra finch males sing during agonistic encounters with other males and when courting females. Male zebra finches castrated soon after hatching imitate the song of adults, though they sing less frequently, the internote intervals tend to be somewhat longer, and song components more variable (Arnold, 1975b). Castration done in adult zebra finch males also reduces the incidence of song (Pröve, 1974; Arnold, 1975a). In such birds the tempo of song tends to be slower, an effect reflected both in the duration of song components and in the duration of the silent intervals between successive song components. This effect disappears when castrate males are given testosterone (Arnold, 1975a). Adult female zebra finches do not sing and cannot be induced to sing even when treated with testosterone (Arnold, 1974).

B. UPTAKE OF STEROID HORMONES BY
   VOCAL CONTROL PATHWAYS

Hormone autoradiography allows us to recognize parts of the brain where the nuclei of neurons concentrate labeled hormone or its metabolites. This nuclear concentration is thought to indicate hormonal access to DNA, on which the hormone presumably acts to induce changes in the nature or quantity of protein synthesis. Access of hormone of its metabolites to the nucleus is thought to depend on the cytoplasmic occurrence of *receptor* proteins. The receptor–hormone complex then is allowed to penetrate the nuclear membrane and to attach to specific sites of the DNA (review in McEwen *et al.*, 1974).

Until recently gonadal hormones had been thought to act predominantly on limbic system structures such as the hypothalamus and septum, and thus influence reproductive behavior (e.g., Morrell *et al.*, 1975). We speculated that a hormone such as testosterone may also act on the various stations of the vocal control pathways. Our first attempt to use tritiated testosterone ($^3$H-T) autoradiography to test this idea focused on nucleus ICo of the chaffinch. This was before we had described HVc and RA and their involvement in song control. At that time various authors had reported that electrical stimulation of ICo induced vocalization and display postures in red-winged blackbirds (Brown, 1971; Newman, 1972), quail (Potash, 1970), and gulls (Delius, 1971). Much to our satisfaction we were able to demonstrate concentration of label in the nuclei of ICo neurons (Zigmond *et al.*, 1973). This was the first time that mesencephalic structures were shown to concentrate a hormone or its metabolites. In due time, however, we came to realize that in canaries ICo was not part of the direct efferent pathway controlling vocalization. As we became aware of the role of HVc, RA, and nXIIts, we were pleased to observe that the motor neurons of nXIIts, virtually without exception, showed nuclear concentration of testosterone (or its metabolites), and that many neurons in HVc also showed this property (Arnold *et al.*, 1976). This work was done with zebra finches. At the time we also noted concentrations of label by nucleus MAN. A later study (Nottebohm and Kelley, 1978 and in preparation) showed that MAN projects to HVc and RA. Recently Arnold (1979) has described nuclear concentration of androgen in RA cells. Thus a total of five brain stations directly or indirectly related to song control (ICo, HVc, MAN, RA, and nXIIts) have been shown to concentrate label following somatic injection of $^3$H-T (summarized in Fig. 15). Label is concentrated by HVc, RA, MAN, and nXIIts in adult zebra finches and canaries following injection of tritiated testosterone but not following injections of tritiated estradiol (Arnold, 1979; D. B. Kelley and F. Nottebohm, pilot observations). Presumably HVc, RA, MAN, and nXIIts neurons have androgen receptors. Label is concentrated by ICo neurons following systemic injection of either tritiated testosterone or tritiated estradiol. ICo may have both androgen and estradiol receptors, or perhaps testosterone is aromatized to estradiol before it can enter the nucleus of ICo neurons.

The occurrence of androgen concentration by *each* of the afferent stations controlling song is remarkable and suggests a pervasiveness of androgen effects that is novel to studies of brain-behavior relations. As we shall see, this influence extends to the very muscles responsible for song.

## C. HIGH-AFFINITY ANDROGEN BINDING PROTEINS IN SYRINGEAL TISSUES OF SONGBIRDS

Very recently we have been able to show that putative androgen receptors are not restricted to the brain pathways controlling song but are also found in the muscles of the syrinx. Syringeal muscles of zebra finches and canaries have specific high-affinity androgen-binding proteins. The levels of binding present in syrinxes from female and castrated male zebra finches (40–50 fmoles/mg protein) are far in excess of those demonstrated to exist in any other striated muscle and are within the range of values observed for classical androgen-sensitive tissues such as the mouse kidney. Canaries do most of their singing via the left syringeal half, but both right and left syringeal halves show a comparable concentration of high-affinity androgen-binding proteins. Clearly the L–R asymmetry in syringeal function is not related to an asymmetric concentration of androgen receptors (Lieberburg and Nottebohm, 1979).

## D. EFFECTS OF TESTOSTERONE ON THE SIZE OF BRAIN CONTROL AREAS

As described earlier, efferent stations of the vocal control pathways are markedly smaller in female than in male canaries. Testosterone treatment of *adult* female canaries over a period of 4 weeks brings these birds into song. When sacrificed at the end of this period HVc and RA has enlarged by 50 and 69%, respectively, as compared with the same structures in untreated birds of the same age. These initial observations were conducted with intact 2-year-old females of which five were controls and six received testosterone. The outcome was so unexpected that we decided to repeat the experiment using females ovariectomized during their first month of life, implanted with testosterone or cholesterol silastics[2] at 11 months. These birds were sacrificed 1 month later. At that time the HVc and RA of the testosterone (T)-treated birds was,

---

[2] Silastic: a synthetic elastomere through which molecules diffuse at a constant rate. In the experiments described here silastic hollow tubes were filled with known amounts of testosterone or cholesterol crystals, then sealed at both ends.

respectively, 90 and 53% larger than that of the cholesterol controls
(Figs. 16 and 17). We do not know whether this increase in volume is due
to recruitment of new neurons from the periphery of HVc and RA, due
to increase in the size of neurons and in particular to growth of their
dendritic tree, due to mitotic events, or even due to differentiation of
cohorts of heretofore undifferentiated cells. However, inspection of
cresyl violet-stained material suggests that T treatment induces a visibly
greater spacing between the somas of neurons in HVc and RA (Fig. 18)
which could result from increases in dendritic arborization. Nonvocal
control areas such as nucleus spiriformis medialis and nucleus rotundus
showed no T-dependent increase in volume. We have here a very striking
and robust gross morphological effect of testosterone, which occurs in
adulthood at a time when the female vocal control stations are assuming
an active involvement in song.

The song of the T-treated females tends to be much simpler than that
of intact males, with a range of 4 to 11 syllable types in T-treated
females vs a range of 15 to 41 in 1-year-old intact males. Interestingly,
though, the female syllables are better structured than those of deaf
males. This suggests that when adult female canaries develop song under
the influence of testosterone, they rely on auditory feedback.

Male canaries castrated during their first month of life and sacrificed

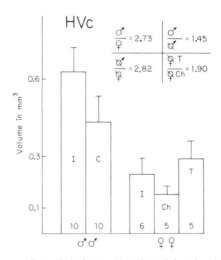

FIG. 16. HVc volume (bilateral) in intact (I) male and female adult canaries, in male
canaries castrated soon after hatching (C), and in female canaries ovariectomized soon
after hatching, then treated during 1 month with cholesterol (Ch) or testosterone (T) at 11
months of age. The volume ratios are self-explanatory; ♂ stands for castrate male; ♀ for
ovariectomized female. For the ♂/♀ ratio used the values of the ovariectomized female
canaries treated with Ch. Nottebohm (1980), reproduced with permission from *Brain Research*.

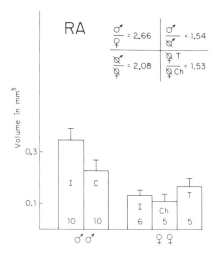

F<small>IG</small>. 17. Explanation same as for Fig. 16, but here corresponding to RA volumes. Nottebohm (1980), reproduced with permission from *Brain Research*.

at 12 months of age do not develop adult song during that first year. Their HVc and RA are 45 and 53% smaller, respectively, than that of intact controls. These results are presented in Figs. 16 and 17. We have not yet tried to correct the effects of early castration by testosterone therapy. Judging from the effect of T on females such treatment might be expected to cancel the behavioral and anatomical deficiencies that follow early elimination of both testis.

The notion that a well-defined nucleus of the *adult* brain can grow substantially following hormone treatment seems novel, yet is a fact. It should be noted, though, that we do not know whether the effects of hormone were mediated directly or indirectly. In terms of data, all we have at this time is a correlation between presence of testosterone, uptake of testosterone or its metabolites by brain stations involved in song control, occurrence of song, and an increase in the gross volume of HVc and RA. However, by a careful choice of species, behavioral test, brain station, and side of brain it should be possible to decide how much of the observed HVc and RA volume change is due to use and disuse, to hormone effects, and to acquisition of new motor skills.

E. E<small>FFECTS OF</small> T<small>ESTOSTERONE ON</small> N<small>EURONS</small>
   <small>AND</small> M<small>USCLE</small>: M<small>OLECULAR</small> S<small>TUDIES</small>

The neurotransmitter used by the motor neurons innervating syringeal muscles is acetylcholine, In joint research with Drs. Victoria Luine, Bruce McEwen, and Cheryl Harding (Luine *et al.,* 1978 and in press)

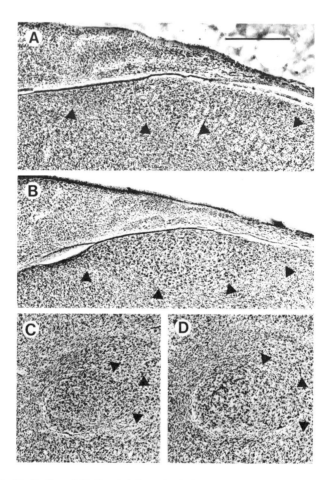

Fɪɢ. 18. (A, B, C, and D) Cresyl violet-stained 50-µm-thick sections from four different female canaries ovariectomized 7–9 days after hatching and sacrificed at 12 months of age. (A·and B) Cross-sections of HVc; (C and D) cross-sections of RA. Birds (A) and (C) received a subcutaneous silastic implant of cholesterol at 11 months. Birds (B) and (D) received a subcutaneous silastic implant of testosterone at 11 months. The anterior-posterior level of sectioning corresponds to that showing the maximal cross-sectional area of HVc or RA for each of these birds. Birds were chosen so as to represent median HVc and RA volumes for each of the two groups compared. The horizontal calibration bar corresponds to 0.5 mm. In (A) and (B) black triangles point to the ventral boundary of HVc. In (C) and (D) black triangles point to the dorsolateral boundary of RA. The remainder of the RA boundary can be recognized as a pale fibrous lamina. Nottebohm (1980), reproduced with permission from *Brain Research*.

we looked at the effects of T on whole syrinx levels of two enzymes: choline acetyltransferase (CAT), responsible for acetylcholine synthesis, and acetylcholinesterase (AChE), responsible for decoupling the acetyl and choline moities soon after acetylcholine is released into the neuromuscular synaptic cleft, thus ensuring that synaptic transmission is narrowly defined in time. Though we are still unclear about the variables affecting CAT levels, we now have strong evidence that the levels of AChE are T dependent. Four weeks after castration the levels of AChE in the syrinx of zebra finch males are approximately one-half those in intact birds. This difference is completely corrected by testosterone therapy. Interestingly, a comparison of the levels of AChE in the left and right halves of the syrinx of canary males indicates that whereas the left has $894 \pm 63 \times 10^{-9}$ moles/hour of AChe, the right side has $592 \pm 52 \times 10^{-9}$ moles/hour, a significant difference of 34% ($n = 10$). This difference in the levels of AChE between the two sides disappears following castration, the left and right syringeal halves showing, respectively, $286 \pm 33$ and $256 \pm 33 \times 10^{-9}$ moles/hour of AChE.

Further work with male zebra finches (Luine *et al.*, 1978 and in press), using sections of tracheosyringealis nerve shows that significantly larger levels of CAT and AChE travel in the nerve of castrates treated with T than in that of castrates treated with cholesterol. We do not know yet whether the T-dependent levels of AChE seen in whole syrinx are fully explained by the flow of AChE from nerve to syringeal muscle, or whether they may result from T acting on both nerve and muscle. Since both the nXIIts motor neurons and syringeal muscle have putative androgen receptors, T may act on either target via classic genomic mechanisms. The difference in AChE levels between the right and left syringeal halves indicates that on top of these genomic effects there may also be an effect of use and disuse, as suggested also by right-left differences in muscle mass (Fig. 2). The problem ahead is to tease apart and understand these interactions between use and disuse and genomic effectiveness of T.

## VI. The Evolution of Song Learning and of
## Its Anatomical Correlates

Some time ago (Nottebohm, 1968) I noted that vocal development in birds falls into three basic categories:

1. No auditory feedback necessary for development of normal vocalizations. Examples: domestic fowl, *Gallus domesticus* (Konishi, 1963), and ring doves, *Streptopelia risoria* (Nottebohm and Nottebohm,

1971). These species do not imitate external models and develop normal vocalizations when deafened soon after hatching. This condition is thought to be represented in a majority of avian orders, which therefore lack vocal learning. From an evolutionary viewpoint this is likely to be the more primitive condition (review in Nottebohm, 1972a, 1975).

2. Auditory feedback necessary but environmental experience not indispensable. Examples: song sparrow, *Melospiza melodia* (Mulligan, 1966; Kroodsma, 1977), and canaries (Metfessel, 1935, 1940; Waser and Marler, 1977). Birds in this group can imitate in a facultative manner. In the absence of external models they can produce well-structured song, though in the case of song sparrows auditory isolates also produce abnormal songs.

3. The development of song is dependent on the availability of auditory feedback and exposure to environmental sources. Examples: chaffinch (Poulsen, 1951; Thorpe, 1958; Nottebohm, 1968), white-crowned sparrow (Marler and Tamura, 1964; Konishi, 1965), and zebra-finch (Immelmann, 1969; Price, 1977). In the absence of conspecific models these species produce grossly aberrant song.

HVc and RA are easily recognizable, cytoarchitectonically discreet brain stations in canaries, white-crowned sparrows, rufous-collared sparrows *(Zonotrichia capensis),* zebra finches, house sparrows *(Passer domesticus),* starlings *(Sturnus vulgaris),* brown thrashers *(Toxostoma rufum),* long-billed marsh wrens *(Cistothorus palustris),* and red-winged blackbirds *(Agelaius phoeniceus).* All these oscine songbirds learn their song by reference to auditory information. HVc and RA are also well developed in another talented vocal mimic, the Australian lyre bird *(Menura novaehollandiae),* thought to be an atypical songbird within the suborder Oscines (Sibley, 1974). In all but two of the species mentioned in the previous listing, the long-billed marsh wren and the lyre bird, area X of lobus parolfactorius was readily recognizable. HVc, RA, and area X are not recognizable in cresyl violet-stained brains of nonoscine Passeriformes such as the Eastern kingbird, *Tyrannus tyrannus,* the furnarid *Asthenes hudsoni,* and the dendrocolaptid *Synallaxis frontalis.* Neither are there nuclei recognizable as HVc, RA, or area X in the very detailed atlas of the pigeon brain (Karten and Hodos, 1967). It is tempting to conclude that HVc, RA, and to a lesser extent area X evolved their present characteristics in oscine passeriformes in response to selective pressures favoring vocal learning. If so, there may be something special about the anatomy and physiology of these centers, or about their inputs and connectivity, that relates to the learning task. The characterization of this "something special" may in turn help us recognize the nature of anatomical and physiological variables which are causally related to vocal learning, or, in a more general manner, related to the learning of new, complex, motor patterns. In time, as areas homologous to the oscine HVc, RA, etc. are identified in other vocal learners such as parakeets and hummingbirds, it will be possible to discover whether the evolutionary strategy followed by these groups has produced similar neural "solutions" for the requirements of vocal learning.

## VII. Overview and Summary

The development of a vocal repertoire by reference to auditory information is one of the traits considered to be symptomatic of human nature. We now have an animal model for the study of vocal learning, where brain processes involved in this task can be studied in considerable detail. This is particularly timely since studies by Marler and his collaborators strongly suggest that song learning in birds and language learning in humans may share basic processes of perceptual abstraction (Marler and Peters, 1977).

Vocal learning in songbirds involves a few well-defined efferent stations that have access to auditory information. These stations develop late in ontogeny, at the time birds are thought to be acquiring the auditory-motor integration that will later enable vocal learning. Vocal control stations are much larger in males, that sing, then in females, that do not. In some of the species tested vocal learning is accompanied by left hemispheric dominance for this task. We do not know whether this is a necessary correlate of vocal learning. In a species such as the canary, the neural plasticity required for vocal learning persists well after sexual maturity, and canaries each year develop a new song repertoire. This neural plasticity in adulthood is manifest in other ways: canaries can shift hypoglossal and hemisperic dominance for song control. A reflection of this persistent plasticity in adulthood is the fact that fully mature female canaries respond to testosterone treatment by developing male-like song, and that this is accompanied by marked growth of telencephalic vocal control stations. The role of testosterone may not be central to the occurrence of vocal learning, as shown by Arnold's work on zebra finches, but pathways for vocal control are very sensitive to this hormone. The effects of testosterone on these pathways are thought at this time to lead to two types of changes: anatomical, controlling the growth of vocal control stations, and physiological, controlling the amount of enzymes involved in neural transmission. These two effects may be related. The relation of testosterone or its metabolites to the performance of vocal control pathways is underscored by the fact that neurons in efferent stations controlling song seem to have receptors that may give the hormone or its metabolites access to genomic material. During the past 10 years we have shown that vocal control pathways of the songbird brain lend themselves well to studying various aspects of vocal learning. This has been merely a beginning. There is a need for broader comparative studies, and for much finer anatomical and physiological descriptions. There is a need for more detailed developmental studies. In particular, there is a need to characterize anatomical and physiological properties of vocal control pathways that may relate specifically to hormonal effects, to effects of use and disuse, to effects of age and, eventually, after all these other variables have been accounted for, to the effects of learning a new motor task. The challenge seems well worth another 10 years of effort!

### Acknowledgments

Research described here was supported by PHS grants 5R01 MH18343 to the author and 5 S07 RR07065 to Rockefeller University. I am also very grateful for support from Rockefeller Foundation Grant RF70095 for Research in Reproductive Biology. Besides these generous sources of assistance, the last 10 years of work reviewed in this chapter owe much to support I have received from Professor Peter Marler.

### References

Andrew, R. J. (1974). Changes in visual responsiveness following intercollicular lesions and their effects on avoidance and attack. *Brain, Behavior and Evolution* 10, 400–424.
Andrew, R. J., and deLanerolle, N. (1974). The effects of muting lesions on emotional behavior and behavior normally associated with calling. *Brain, Behavior and Evolution* 10, 377–399.
Arnold, A. P. (1974). Behavioral Effects of Androgen in Zebra Finches *(Poephila guttata)* and a Search for Its Site of Action. Ph.D. Thesis, Rockefeller University.
Arnold, A. P. (1975a). The effects of castration and androgen replacement on song, courtship and aggression in zebra finches *(Poephila guttata). Journal of Experimental Zoology* 191, 309–326.
Arnold, A. P. (1975b). The effects of castration on song development in zebra finches *(Poephila guttata). Journal of Experimental Zoology* 191, 261–278.
Arnold, A. P. (1979). Hormone accumulation in the brain of the zebra finch after injection of various steroids and steroid competitors. *Society for Neuroscience Abstracts* 5, 437.
Arnold, A. P., Nottebohm, F., and Pfaff, D. W. (1976). Hormone concentrating cells in vocal control and other areas of the brain of the zebra finch *(Poephila guttata). Journal of Comparative Neurology* 165, 487–512.
Baldwin, F. M., Goldin, H. S., and Metfessel, M. (1940). Effects of testosterone propionate on female Roller canaries under complete song isolation. *Proceedings of the Society of Experimental Biology and Medicine* 44, 373–375.

Boord, R. L. (1968). Ascending projections of the primary cochlear nuclei and nucleus laminaris in the pigeon. *Journal of Comparative Neurology* 133, 523-530.

Boord, R. L. (1969). The anatomy of the avian auditory system. *Annals of the New York Academy of Science* 167, 186-198.

Boord, R. L., and Rasmusen, G. L. (1963). Projection of the cochlear and lagenar nuclei in the pigeon. *Journal of Comparative Neurology* 120, 463-475.

Brisson, P., and Vaugien, L. (1957). Testes stimulation of the Chaffinch obtained in winter by artificial illumination, gonadotrophin and thyroxin. *Compte Rendu de l'Académie des Sciences (Paris)* 245, 354-366.

Broca, P. (1865). Sur la faculté du langage articulé *Bulletin de la Societé de Anthropologie de Paris* 6, 377-393.

Brown, J. L. (1965). Vocalization evoked from the optic lobe of a songbird. *Science* 149, 1002-1003.

Brown, J. L. (1971). An exploratory study of vocalization areas in the brain of the redwinged blackbird *(Agelaius phoeniceus)*. *Behavior* 24, 91-127.

Catchpole, C. K. (1973). The functions of advertising song in the Sedge Warbler *(Acrocephalus schoenobaenus)* and the Reed Warbler *(A. scirpaceus)*. *Behavior* 46, 300-320.

Collard, J., and Grevendal, L. (1946). Etudes sur les caractères sexuels des Pinsons, *Fringilla coelebs* et *F. montifringilla*. *Gerfaut* 2, 89-107.

Corballis, M. C., and Morgan, M. J. (1978). On the biological basis of human laterality. I. Evidence for a maturational left-right gradient. II. The mechanisms of inheritance. *Behavior Brain Sciences* 2, 261-336.

deLanerolle, N., and Andrew, R. J. (1974). Midbrain structures controlling vocalization in the domestic chick. *Brain, Behavior and Evolution* 10, 354-376.

Delius, J. D. (1971). Agonistic behavior of juvenile gulls, a neuroethological study. *Animal Behavior* 21, 236-246.

Dewson, J. H. (1977). Preliminary evidence of hemispheric asymmetry of auditory function in monkeys. *In* "Lateralization in the Nervous System" (S. Harnad, R. W. Doty, L. Goldstein, J. Jaynes, and G. Krauthamer, eds.), pp. 63-71. Academic Press, New York.

Feder, H. H., Storey, A., Goodwin, D., Reboulleau, C., and Silver, R. (1977). Testosterone and "5α-dihydrotestosterone" levels in peripheral plasma of male and female ring doves *(Streptopelia risoria)* during the reproductive cycle. *Biology of Reproduction* 16, 666-677.

Follett, B. K., and Farner, D. S. (1966). The effect of the daily photoperiod on gonadal growth, neuro-hypophysial hormone content and neurosecretion in the hypothalamo-hypophysial system of the Japanese quail (*Coturnix coturnix japonica*). *General and Comparative Endocrinology* 7, 111-124.

Gazzaniga, M. S. (1970). "The Bisected Brain." Appleton-Century-Crofts, New York.

Gazzaniga, M. S., and LeDoux, J. E. (1978). "The Integrated Mind." Plenum, New York.

Geschwind, N. (1970). The organization of language in the brain. *Science* 170, 940-944.

Greenwalt, C. H. (1968). "Bird Song: Acoustics and Physiology." Smithsonian Inst. Press, Washington, D. C.

Hooker, B. I. (1968). Birds, *In* "Animal Communication" (T. A. Sebeok, ed.), pp. 311-337. Indiana University Press, Bloomington.

Howard, H. E. (1920). "Territory in Bird Life." Murray, London.

Immelman, K. (1969). Song development in the zebra finch and other estrildid finches. *In* "Bird Vocalizations" (R. A. Hinde, ed.), pp. 61-74. Cambridge Univ. Press, Cambridge.

Karten, H. (1967). The organization of the ascending auditory pathway in the pigeon

*(Columba livia)*. I. Diencephalic projections of the inferior colliculus (nucleus mesencephalius lateralis pars dorsalis). *Brain Research* 6, 409–427.

Karten, H. (1968). The ascending auditory pathway in the pigeon *(Columba livia)*. II. Telencephalic projections of the nucleus ovoidalis thalami. *Brain Research* 11, 134–153.

Karten, H. J., and Hodos, W. (1967). "A Stereotaxic Atlas of the Brain of the pigeon *(Columbia livia)*. Johns Hopkins Press, Baltimore.

Kelley, D. B., and Nottebohm, F. (1979). Projections of a telencephalic auditory nucleus—field L—in the canary. *Journal of Comparative Neurology* 183, 455–470.

Konishi, M. (1963). The role of auditory feedback in the vocal behavior of the domestic fowl. *Zeitschrift für Tierpsychologie* 20, 349–367.

Konishi, M. (1965). The role of auditory feedback in the control of vocalization in the white-crowned-sparrow. *Zeitschrift für Tierpsychologie* 22, 770–783.

Konishi, M., and Nottebohm, F. (1969). Experimental studies in the ontogeny of avian vocalizations. *In* "Bird Vocalizations" (R. A. Hinde, ed.), pp. 29–48. Cambridge Univ. Press, Cambridge.

Krebs, J. (1976). Bird song and territorial defense. *New Scientist* (June 3), 534–536.

Kroodsma, D. E. (1976). Reproductive development in a female songbird: Differential stimulation by quality of male song. *Science* 192, 574–575.

Kroodsma, D. E. (1977). A reevaluation of song development in the song sparrow. *Animal Behavior* 25, 390–399.

Lemon, R. E. (1973). Nervous control of the syrinx in white-throated sparrows *(Zonotrichia albicollis)*. *Journal of Zoology (London)* 171, 131–140.

Levy, J. (1972). Lateral specialization of the human brain: Behavioral Manifestations and possible evolutionary basis. *In* "The Biology of Behavior" (J. A. Kiger, ed.), pp. 159–180. Oregon State Univ. Press, Corvallis, Oregon.

Levy, J. (1977). The origins of lateral asymmetry. *In* "Lateralization in the Nervous System" (S. Harnad, R. W. Doty, L. Goldstein, J. Jaynes, and G. Krauthamer, eds.), pp. 195–209. Academic Press, New York.

Lieberburg, I., and Nottebohm, F. (1979). High-affinity androgen binding proteins in syringeal tissues of songbirds. *General and Comparative Endocrinology* 37, 286–293.

Lofts, B., Follett, B. K., and Murton, R. K. (1970). Temporal changes in the pituitary-gonadal axis. *Memoires of the Society for Endocrinology* 18, 545–575.

Luine, V., Lieberburg, I., Nottebohm, F., Harding, C., and McEwen, B. (1978). The avian syrinx: An androgen sentitive motor organ? *Society for Neuroscience Abstracts* p. 371.

Luine, V., Nottebohm, F., Harding, C., and McEwen B. S. Androgen affects cholinergic enzymes in syringeal motor neurons and muscle. *Brain Research* (in press).

McEwen, B. S., Deneg, C. J., Gerlach, J. L., and Plapinger, L. (1974). Chemical studies of the brain as a steroid hormone target tissue. *In* "The Neurosciences: Third Study Program" (F. O. Schmitt and F. G. Worden, eds.) pp. 599–620. MIT Press, Cambridge.

Marler, P. (1956). The voice of the Chaffinch and its function as a language. *Ibis* 98, 231–261.

Marler, P. (1960). Bird songs and mate selection. *In* "Animal Sounds and Communication" (W. Lanyon and W. Tavolga, eds.). Amer. Inst. Biol. Sci., AIBS Publ. No. 7, Washington, D.C.

Marler, P., and Peters, S. (1977). Selective vocal learning in a sparrow. *Science* 198, 519–521.

Marler, P., and Tamura, M. (1964). Culturally transmitted patterns of vocal behavior in sparrows. *Science* 146, 1483–1486.

Menaker, M., and Keatts, H. (1968). Extraretinal light perception in the sparrow.

II. Photoperiodic stimulation on testis growth. *Proceedings of the National Academy of Science* **60**, 146–151.

Metfessel, M. (1935). Roller canary song produced without learning from external sources. *Science* **81**, 470.

Metfessel, M. (1940). Relationships of heredity and environment in behavior. *Journal of Psychology* **10**, 177–198.

Morrell, J. I., Kelley, D. B., and Pfaff, D. W. (1975). Sex steroid binding in the brains of vertebrates. *In* "Brain-Endocrine Interaction II" (K. M. Knigge, D. E. Scott, and H. Kobayashi, eds.), pp. 230–256. Karger AG, Basel.

Mulligan, J. A. (1966). Singing behavior and its development in the Song Sparrow, *Melospiza melodia*. *University of California, Berkeley, Publ. Zoology* **81**, 1–76.

Newman, J. D. (1972). Midbrain control of vocalizations in redwinged blackbirds *(Agelaius phoeniceus)*. *Brain Research* **48**, 227–242.

Nottebohm, F. (1966). The Role of Sensory Feedback in the Development of Avian Vocalizations. Ph.D. dissertation, Univ. of California, Berkeley.

Nottebohm, F. (1967). The role of sensory feedback in the development of avian vocalizations. *In* "Proceedings of the XIV International Ornithological Congress" (D. W. Snow, ed.). Blackwell, Oxford.

Nottebohm, F. (1968). Auditory experience and song development in the Chaffinch, *Fringilla coelebs*. *Ibis* **110**, 549–568.

Nottebohm, F. (1969). The "critical period" for song learning. *Ibis* **111**, 386–387.

Nottebohm, F. (1970). Ontogeny of bird song. *Science* **167**, 950–956.

Nottebohm, F. (1971). Neural lateralization of vocal control in a passerine bird. I. Song. *Journal of Experimental Zoology* **177**, 229–261.

Nottebohm, F. (1972a). The origins of vocal learning. *American Naturalist* **106**, 116–140.

Nottebohm, F. (1972b). Neural lateralization of vocal control in a passerine bird. II. Subsong, calls, and a theory of vocal learning. *Journal of Experimental Zoology* **179**, 35–49.

Nottebohm, F. (1975). Vocal behavior in birds. *In* "Avian Biology" (J. R. King and D. S. Farner, eds.), Vol. 5, Chap. 5, pp. 287–332. Academic Press, New York.

Nottebohm, F. (1976). Phonation in the Orange-winged Amazon Parrot, *Amazona Amazonica*. *Journal of Comparative Physiology (Series A)* **108**, 157–170.

Nottebohm, F. (1977). Asymmetries in neural control of vocalization in the canary. *In* "Lateralization in the Nervous System" (S. Harnad, R. W. Doty, L. Goldstein, J. Jaynes, and G. Krauthamer, eds.), pp. 23–44. Academic Press, New York.

Nottebohm, F. (1979). Origins and mechanisms in the establishment of cerebral dominance. *In* "Handbook of Behavioral Neurobiology" (M. S. Gazzaniga, ed.), pp. 295–344. Plenum, New York.

Nottebohm, F. (1980). Testosterone triggers growth of brain vocal control nuclei in adult female canaries. *Brain Research* (in press).

Nottebohm, F., and Arnold, A. P. (1976). Sexual dimorphism in vocal control areas of the songbird brain. *Science* **194**, 211–213.

Nottebohm, F., and Kelley, D. B. (1978). Projections to efferent vocal control nuclei of the canary telencephalon. *Society for Neuroscience Abstracts* **4**, 101.

Nottebohm, F., and Nottebohm, M. (1971). Vocalizations and breeding behavior of surgically deafened ring doves, *Streptopelia risoria*. *Animal Behavior* **19**, 313–327.

Nottebohm, F., and Nottebohm, M. (1976). Left hypoglossal dominance in the control of canary and white-crowned sparrow song. *Journal of Comparative Physiology Series A* **108**, 171–192.

Nottebohm, F., and Nottebohm, M. (1978). Relationship between song repertoire and age in the canary, *Serinus canarius*. *Zeitschrift für Tierpsychologie* **46**, 298–305.

Nottebohm, F., Stokes, T. M., and Leonard, C. M. (1976). Central control of song in the canary, *Serinus canarius*. *Journal of Comparative Neurology* **165**, 457–486.

Nottebohm, F., Manning, E., and Nottebohm, M. (1979). Reversal of hypoglossal dominance in canaries following unilateral syringeal denervation. *Journal of Comparative Physiology* **134**, 227–240.

Penfield, W., and Roberts, L. (1959). "Speech and Brain Mechanisms." Princeton University Press, Princeton.

Petersen, M. T., Beecher, M. D., Zoloth, S. R., Moody, D. B., and Stebbins, W. C. (1978). Neural lateralization of species-specific vocalizations by Japanese macaques *(Macaca fuscata)*. *Science* **202**, 324–327.

Potash, L. M. (1970). Vocalization elicited by electrical brain stimulation in *Coturnix coturnix japonica*. *Behavior* **36**, 149–167.

Poulsen, H. (1951). Inheritance and learning in the song of the Chaffinch *(Fringilla coelebs L.)*. *Behavior* **3**, 216–227.

Price, P. H. (1977). Determinants of Zebra Finch Song: Studies of Species Song Uniformity, Bases of Physiological Determination, and Developmental Plasticity. Ph.D. dissertation, Univ. of Pennsylvania.

Pröve, E. (1974). Der Einfluss von Kastration und Testosterone substitution auf das Sexualverhalten männlicher Zebrafinken *Taeniopygia guttatd castanotis*. *Gould. Journal of Ornithology* **115**, 338–347.

Pröve, E. (1978). Quantitative Untersuchungen zu Wechselbeziehungen zwischen Balzaktivität und Testosterontitern bei männlichen Zebrafinken *(Taeniopygia guttata castanotis)*. *Zeitschrift für Tierpsychologie* **48**, 47–67.

Robinson, R. G. (1978). Differential behavioral effects of right vs. left cerebral infarction: Evidence for cerebral lateralization in the rat. *Society for Neuroscience Abstracts* p. 79.

Rogers, L. J., and Anson, J. M. (1979). Lateralisation of Function in the chicken forebrain. *Pharmacology Biochemistry and Behavior* **10**, 679–686.

Rowan, W. (1926). On photoperiodism, reproductive periodicity, and the annual migration of birds and certain fishes. *Proceedings of the Boston Society of Natural History* **38**, 147–189.

Shoemaker, H. H. (1939). Effect of testosterone propionate on the behavior of the female canary. *Proceedings of the Society of Experimental Biology and Medicine* **41**, 229–302.

Sibley, C. G. (1974). The relationships of the lyrebirds. *Emu* **74**, 65–79.

Silver, R. (1978). The parental behavior of ring doves. *American Scientist* **66**, 209–215.

Sperry, R. W. (1974). Lateral specialization in the surgically separated hemispheres. *In* "The Neurosciences: Third Study Program" (F. O. Schmitt and F. G. Worden, eds.), pp. 5–19. MIT Press, Cambridge.

Stokes, T. C., Leonard, C. M., and Nottebohm, F. (1974). A stereotaxic atlas of the telencephalon, diencephalon, and mesencephalon of the canary, *Serinus canarius*. *Journal of Comparative Neurology* **156**, 337–374.

Thorpe, W. (1958). The learning of song patterns by birds, with special reference to the song of the chaffinch, *Fringilla coelebs*. *Ibis* **100**, 535–570.

Thorpe, H. W., and Pilcher, P. M (1958). The nature and characteristics of subsong. *British Birds* **51**, 509–514.

Waser, M. S., and Marler, P. (1977). Song learning in canaries. *Journal of Comparative and Physiological Psychology* **91**, 1–7.

Wernicke, C. (1874). "Der aphasische symptomen complex." Max, Cohn and Weigert, Breslau.

Wilson, D. W., and Wyman, J. (1965). Motor output patterns during random and rhythmic stimulation of locust thoracic ganglia. *Biophysical Journal* **5**, 121–143.

Zigmond, E., Nottebohm, F., and Pfaff, D. W. (1973). Androgen-concentrating cells in the midbrain of a songbird. *Science* **179**, 1005–1007.

PROGRESS IN PSYCHOBIOLOGY AND PHYSIOLOGICAL PSYCHOLOGY, VOL. 9

# Neuronal Activity of Cingulate Cortex, Anteroventral Thalamus, in Hippocampal Formation and Discriminative Conditioning: Encoding and Extraction of the Significance of Conditional Stimuli

Michael Gabriel, Kent Foster, Edward Orona,
Steven E. Saltwick, and Mark Stanton

*Department of Psychology*
*University of Texas*
*Austin, Texas*

Copyright © 1980 by Academic Press, Inc.
All rights of reproduction in any form reserved.
ISBN 0-12-542109-5

# I. Introduction

A paradox has existed since the early 1960s in relation to studies directed toward identification of critical neural substrates for learning and memory. On the one hand, studies of human neuropathology of memory have indicated that structures of the limbic system are essential mediators of these processes. This attribution of function to limbic structures is based on observations of deficiency of recall and memory acquisition in patients with bilateral surgical damage to the medial temporal lobe, including the hippocampal formation (Scoville, 1954; Scoville and Milner, 1957; Penfield and Milner, 1958). Similar defects have been shown in chronic alcoholic patients with Korsakoff's disease to be correlated with tissue damage in diencephalic limbic structures such as the mammillary bodies (Malamud and Skillicorn, 1956; Barbizet, 1963; Angelergues, 1969; Victor *et al.,* 1971; Kahn and Crosby, 1972), the anterior group of thalamic nuclei (Sweet *et al.,* 1959; Angelergues, 1969), and the mediodorsal nucleus of the thalamus (Victor *et al.,* 1971; Adams, 1969).

On the other hand, studies of the effects of brain damage in infrahuman mammals have not clearly implicated the limbic system in mediation of associative processes.

It is true that performance of learned behavior is impaired by damage to infrahuman limbic structures (see reviews by McCleary, 1966; Douglas and Pribram, 1966; Douglas, 1967; Thomas *et al.,* 1968; Isaacson, 1974; Altman *et al.,* 1973; Nadel *et al.,* Black, 1975; Horel, 1978). For example, deficit in acquisition of aversively motivated behavior follows damage to the cingulate cortex (McCleary, 1961; Pribram and

Weiskrantz, 1957; Lubar, 1964; Schreiner and Kling, 1953; Lubar and Perachio, 1965; Thomas and Slotnick, 1962; Thomas and Otis, 1958; Trafton *et al.,* 1969; Kimble and Gostnell, 1968; Eckersdorf, 1974; Ursin *et al.,* 1969; Trafton, 1967). Bilateral destruction in the hippocampal formation yields performance deficit in complex mazes (e.g., Winocur and Breckenridge, 1973; Kimble and Dannen, 1977), serial patterning tasks (Kimble and Pribram, 1963), alternation behavior (e.g., Means *et al.,* 1971), and extinction (e.g., Jarrard *et al.,* 1964; Jarrard and Isaacson, 1965). These results are compatible with the idea of limbic system involvement in associative processes. Nevertheless, such a conclusion is not compelled by the evidence, and a substantial consensus based on these studies attributes the behavioral deficits to disruption of processes other than learning or memory.

For one thing, animals with lesions of the hippocampal formation are capable of normal learning and retention in a variety of experimental situations (e.g., Mishkin and Pribram, 1954; Orbach and Fantz, 1958; Correll and Scoville, 1967; Schmaltz and Theios, 1972; Solomon and Moore, 1975; Means *et al.,* 1970). Certainly these latter results do not support the hypothesis that infrahuman hippocampal function is essential to formation of permanent memory, as argued by Milner (1970, 1972) on the basis of her studies of brain-damaged humans.

Moreover, the view that the hippocampal formation and other limbic structures are critically involved in infrahuman learning and memory has suffered because other hypotheses seem to account for the results of studies of the behavioral relevance of these structures in infrahumans with more power and parsimony than the learning hypothesis. Thus, certain authors have published well-documented arguments implicating the hippocampal formation in mediation of arousal reactions, and orientation, which occur to novel and/or meaningful stimuli (Grastyan *et al.,* 1959; Green and Arduini, 1954; Routtenberg, 1971; Bennet, 1975; Kesner and Wilburn, 1974). Other well-integrated accounts have been presented implicating limbic structures in modulation (e.g., inhibition, facilitation) of behavioral responses (McCleary, 1966; Douglas, 1967; Vanderwolf, 1971; Vanderwolf *et al.,* 1973; Dickenson, 1974; Altman *et al.,* 1973; Thomas *et al.,* 1968). Theories of this kind considered collectively have as many or more adherents than theories which postulate a critical role for infrahuman limbic structures in learning and memory.

These considerations give rise to the inference that there has been a progressive divergence through evolution, of the function subserved by human limbic structures, from that subserved by infrahuman structures. Perhaps human limbic structures are major substrates of learning and memory, but nonlimbic structures mediate learning and memory in the infrahuman system.

We will refer to this proposition as the divergence hypothesis, in the remainder of this essay. Thus far we have summarized evidence that is basically supportive of the hypothesis. We now offer arguments and data which in our view weigh against it.

Reasons for caution in relation to the divergence hypothesis have been voiced by Iverson (1973) and by Gaffan (1974), who have pointed out that the apparent conflict between the human and animal literatures may be a result of attempts to compare human and animal performances directly, on tasks that are incommensurate. Perhaps the behavioral relevance of infrahuman limbic structures would resemble that of the human structures if their roles could be assessed in the context of behavior which is common to both kinds of subject. In fact, evidence supporting commonality of limbic functioning between humans and infrahumans has been obtained in studies indicating that manipulation of certain task variables produces similar effects in humans and in infrahumans with limbic system damage (see reviews by Warrington and Weiskrantz, 1973; Weiskrantz, 1978; see also Gaffan, 1974; Jarrard, 1975; Winocur and Black, 1978; Winocur and Olds, 1978). For example, irrelevant experiences interposed between initial learning and tests for retention are detrimental to retention performance in animals with hippocampal lesions (e.g., Jarrard, 1975; Winocur, 1979). Such susceptibility to interposed disruption is the defining characteristic of the classic human amnesia produced by bilateral hippocampectomy (Scoville and Milner, 1957; Penfield and Milner, 1958). An additional instance of this kind is provided by findings indicating that provision of extra cues during recall enhances retention performance of hippocampectomized animals (e.g., Winocur and Black, 1978) and humans (Warrington and Weiskrantz, 1968).

A second source of information weighing against the divergence hypothesis is the view of infrahuman limbic functioning provided by a growing body of evidence obtained with a methodology fundamentally different from the lesion method. These studies have involved the observation of limbic neuronal correlates of classical and instrumental conditioning in intact, awake, and behaving animal subjects (Olds *et al.*, 1972; Segal and Olds, 1972; Linesman and Olds, 1973; Berger and Thompson, 1977, 1978; Segal, 1973; Gabriel *et al.*, 1973a,b, 1977a,b).

Our own studies are representative of this approach. Section II will be devoted primarily to description and interpretation of our results. Special emphasis shall be placed upon aspects of the data which seem to have relevance to the divergence hypothesis.

## II. Neuronal Activity of Limbic Structures in Relation to Discriminative Avoidance Learning and Performance in the Rabbit

A. BRIEF HISTORY OF THE STUDIES

Our initial work on the role of limbic structures in behavioral learning was stimulated by the prior work of Professor Richard F. Thompson and his colleagues who had definitively mapped the polysensory "association areas" of the cerebral cortex in cats (Thompson *et al.,* 1963), and who had shown these areas to be involved in mediating a variety of associatively based behavioral phenomena including habituation (Thompson and Shaw, 1965), sensory preconditioning (Thompson and Kramer, 1965) and discriminative learning (Thompson and Smith, 1967).

The link leading from the work of Thompson and his colleagues to the study of the possible associative functions of rabbit limbic system was provided by collaborative studies carried out while the senior author was a postdoctoral fellow in Dr. Thompson's laboratory. The collaborative studies indicated that medially situated areas of the rabbit cerebral cortex, including the cingulate cortex of the hemispheric medial wall, manifested polysensory evoked responsiveness, similar to that shown by association cortex of the cat (see Gabriel *et al.,* 1973a). In addition, other studies had documented the polysensory properties of rabbit cingulate cortex (e.g., Vinogradova, 1970). These outcomes suggested that cingulate cortex would be importantly involved in mediating associatively based behaviors of the rabbit.

The latter suggestion was supported by additional collaborative studies which involved recording of neuronal activity from rabbit cingulate cortex during acquisition of acoustically cued, locomotory avoidance behavior. These studies demonstrated development of short-latency conditioned neuronal responses in cingulate cortex, during the acquisition of behavioral avoidance responses (CRs) (Gabriel *et al.,* 1973a). The conditioned neuronal activity manifested significant gradients of stimulus generalization, during the extinction test given on the day after acquisition (Gabriel *et al.,* 1973b).

The fact that the neuronal activity observed in these studies manifested the same basic associative properties (acquisition, stimulus control) as the conditioned behavior itself suggested that the neuronal activity served as a basis for the rabbit's evaluation of, and behavioral response to, the conditional stimulus.

On the other hand, certain observations indicated that the neuronal activity was not directly tied to the animal's behavior. The neuronal activity seemed to provide information not conveyed by the behavior, concerning the rabbit's associative status. These extra signs were manifested during the extinction-generalization test (Gabriel *et al.*, 1973b).

It should be mentioned that the decline of CRs in a single extinction session (within-session CR-extinction) is partially a "performance effect." This assertion is based on the observations of savings and spontaneous recovery (see Kimble, 1961, chap. 10) which indicate that a conditioned habit is not lost after a CR undergoes extinction. Presumably, performance factors (e.g., behavioral response habituation) operate in the extinction situation to produce cessation of behavioral CRs despite considerable residual habit strength, following a single extinction session. What was interesting in our data was the absence of within-session extinction of the associative neuronal response of cingulate cortex. The neuronal response persisted without decline throughout the entire session in which behavioral responses extinguished. Because of its persistence, and given the associative properties of stimulus control that it showed, the neuronal response seemed to reflect a fundamentally different kind of retention phenomenon, relative to the behavioral CR. A similar finding had been reported by Segal who showed persistence of appetitively conditioned neuronal activity of the cingulate cortical area accompanying extinction of behavioral responding (Segal, 1973). Analogously, Buchwald and Brown (1973) reported persistence of conditioned gamma motorneuronal activity accompanying extinction of a classically conditioned leg-flexion response in the cat.

An additional finding of our own study suggested that the activity of the cingulate cortex provided a different measure of retention than that provided by the behavioral CR. Separate generalization gradients were constructed for successive stages of the extinction test. The gradients based on behavioral CRs were not significant in the initial test stage. The absence of significant gradients was the result of a ceiling effect; the rabbits responded behaviorally to every stimulus, whether CS or test, early in extinction. However, CR-extinction occurred at a more rapid rate to test tones, compared to the CS. Thus, significant behavioral gradients were obtained in the later stages of the test.

The test-stage by gradient interaction is a finding of interest in its own right,[1] however, the critical observation for the present discussion was

[1]This effect has been obtained previously using a species and test situation different from our own (Hoffman, 1966). We would like to propose tentatively that performance factors operating in early test stages, and dissipating as the test progressed, were responsible for the effect. For example, consider the possibility that arousal may produce a low CR criterion and, therefore, high "hit" and "false alarm" rates, in initial stages of an

the absence of a test-stage by gradient effect for gradients based on neuronal activity of cingulate cortex. The early-trial ceiling effect seen in the behavioral data was not present in the neuronal data. The neuronal gradients were significant in all stages of the test, early and late. Again, the neuronal response of the cingulate area was independent of the behavioral CR. In fact, the neuronal response seemed a more *sensitive* index than the behavior, since it manifested stimulus-control early in the extinction test, and it persisted throughout the test, whereas the behavior showed neither of these effects.

These findings raised the interesting possibility that the assessment of neuronal activity in cingulate cortex during conditioning would provide a relatively direct measure of the status of the rabbit's avoidance habit — one that was independent of performance factors such as habituation and ceiling effects. In order to explore this idea we adopted a behavioral paradigm involving the procedures of differential conditioning and reversal. We felt that these procedures would permit more extensive and varied observation of the relationships between learned behavior and neuronal activity in the cingulate cortex. The results obtained from our most recent work on correlates of differential conditioning and reversal are described next (Gabriel *et al.,* 1977a,b, 1980a,b,d; Foster *et al.,* 1980).

B. RECENT STUDIES: NEUROANATOMICAL FOCUS

In our recent studies we focused on neuronal activity of the cingulate cortex of the rabbit hemispheric medial wall. To date we have obtained results from a total of 50 locations within cingulate cortex ranging from 3.0 to 9.0 mm posterior to bregma at depths ranging from 0.2 to 4.0 mm beneath the dorsal surface, and from 0.2 to 2.0 mm lateral to the midline. A majority of these placements (37) were located in a restricted area from 3.0 to 4.0 mm posterior to bregma. However, we have seen, to date, no significant difference between the activity of these placements, and activity of the remaining placements located more posteriorly.

The term cingulate cortex refers to the dorsally situated tissue of the medial wall, whereas more ventrally situated tissue is properly referred to as retrosplenial cortex (see Rose and Woolsey, 1948). Our electrodes

---

avoidance retention test. The observations of incubation of avoidance CRs (hits) and increased intertrial responses (false alarms) in the first 10–15 minutes of avoidance extinction compared to the remaining 15-minute periods (Gabriel, 1970) is compatible with this interpretation.

occupied both cingulate and retrosplenial regions, and we have not seen significant differences in the activity recorded from them. Thus, for convenience we will use "cingulate" to refer to both regions.

An additional target in our studies has been the anteroventral (AV) nucleus of the thalamus. Neuronal cell bodies in the AV nucleus of rabbit and rat send axonal fibers to the cingulate cortex (Rose and Woolsey, 1948; Domesick, 1972).

Other results indicate that a corticothalamic pathway exists connecting the regions of our cortical electrode placements with the AV nucleus. The existence of such a projection has been documented by Domesick for the rat (Domesick, 1969). In addition, Berger et al. (1979) have demonstrated a projection from the rabbit AV nucleus to laminae I and IV of cingulate cortex, and a projection back to the AV nucleus from laminae V and VI of cingulate cortex.

## C. RECENT STUDIES: BEHAVIORAL PROCEDURES AND RESULTS

The behavioral procedures involved instrumental conditioning of the locomotory response of the rabbit, using a rotating wheel apparatus (Brodgen and Culler, 1936). During conditioning a pure tone (CS + ) was followed after 5 seconds by onset of a footshock (UCS) delivered through the grid floor of the wheel apparatus. A second tone of a different frequency (CS − ) was interspersed with the CS + , but it was never followed by footshock. Sixty trials with each stimulus were given in each daily session. The interval between the end of a trial to the onset of a new trial was 10, 15, 20, or 25 seconds, these values occurring in a random sequence. Locomotion reset this interval. The order of the stimuli was randomized so that the subjects could not "predict" which would occur on a given trial. Locomotion elicited by the UCS terminated it, and locomotion during the CSs terminated them and prevented delivery of the UCS on CS + trials. Each rabbit was given daily sessions of conditioning until he attained a criterion requiring that the percentage of avoidances exceed the percentage of responses to the CS − by 60, in two consecutive sessions. A subgroup of rabbits experienced three or six sessions of overtraining (conditioning beyond criterion), and all rabbits experienced reversal training to the criterion. Further details of these procedures are provided elsewhere (Gabriel et al., 1976, 1977b).

Prior to conditioning, each rabbit received a session of pretraining, in which the tone signals and the shock UCS were presented in an unpaired fashion to control for possible nonassociative effects of the stimuli. [See Gabriel and Saltwick (1977) for the detailed procedure of pretraining.]

The mean number of sessions prior to the acquisition criterion was 3.06, and the mean number prior to reversal criterion was 9.30. Frequency and latency of responding to CS+ and CS− are plotted as a function of task stages in Fig. 1. The stages are pretraining (PT), first exposure to conditioning (FE), session in which first significant behavioral discrimination was achieved (FS), session in which criterion was attained (CR), and the beginning, middle, and end sessions of overtraining (OTB, OTM, and OTE, respectively).[2] The stages of reversal are the first session (R1), the session before the first significant reversal (BR), the session of first significant reversal (FR), and the session of reversal criterion (RC). Analysis of variance revealed robust ($p < 0.001$) behavioral discrimination in FS, CR, OT, and reversal for both percentage and latency of conditioned responding. Also, small but significant ($p < 0.05$) discrimination was detected in FE for the percentage measure but not for latency. There was no significant discrimination in PT.

**BEHAVIOR**

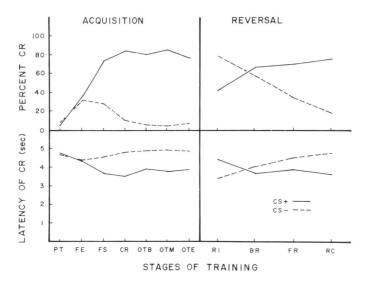

FIG. 1. The mean percentage of behavioral conditioned responses (CR, upper half of figure) and latency of CR in seconds (lower half of figure) is plotted as a function of stage of acquisition, overtraining, and reversal training. See (Section II,C) for the definitions of the stages.

[2]It was necessary, for instances in which rabbits met criterion in the first or second sessions of conditioning, to divide the first session of conditioning into quarters or halves to obtain behavioral and neuronal values for FE and FS. This happened for 11 of the 50 rabbits contributing data to the present report.

## D. RECENT STUDIES: ELECTROPHYSIOLOGICAL
TECHNIQUES

Throughout all stages of behavioral training neuronal activity from three brain regions was recorded on magnetic tape and processed by a computer. Details of the techniques of electrode construction, implantation, recording, and data reduction have been presented elsewhere (e.g., Gabriel *et al.*, 1976, 1977b). Representative neuronal records obtained with these techniques are shown in Fig. 2. These records may be categorized as multiple unit records, consisting of the combined action potentials from a population of neurons surrounding the electrode. The two records shown in Fig. 2 were obtained from cingulate cortex during

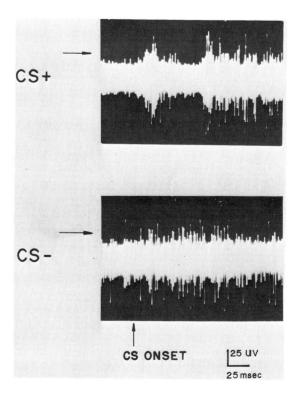

FIG. 2. Representative neuronal records obtained from lamina II of cingulate cortex, during discriminative performance at criterion, by an individual rabbit. The display was obtained by photographing the oscilloscope trace of the record during presentation of the CS+ (upper trace) and the CS− (lower trace). The vertical arrow (lower left) indicates CS-onset, and the horizontal arrows (left of each trace) indicate the Schmitt trigger level.

presentation of the CS+ and CS− to a trained rabbit. Note the triphasic nature of the neuronal response to the CS+. That is, there is an initial excitation at 15–25 milliseconds following tone onset. This excitation is followed by a cessation of neuronal firing in the interval from 35 to 75 milliseconds, and a second excitation at 75 milliseconds, which peaks at approximately 100 milliseconds and declines slowly through the remainder of the trial. This triphasic response pattern is consistently obtained in cingulate cortex and in the AV thalamus. Others have observed similar triphasic patterns from the visual and somatosensory areas of the cortex, during conditioning of chronically implanted, awake, behaving rabbits (Shvyrkov and Aleksandrov, 1973).

In order to minimize the size of the neuronal population contributing data to the analysis, outputs from the preamplifiers were fed into Schmitt triggers whose levels were set independently so as to be exceeded by only the largest three or four neuronal spikes on each record. The Schmitt trigger levels are indicated by the arrow at the left of each trace in Fig. 2. Each Schmitt trigger produced an output pulse each time a neuronal spike exceeded its level. The output pulses were fed into a PDP-8 computer programmed to process the neuronal data and to control the behavioral experiment, on-line.[3]

The computer used the outputs from the Schmitt triggers to construct peristimulus histograms. Each histogram reflected the frequency, summed over trials in a session, of neuronal firing in consecutive 10-millisecond intervals (bins) preceding and following the onsets of the CSs. Separate histograms were constructed from the trials with the CS+, and from the trials with the CS−. Thus, two histograms were obtained from each session, each from a total of 60 trials.

Standard scores (z-scores), based on the frequency of firing in each bin, were computed for each of the first 20 bins after CS-onset. To compute the z-scores, the mean frequency in 30 pre-CS (baseline) bins was subtracted from the frequency in each of the 20 bins which followed CS-onset. The difference in each case was divided by the standard deviation of the pre-CS bins. In addition, the mean frequency of counts in the eleventh through the twentieth bins following CS-onset was computed. The mean of the pre-CS bins was subtracted from it, and the difference was divided by the standard error of the pre-CS mean, yielding a single score (T-score), which served as our measure of neuronal response in the second period of 100 milliseconds after CS-onset. Additional T-scores

[3]We wish to acknowledge the invaluable contribution of Mr. Steven E. Saltwick, who wrote the programs which controlled the behavioral experiment and constructed the neuronal peristimulus histograms.

were computed for the third through the sixth periods of 100 milliseconds following the CS-onset. Thus, in all cases our scores reflected the magnitude of CS-evoked neuronal response, normalized with respect to the pre-CS baseline. All neuronal records obtained during training were stored permanently using a magnetic tape system. Figure 3 illustrates the system utilized for the collection of the neuronal data.

E. RECENT STUDIES: NEURONAL CORRELATES OF
   DISCRIMINATIVE ACQUISITION AND OVERTRAINING IN
   CINGULATE CORTEX AND ANTEROVENTRAL THALAMUS

Neuronal activity accompanying discriminative behavioral conditioning is shown in Figs. 4 and 5. These data represent average results obtained from all placements in cingulate cortex. Figure 4 shows the magnitude of the cortical neuronal responses, in the form of $z$-scores, evoked by the CS+ and the CS− over 19 consecutive 10-millisecond bins following CS onset. Figure 5 shows response magnitudes, in the form of $T$-scores, for five consecutive periods of 100 milliseconds each. Thus, Fig. 5 indicates effects at a relatively great range of latencies, whereas Fig. 4 illustrates short-latency changes with relatively fine temporal grain. The separate panels of the figures show the neuronal response magnitudes in pretraining, and in the six behaviorally defined stages of discriminative conditioning (see Section II, C).

Note that the neuronal response profiles evoked by the conditional stimuli (Fig. 4) were triphasic in form, yielding an increase in activity above the pretone baseline in the initial 15–25 milliseconds following tone onset, decreased activity to a level equivalent to the pretone baseline or below the pretone baseline in the interval from 35 to 75 milliseconds, and increased activity once again beginning at 75 milliseconds and continuing until the end of the 200-millisecond period of analysis. These triphasic profiles reflected the periodicity of the evoked response of cingulate cortex, illustrated in the photographic record (Fig. 2).

A salient feature of these data was the development with conditioning of a discriminative neuronal response, defined as a significantly greater neuronal response to the CS+, relative to the CS−, within the third component (100–200 milliseconds) of the triphasic response and at greater latencies.[4] This significant neuronal discrimination was present

---

[4]In all cases, the references in the text to statistical significance are based upon individual comparisons of mean neuronal response magnitudes associated with the CS+, with means associated with the CS−. The procedure used for the comparisons was the $t$ test carried out following a significant overall $F$ in the analysis of variance (Winer, 1962, p. 210).

## RECORDING SYSTEM FOR
## STUDY OF NEURONAL ACTIVITY

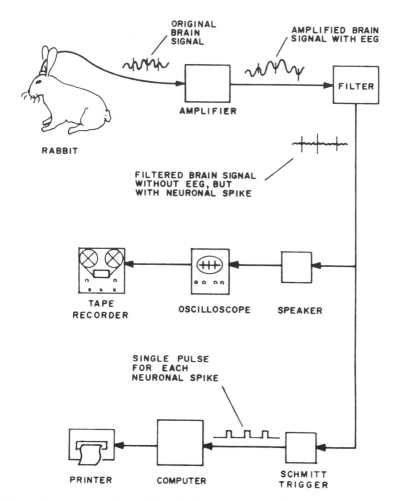

FIG. 3. The system used for on-line collection and analysis of neuronal data.

during the session of first significant (FS) behavioral discrimination, the day of criterion (CR) attainment, and throughout all stages of overtraining.

It is of interest to note that the discriminative effect in cingulate cortex was produced by a drop in the magnitude of neuronal response to the CS− during FS, CR, and all sessions of overtraining, relative to the response elicited by the prospective CS− in pretraining.

138                                    Michael Gabriel *et al.*

CINGULATE CORTEX

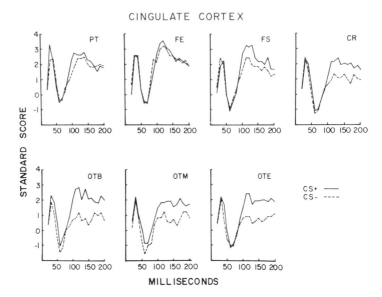

Fig. 4. In each panel the average neuronal response of limbic cortex to CS+ and CS−
is plotted for 19 consecutive 10-millisecond bins after tone-onset. Each panel shows data of
a different behaviorally defined stage of acquisition (see Section II,C for definitions of the
stages). The ordinate values are in standard score (*z*-score) units reflecting response
magnitude relative to the pre-CS baseline (see Section II,D for further details). Because
neuronal responses did not occur in the first 10-millisecond interval after tone onset, the initial bin was omitted from the analysis and from the figure. Thus, the left-most bin in each
panel of the figure represents the interval from 10 to 20 milliseconds after tone-onset. The
millisecond values on the abscissa represent elapsed time relative to tone-onset. Reprinted
with permission from Foster *et al.* (1980).

A configuration of findings similar to those obtained for cingulate
cortex was also obtained for the AV thalamus. Thus, the profile of the
neuronal response was a triphasic one, and discriminative neuronal activity occurred within the third component of the triphasic response, as
well as at all greater latencies (see Figs. 6 and 7). In addition, the AV
nucleus showed no change in overall response magnitudes or in the
magnitudes of the discriminative effects as a function of stage of overtraining.

There were three interesting differences in the results obtained from
the AV nucleus, compared to cingulate cortex. First, a significant
neuronal discrimination occurred in the first, short-latency component
of the triphasic response of AV thalamic neurons during the criterial
stage and overtraining. Cingulate cortex activity showed discrimination
only in the third component of the triphasic response, beginning at 75
milliseconds.

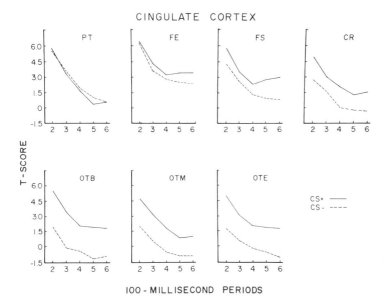

CINGULATE CORTEX

100 - MILLISECOND PERIODS

FIG. 5. In each panel, the average neuronal response of the cingulate cortex to CS+ and CS− is plotted for five consecutive intervals of 100 milliseconds following tone-onset. Each panel shows data of a different behaviorally defined stage of acquisition (see Section II,C for definition of the stages). The ordinate values are in *T*-score units reflecting response magnitude relative to the pre-CS baseline (see Section II,D for further details). The numeral 2 at the leftmost position on each abscissa represents the interval from 100 to 200 milliseconds. The numeral 3 represents the interval from 200 to 300 milliseconds, etc. Reprinted with permission from Foster et al. (1980).

The most striking difference between activity of the AV nucleus and cingulate cortex was the difference in the stage of conditioning at which significant discriminative neuronal activity first occurred. Thus, the AV nucleus first manifested a significant discriminative effect during the criterial stage (CR). There was no trace of a discriminative effect in the two earlier stages (FE and FS) in which cingulate cortex showed discrimination.

The AV nucleus also differed from cingulate cortex in terms of the relative effect of CS+ and CS−. Thus, whereas the discrimination in cortex was produced entirely by a drop relative to earlier stages of conditioning in response to the CS−, the discrimination in the AV nucleus resulted primarily from significant increase in response to the CS+. This effect may be noted by comparing the results which occurred in the criterial session to those of the session of first significant behavioral discrimination (Fig. 7).

In summary, we have seen that neuronal activity in cingulate cortex

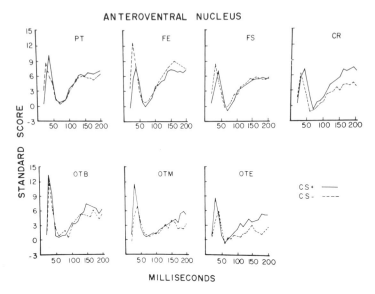

FIG. 6. Average neuronal response of anteroventral thalamus (AV) to CS + and CS − for the initial 19 10-millisecond bins following tone-onset. All labels are as defined in the legend to Fig. 4 and in Section II,C. Reprinted with permission from Foster *et al.* (1980).

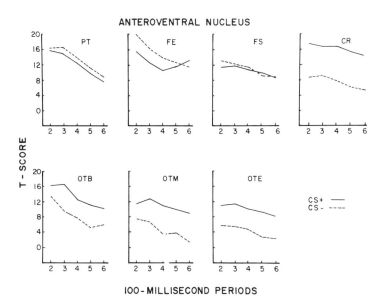

FIG. 7. Average neuronal response of anteroventral thalamus (AV) to CS + and CS − for five consecutive periods of 100 milliseconds beginning 100 milliseconds from tone-onset. All labels are as defined in the legend to Fig. 5 and in Section II,C. Reprinted with permission from Foster *et al.* (1980).

and in the AV nucleus of the rabbit becomes discriminative in character during training in a discriminative avoidance task. The discriminative effect in cingulate cortex occurred at a relatively early stage of training—a stage in which the rabbits' behavioral discrimination was incipient. The discriminative effect in the AV nucleus occurred at a later stage of training—a stage in which the rabbits displayed a high level of behavioral discrimination.

F. HETEROGENEITY AND LAMINAR SPECIFICITY
   OF DISCRIMINATIVE NEURONAL ACTIVITY
   IN CINGULATE CORTEX

## 1. Heterogeneity of Activity

Informal inspection of the neuronal responses of individual subjects revealed that not every record conformed to the pattern shown in the overall response profiles of Figs. 4 and 5. To examine this more systematically, the neuronal records from each stage of behavioral acquisition and overtraining were classified in terms of presence versus absence of neuronal discrimination, defined as a neuronal response to the CS+ greater than the response to the CS−.[5] The results of this analysis are summarized in Table I.

The results showed a substantial number (14) of the records to be in conformity with the overall group-based pattern of neuronal discrimination in cingulate cortex (Figs. 4 and 5). For these records neuronal discrimination was first detected during FE and/or during FS, and it continued to be manifested during CR and overtraining. Because they showed neuronal discrimination early in training, and because the discrimination persisted throughout training, we refer to these records as

[5]Discrimination was judged to be present in a given session of training if at least two of the five consecutive T-scores obtained from the CS+ histogram exceeded their respective CS− T-scores by a minimum of three T units. This criterion had to be met after the corresponding T-score difference, obtained during pretraining, was subtracted from the difference in training. Thus, the presence of neuronal discrimination during training was assessed relative to the differential responsiveness observed prior to training. The five consecutive T-scores were those associated with the five consecutive 100-millisecond intervals, beginning at 100 milliseconds following CS-onset. The T-score for the interval from 0 to 100 milliseconds was not used for this analysis because of the complexities introduced by the presence of the triphasic neuronal response in this interval, and because neuronal discrimination did not occur in this interval, by the overall analysis. The results obtained with this criterion were essentially replicated when a different criterion (a difference of three T-units at three or more 100-millisecond intervals) was used. Therefore, the findings were not specific to a particular criterion.

Michael Gabriel et al.

TABLE I
CATEGORIES OF NEURONAL DISCRIMINATION
DURING BEHAVIORAL ACQUISITION[a]

|  | EARLY FADERS | EARLY PERSISTERS | LATE DISCRIMINATORS | NON- DISCRIMINATORS | TOTAL |
|---|---|---|---|---|---|
| CINGULATE CORTEX | 8 | 14 | 11 | 13 | 46 |
| AV NUCLEUS | 0 | 3 | 9 | 1 | 13 |

[a]The number of neuronal records is shown from cingulate cortex and from the AV nucleus classified as early fader, early persister, late discriminator, or nondiscriminator. The classification was performed on the basis of the nature of the discriminative neuronal activity displayed during acquisition. (See Section II,F,1 and footnote 5) for a description of the criteria used to perform the classification.

early persistent discriminators. An individual record (R 72–5) manifesting early persistent discrimination is shown in Fig. 8.

The early category of neuronal discrimination included all records which showed neuronal discrimination during FE and/or during FS. A subset ($N = 8$) of the early discriminating records did not continue to show neuronal discrimination beyond FE and/or FS. We refer to records of this kind as early fading discriminators.

Eleven of the records obtained from cingulate cortex showed late neuronal discrimination. In these cases, neuronal discrimination occurred during CR and/or during OT, but not during FE or FS (Fig. 8B).

Finally, 13 of the records yield no evidence for neuronal discrimination at any stage of training.

It is interesting to note the relative frequencies of each of the three categories of neuronal discrimination illustrated in Table I. The most populous category was the early persisting category, which conforms to the overall pattern of the averaged data. This category accounted for

31% of the cases. Each of the remaining patterns (early fading and late) is represented by a smaller proportion of the cases (17% and 25%, respectively).

This distribution of cases may be accounted for by assuming the existence of two cellular populations in cingulate cortex, one population consisting of neurons which show discriminative activity early in training and a second consisting of late-discriminating neurons. Since the multiple unit recording technique involves sampling of small groups of neurons, a considerable number of our samples may be assumed to have been "mixed." That is, they involved simultaneous recording from members of early and late discriminating populations. We assume that mixed neuronal samples yielded the early persistent pattern of neuronal discrimination. Carrying this reasoning further, one could assume that a proportion of our neuronal samples were "pure." That is, they were composed either of pure early or pure late discriminating elements. We suggest that the pure records yielded the response patterns in the late category, and in the early fading category.

It is interesting to note that certain of the records were bimodal in character, showing transient early discrimination, and late discrimination, with no discrimination in the mid-stages of acquisition (e.g., Fig. 8A, R61-4). We interpret records of this kind as "mixed" records, in which the early discriminating elements underwent fading before onset of discrimination in the late elements.

## 2. Neuroanatomical Correlates of the Categories of Neuronal Discrimination

*a. Cingulate Cortex and the AV Thalamus.* The data shown in Table I indicate that there was a prevalence of early discriminating records relative to late discriminating records in cingulate cortex. However, the reverse was true in the AV nucleus. A $\chi^2$ test revealed a significant relationship ($p < 0.05$) between category (early versus late discrimination) and brain locus (cingulate cortex versus AV nucleus), supporting the idea that early discrimination prevailed within cingulate cortex whereas late discrimination prevailed in the AV nucleus. This result was to be expected on the basis of the overall analyses (Figs. 4, 5, 6, and 7), but it goes beyond the overall analyses in emphasizing that there was heterogeneity of neuronal discrimination within cingulate cortex and within the AV nucleus. Each structure manifested both early and late neuronal discrimination.

*b. Cortical Laminar Specificity of Early and Late Neuronal Discrimination.* Inspection of the photographs of brain sections containing

# PATTERNS OF NEURONAL DISCRIMINATION
# IN INDIVIDUAL SUBJECTS

## A. EARLY DISCRIMINATORS

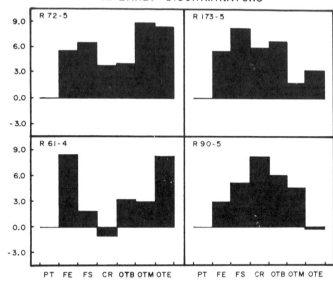

## B. LATE DISCRIMINATORS

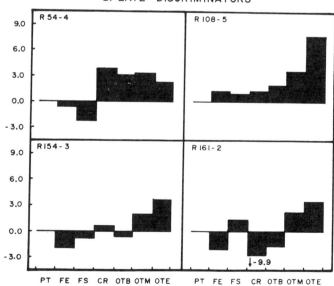

STAGES OF ACQUISITION

the electrode tracks revealed that placements were present in each of the six laminae that have been distinguished within the regions of cingulate cortex monitored in our studies (see Rose, 1933; see also Fig. 9). Discussion provided by Ranson and Clark (1959) based on the work of Kappers (1909) indicates that the internal granular lamina (IV) and the supragranular laminae (II and III) are receptive laminae of cortex. That is, most of the afferents from thalamus and from other brain regions terminate in these laminae. More recently, it has been recognized that lamina I may also be a site of termination of fibers from thalamic nuclei (e.g., Carey *et al.,* 1979). On the other hand, the infragranular laminae (V and VI) contain primarily efferent neurons—neurons which are the origins of axonal projections to thalamus and to other parts of the brain (Ranson and Clark, 1959).

Available data (see Section II,B) suggest that the rabbit cingulate cortex is organized in accord with the general principles espoused in Ranson and Clark. In other words, it is likely that the superficial laminae (I–IV) of cingulate cortex are receptive laminae and the deep laminae (V and VI) of cingulate cortex are efferent laminae.

Since the superficial and deep laminae may be distinguished functionally as input and output regions, respectively, we felt it reasonable to use the distinction between superficial and deep laminae in conceptualizing a two-level "cortical depth" factor. There were 18 electrode placements in one of the four superficial laminae and 28 placements in one of the two deep laminae. Four of the total 50 cortical placements could not be classified in this way.

In relating category of neuronal discrimination to cortical depth we found the following significant association: early discriminating records predominated in the deep cingulate laminae and late discriminating

---

FIG. 8. The bars in each panel of the figure represent the magnitude of neuronal discrimination that was present at a particular stage (i.e., PT, FE, FS, etc.) of acquisition, for an individual rabbit (see Section II,C for definition of stages). The bar values were obtained by subtracting the average of the $T$-scores reflecting the neuronal response to the CS+ from the average reflecting the neuronal response to the CS− at each stage of acquisition. To obtain each $T$-score average, $T$-scores two through six, reflecting neuronal response from 100 to 600 milliseconds following tone-onset were used. The $T$-score differences for each session were adjusted for pretraining differences. That is, each difference present in pretraining for a given rabbit was subtracted from the difference in each session. Thus, the difference present in PT was arbitrarily defined as zero and differences at the various stages of acquisition were adjusted accordingly. The upper portion of the figure (A) illustrates individual records classified as early discriminators (records which showed neuronal discrimination in FE and/or FS). The lower portion of the figure (B) shows neuronal records classified as late discriminators (records which yielded discrimination in CR or in OT, but not in FE and/or FS). Details of the method used to classify the records are described in footnote 5. Reprinted with permission from Foster *et al.* (1980).

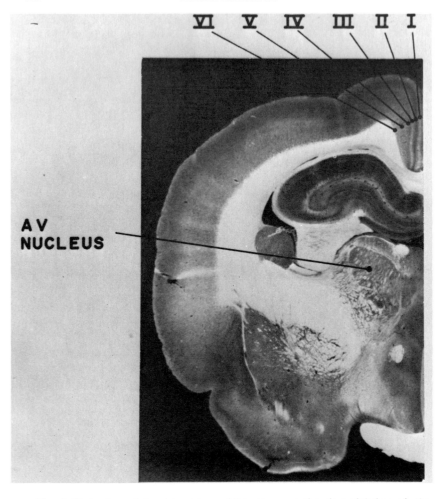

FIG. 9. Six laminae of cingulate cortex and the anteroventral nucleus of thalamus in the rabbit. Designation of the laminae was based on the atlas of Rose (1933).

records predominated within the superficial laminae [$\chi^2(1) = 11.50$, $p < 0.001$]. This outcome is illustrated in Fig. 10.

As a further step in examining the relation between cortical depth and category of neuronal discrimination, we performed analysis of variance on data of the discriminating cortical records using depth of cortical placement as a two-level factor. The analysis on the $T$-score data yielded a significant interaction of stage of training, stimulus, and the depth factor (see Figs. 11 and 12). Subsequent individual comparisons computed

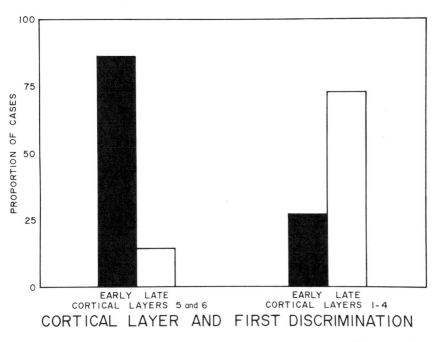

CORTICAL LAYER AND FIRST DISCRIMINATION

FIG. 10. Proportion of cingulate cortical neuronal records classified as early discriminators (dark bars) or late discriminators (light bars), localized in either the superficial laminae (right half of the figure) or in the deep laminae (left half of the figure). The superficial laminae (I–IV) and the deep laminae (V and VI) are shown in Fig. 9. A $\chi^2$ test revealed a significant association ($p < 0.001$) between classification of the records as early or late discriminators, and presence in either superficial or deep cortical laminae. Reprinted with permission from Gabriel et al. (1980d).

on the means of this interaction revealed that significant neuronal discrimination in the deep laminae first occurred in FE and FS, prior to and simultaneously with the initial-most behavioral discrimination. However, significant neuronal discrimination in the superficial laminae first occurred during the critical session, when the behavioral discrimination was being performed at its maximum level. These results indicated that the deep cortical laminae manifested predominantly early-forming neuronal discrimination, whereas the superficial laminae manifested predominantly late-forming neuronal discrimination, during the course of behavioral discrimination learning.

An interesting relationship revealed by the group-based analysis was the similarity of the pattern of acquired neuronal discrimination shown

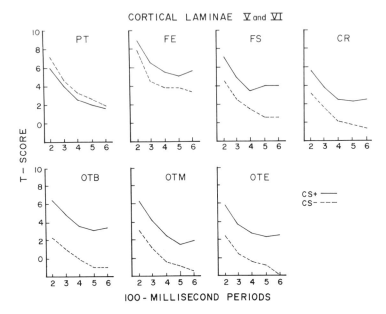

FIG. 11. Average neuronal response of the deep laminae (V and VI) of cingulate cortex during acquisition in five consecutive periods of 100 milliseconds following tone-onset. All labels are as defined in the legend to Fig. 5 and in Section II,C. Note that neuronal discrimination develops in the early stages of acquisition. Reprinted with permission from Foster *et al.* (1980).

by neurons in the superficial laminae of cingulate cortex and in the AV nucleus. Neither region showed neuronal discrimination until CR. In other words, both regions yielded the late-forming variety of neuronal discrimination.

The assumptions that we have tentatively adopted in thinking about these laminar differences are that neuronal discrimination forms in the deep (output) laminae of cingulate cortex in the early stages of discriminative behavioral acquisition. This early discrimination is conveyed to the AV nucleus via the corticothalamic pathway. After the discriminative input from cortex acts upon principal neurons of the AV nucleus for some time, the latter set of neurons form their own discriminative response, which is relayed immediately back to the superficial cortical laminae via the thalamocortical pathway.

Thus, we propose that there is a serial progression of discriminative neuronal activity from cingulate cortex to the AV nucleus during the course of behavioral discrimination learning. It is as though the activity of

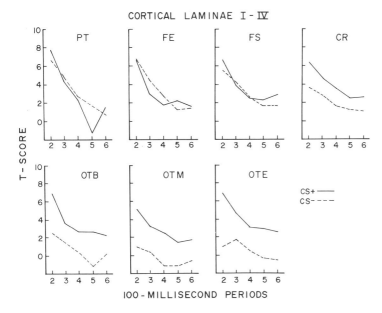

CORTICAL LAMINAE I - IV

100 - MILLISECOND PERIODS

FIG. 12. Average neuronal response of the superficial laminae (I–IV) of cingulate cortex during acquisition in five consecutive periods of 100 milliseconds following tone-onset. All labels are as defined in the legend to Fig. 5 and in Section II,C. Note that neuronal discrimination develops in the late stages of acquisition. Reprinted with permission from Foster *et al.* (1980).

the cortical projection neurons is involved in "teaching" the projection neurons of the AV nucleus how to discriminate between the CS+ and the CS−. Once neurons of the AV nucleus begin to manifest their own discrimination, the resultant discriminative activity in AV principal neurons is conveyed to the superficial cortical laminae via the thalamocortical axons. It may also be carried to other sites (e.g., presubiculum) which are regions of termination of AV thalamic neurons (Shipley and Sorensen, 1975).

The proposed serial flow of neuronal discrimination suggested by our findings is portrayed by the left-most (serial) model shown in Fig. 13. The figure also contains portrayals of a "parallel" model and an "independent" model, which represent other sets of assumptions logically compatible with the data. At present, we believe the serial model to represent the most plausible interpretation of the data because it is most appropriate to known cortical and thalamic neuroanatomical relationships.

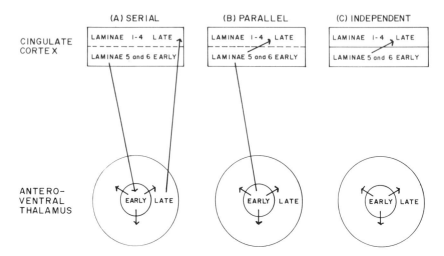

Fig. 13. Three models of cingulate cortical and AV thalamic interaction during discriminative conditioning are illustrated here. The left-most (serial) model involves the assumption that discriminative neuronal activity is relayed from the deep laminae of cingulate cortex to the AV nucleus, via the corticothalamic pathway (see Section II,B). The input from cortex is instrumental in bringing about late-forming (relegated) neuronal discrimination in principal neurons of the AV nucleus (see Section II,E). The discriminative activity is relayed immediately via the thalamocortical path back to the superficial laminae of cingulate cortex providing a signal which initiates disengagement of cortex from task processing. The middle (parallel) model and the right-hand (independent) model represent other logical alternatives for conceptualizing the neuronal data. The parallel model assumes that neuronal discrimination formed in the deep cingulate laminae acts to bring about relegated neuronal discrimination in the AV nucleus, as well as in the superficial cortical laminae. This model envisions no role for the thalamocortical path in production of late-forming discrimination in the superficial cortical laminae. The independent model envisions no instrumentality at all for the early cortical discrimination in bringing about discrimination in the AV nucleus.

## III. Functional Interpretation of Discriminative Neuronal Activity in Cingulate Cortex and in the AV Thalamus

A. Basic Functional Attribute of the Activity:
Neuronal Code for Stimulus Significance

In our experiments rabbits were trained to avoid footshock by performing a locomotory response to a CS+. They also learned nonresponse to a CS−. For such learning to have been manifested behaviorally, the CS+ and CS− must have acquired the ability to elicit unique forms of activity within the nervous system—activity which would reflect the unique significance of these two stimuli and which would serve as a causal precursor to the discriminative behavior. In other words, one of several component modifications that must have occurred within the animal to account for discriminative behavioral learning is the occurrence of precursive discriminative activity in some tissue substrate of the brain.

Our studies have indicated that discriminative neuronal activity comes to be manifested within the deep laminae of cingulate cortex, and later within the AV thalamic nucleus, during discriminative avoidance acquisition. Our fundamental assertion is that the discriminative neuronal activity in these structures is an acquired representation within the rabbits' CNS, of the differential significance of the conditional stimuli. In other words, the discriminative neuronal activity is an acquired neuronal code for stimulus significance. We hypothesize further that the neuronal code for significance operates in various CNS localities at which it may serve to initiate processes associated with the output of adaptive (e.g., avoidance) behavior. In the absence of such a code, the rabbit would have no means at its disposal for performance of selective, stimulus-cued, discriminative behavior.

## Corollary Attributes of the Acquired Neuronal Code for Stimulus Significance

*a. The Acquired Neuronal Code is a Truly Associative Change.* Behavior is said to have undergone associative modification when stimuli acquire control over it. Acquisition of stimulus control of behavior must be shown to have resulted from the occurrence of stimulus contingency, such as the pairing of a CS with a UCS in the Pavlovian conditioning paradigm.

It is not our intention here to attempt to spell out in detail considerations related to criteria and methods for establishing behavioral modifications as associative. Thorough discussion of these ideas is provided elsewhere (e.g., Kimble, 1961; Rescorla, 1967), but we do wish to emphasize here that the principles involved in producing and identifying associative behavior may be applied as well to any activity of an animal, including activity such as neuronal action potentials—activity not traditionally defined as behavior.

In addition, we wish to convey the idea that the discriminative neuronal activities of cingulate cortex and the AV nucleus represent associative activities of the animal. This assertion is based on the observation that the CS+ and the CS− came to evoke distinctive neuronal responses, after these stimuli were placed into contingency relationships (pairing and explicit unpairing, respectively) with the footshock UCS.

The contingency-specific associative character of the neuronal activity is the central empirical property underlying its designation as a neuronal code for stimulus significance. The prime function of the significance code is to reflect within the CNS the existence of an external signal foretelling the occurrence of an important event (footshock, in our studies), and requiring a behavioral response. Such a function could not be realized if the neuronal activity reflected only the physical properties of the stimuli, and not their associative significance.

*b. The Neuronal Code Is Acquired during the First Exposure to Conditioning.* Discriminative neuronal activity did not occur during pretraining but it did occur shortly after the initiation of training, during the session of first exposure (FE) to the CS–UCS contingencies. The discriminative effect in FE was present from 200 to 600 milliseconds for average data of the deep cingulate laminae (Fig. 12). This rapid acquisition of the significance code is in all likelihood of great adaptive value in that it rapidly endows the rabbit with the capacity to form unique internal representations of signals predicting danger, and thus to acquire rapidly the ability to respond to the danger adaptively in anticipatory fashion.

In discussing the rapidity with which the discriminative neuronal activity was acquired, it seems appropriate to mention that in addition to discriminative neuronal activity, there were two other rapidly acquired changes in neuronal activity that occurred during conditioning. One of these took the form of a significant enhancement of the tone-evoked neuronal response of cingulate cortex and of the AV nucleus in pretraining with shock, relative to pretraining without shock (Gabriel and Saltwick, 1977; Fig. 14). The enhanced response was evident almost immediately after onset of the pretraining session in which footshocks accompanied tone presentations, noncontingently. The enhancement in pretaining was nondifferential, occurring equally to the tone that would serve as CS +, and to the tone that would serve as CS −, in subsequent training sessions.

In addition to this generalized enhancement effect which resulted from adding noncontingent footshock to the tone presentations, there was a second enhancement of the tone-evoked neuronal response—an enhancement which occurred in the session of first exposure to conditioning, relative to the pretraining session with noncontingent footshock. That is, this additional enhancement effect was over and above that which occurred in the pretraining session. Moreover, the enhancement which occurred during the session of first exposure to conditioning was specific to the deep laminae of cingulate cortex. It did not occur in the superficial laminae, or in the AV nucleus (Fig. 12).

We would offer the hypothesis that the pretraining enhancement effect was the result of generalized arousal. In other words, the occurrence of footshock through the elicitation of a generalized arousal reaction potentiated the evoked neuronal response to any incoming phasic stimulus.

Because in the first exposure to conditioning in our studies auditory stimuli were paired with footshock, we think it likely that the further enhancement of neuronal response that occurred in the deep cingulate laminae during first exposure was an enhancement specific to the auditory modality. We are currently planning to carry out studies to attempt to evaluate these speculations. Thus, we expect that the addition of noncontingent footshock will potentiate the neuronal response to a visual stimulus as well as to auditory stimuli in cingulate cortex and in the AV nucleus. However, we do not expect to find an even greater enhancement of the neuronal response to the visual stimulus in the deep cingulate laminae during first exposure to conditioning. If these expectations are realized it would support our hypothesis that the pretraining enhancement is due to a completely nonspecific arousal evoked by the footshock. However, the further enhancement that occurs in first exposure would be interpreted by us as an effect specific to the modality of the stimulus paired with footshock during first exposure. As such, it would seem appropriate to regard the further, modality-specific enhancement effect as the very first reflection of acquired neuronal code for stimulus significance. Nevertheless, until the results of these studies are known, we wish to reserve the phrase "neuronal code for stimulus significance" as a denotation for the clearly *discriminative* neuronal activity.

*c. Training Specifies the Neuronal Code for Significance.* We have just seen that cingulate neurons showed an increase during FE, in the magnitude of their response to CS+ and CS−, relative to the response of the previous (pretraining) session. Nevertheless, as training continued, the cingulate neuronal response showed acquisition of discrimination between CS+ and CS−. This discrimination took the form of a progressive dropping-out of the neuronal response to the CS−, with maintenance of the response to the CS+ that was acquired during FE. Viewed within the context of the idea that the neuronal activity is a code for stimulus significance, these observations suggest that

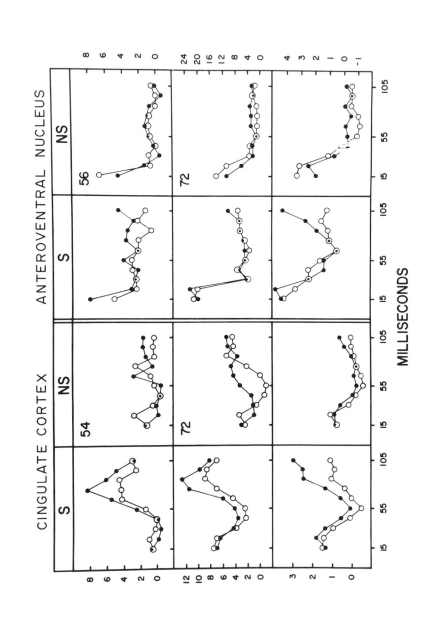

whereas the code is initially rather generalized, it acquires specificity with training, and eventually it is evokable only by stimuli which truly predict aversive consequences. The functional value of such specification of significance code is conservation of the metabolically costly flight and/or fight response as well as utilization of discrete environmental information for the precise timing of well-directed adaptive behavior.

*d. Relegation of the Neuronal Code for Significance.* The acquisition of discriminative activity by neurons in the deep laminae of cingulate cortex is the empirical phenomenon that we have proposed to be reflective of specification of significance code. Given that the cortical significance code has been specified, an additional process which we define as *relegation* takes place. That is to say, discriminative neuronal inputs conveyed to the AV nucleus via axons originating in the deep laminae of cingulate cortex are involved in the construction of changes in the AV nucleus. The changes are the cellular modifications which produce discriminative activity in AV neurons. The relegation process is depicted by the descending arrow of the serial model in Fig. 13.

Given that neurons of the AV nucleus are able to manifest the significance code, then this function need not be carried on further by cingulate neurons. Cingulate neurons are free to build other rapid discriminations, should the need arise. Thus, one facet of the adaptive role of the relegation process may concern the release or freeing of deep cingulate cortex from participation in the mediation of the significance code. A different term applicable to contexts similar to the present one is the concept of automatization, which has been used to characterize the relatively automatic and stereotyped properties of well-practiced as opposed to newly formed behavioral and linguistic adaptations (see Schiffrin and Schneider, 1977). It would be consistent with the present account to assert that the late-forming neuronal discriminations observed in the AV nucleus represent an automatization of the significance coding process.

The idea that relegation permits the disengagement of deep cingulate cortical involvement in production of the code for stimulus significance

FIG. 14. Magnitude of the neuronal response of the cingulate cortex (left half of figure) and of the anteroventral nucleus of the thalamus (AV, right half of the figure) is plotted for the first (●) and the second (○) session-halves. The ordinates are in $z$-units, and the scale of the abscissa is in units of consecutive 10-millisecond bins, begining at 10 milliseconds after tone-onset. The upper two rows of the figure show the data of two individuals (54 and 72) for cingulate and two (56 and 72) for the AV nucleus. The lower most row shows averaged results obtained by pooling the data of all individuals. Reprinted with permission from Gabriel and Saltwick (1977).

implies that there will be a lessening with extended training of discriminative activity in the deep laminae. Our group-based statistical analyses did not show such lessening in the deep laminae. Rather, the discriminative response of the deep laminae achieved its maximum magnitude in CR, and it remained at that magnitude throughout over-training (Figs. 4 and 5). Nevertheless, a considerable number of neuronal records obtained from the deep laminae manifested a decline over stages of training in the magnitude of the discriminative effect (examples are provided in Fig. 8). We offer the suggestion that the fading pattern of discrimination seen in these records represents cortical disengagement from significance coding, which occurs in conjunction with relegation of coding to neurons of the AV nucleus.

We would suggest that the absence of decline in discriminative activity that characterized the group-based data may have reflected the mixed character of many of the deep cortical records—records which contained both early and late discriminating elements. In other words, for these records early fading discrimination is presumed to have occurred in one subset of neurons, but the fading discrimination of this subset was replaced by the late discrimination of a different subset of neurons, present at the tip of the electrode. This view is compatible with the finding that several of the records showed a bimodal pattern of discrimination, characterized by an early discriminative response which faded quickly, only to be supplanted by a second discriminative effect, developing at a later stage of the task. Also, certain of the early discriminating records showed a substantial added increment of neuronal discrimination in the late stages of training (see Fig. 8, R 72-5).

It should be noted that the discriminative activity observed in the deep cortical laminae was of a rather generalized variety. That is, both CS+ and CS− evoked similar excitatory neuronal responses at the outset of training and progress in acquisition was reflected by a gradual drop in the response to the CS−. In the contrast, the advent of relegated discriminative activity in the AV nucleus was characterized by a dramatic step-up in neuronal excitation to the CS+, with no change in response to the CS− (Fig. 7). These results suggest that the relegated response in the AV nucleus may reflect an improvement in the precision of the significance code, relative to the coding process carried out in cingulate cortex. Viewed in this way, it may not be unreasonable to propose that the AV nucleus represents a locus of complex or hypercomplex feature extraction. However, in contrast to the idea of feature extraction that has frequently been applied to functioning of sensory systems— usages which have stressed the built-in nature of information extraction mechanisms—here we refer to extraction of features that have acquired significance through associative learning. We would propose that the term *significance extraction* be used in making reference to this aspect of the relegated code.

It has been proposed that training in a discrimination problem involves eventual "switching-in of stimulus analyzers" for the behaviorally relevant stimulus dimension (see the formulation of Sutherland and Mackintosh, 1971, chap. 10; Mackintosh, 1974). Tonal frequency would be the relevant dimension in our own task. When appropriate analyzers have been switched in, it is argued, then the subject is said to be focused upon or attentive to the relevant dimension. We would offer the suggestion that the late development of relegated code in thalamus, as observed in our studies, may represent such switching-in.

We would point out that the advent of late relegated code in the AV nucleus occurred during the criterial session of training—a session in which the first ample behavioral discrimination took place. The correspondence of ample discriminative neuronal activity and ample behavioral discrimination suggests that the relegated code may represent a neuronal process that is essential for performance of ample behavioral discrimination.

Finally it is reasonable to consider a possible role of relegated code of the AV nucleus in long-term retention of the behavioral discrimination. We have seen that associative modification of neurons in cingulate cortex occurs very quickly following the initiation of training procedures, whereas considerable exposure to training is necessary for associative modification of neuronal activity of the AV nucleus. It is reasonable to infer from this observation that the very rapid associative modifications of cingulate cortex would be highly susceptible to disruption and interference due to brief exposures of this substrate to the occurrence of new and conflicting stimulus contingencies. On the other hand, the AV nucleus would appear to have *temporal isolation* from the influence of briefly acting contingencies. One would not expect such contingencies to interfere with the code already established in the AV nucleus, since the AV nucleus seems to require relatively enduring input as a prerequisite to the development of a significance code. The essential point here is that short-term exposure to new stimulus contingencies should weaken or disrupt the cortical significance code but such exposure should leave intact the code acquired at the level of the AV nucleus. Thus, the significance code acquired in the AV nucleus should have considerable persistence, even in the absence of continuing task involvement. Ultimately, these considerations suggest that relegation of the significance code to neurons of the AV nucleus may be an important component process in the formation of long-term memory for the significance of environmental signals, and for long-term behavioral retention. This suggestion is consistent with results obtained from studies of the effects of AV thalamic damage on human and animal memorial performance (Angelergues, 1969; Sweet *et al.*, 1959; Rich and Thompson, 1965).

One proposed aspect of the functional relevance of relegation is the freeing of the cortical system from continuing involvement in production of the neuronal code, given completion of acquisition and code specification. It is necessary now to address the functional relevance of the late neuronal discriminations that occur in the superficial laminae of cingulate cortex—discriminations which we have attributed to inputs to the cingulate, conveyed by thalamocortical axons originating from principal neurons of the AV nucleus.

We would offer the tentative hypothesis that the discriminative activity which is relayed from the AV nucleus back to cingulate cortex may represent a feedback signal informing the cortical elements as to the discriminative status of the AV nucleus. This feedback signal may allow the cortex to "know" when the AV nucleus has finally formed its own discrimination. Thus, it provides information which allows the cortex to initiate disengagement from the significance coding process. Stated another way, the feedback signal may serve to inhibit the population of cortical elements which had participated in the early formation of the significance code. We are now attempting to test this assumption experimentally. Destruction of the AV nucleus is expected to abolish the early fading and the late categories of cortical neuronal discrimination. Thus, the only kind of discrimination that should occur in lesioned subjects is early persistent neuronal discrimination.

B. Relevance of the Code for
   Significance to Acquisition and Performance
   of Avoidance Behavior

*Interpretation of Results from Studies of the Effects
of Damage Induced in Cingulate Cortex
and in the AV Nucleus*

We have argued that discriminative neuronal activity acquired within the cingulate cortex and the AV nucleus is a code for stimulus significance. This proposition involves two fundamental subassertions about the relevance of the discriminative activity to acquisition and performance of avoidance behavior.

The first subassertion is that the significance code is a representation in the nervous system of the differential significance of the conditional stimuli. Thus, the code is not directly tied to the output of the behavioral avoidance response. Rather, the significance code may be present in certain circumstances, without the occurrence of behavioral avoidance. We have referred previously to observations illustrating this point [e.g., the persistence of stimulus-specific discriminative neuronal activity in cingulate cortex through a series of extinction trials in which the avoidance response ceases to occur (see Section II,A)].

The second subassertion implicit in the idea of a code for significance is that such a code represents an internal neuronal message indicating the external presence of critical stimuli (e.g., the CS + ). Thus, the code for significance is assumed to be critical for the subject's ability to predicate its avoidance performance upon the occurrence of a discrete, phasically presented external cue.

Our own studies support this subassertion by showing a correspondence of acquisition of the discriminative behavioral response, by acquisition of discriminative neuronal activity. In addition, support is forthcoming from a substantial body of experimental literature involving studies of avoidance acquisition and performance in animals with induced lesions of cingulate cortex and the AV nucleus. In the following text we shall describe the major outcomes of these studies—outcomes which seem to us to be compatible with the assertions made here on the functional relevance of the code for significance.

a. *Lesions of Cingulate Cortex.* There exist a substantial number of studies reporting impaired acquisition of discrete trial, cued, aversively motivated behavior in animals (cats, dogs, rats) with lesions in cingulate cortex (McCleary, 1961; Thomas and Otis, 1958; Thomas and Slotnick, 1962; Lubar and Perachio, 1965; Kimble and Gostnell, 1968; Trafton, 1967; Trafton *et al.*, 1969; Ursin *et al.*, 1969; Eckersdorf, 1974). Data from these studies are fundamentally compatible with the idea that the significance code acquired in cingulate cortex is critical for behavioral acquisition. Nevertheless, it is surprising to observe that none of the authors who have studied the effects of cingulate cortical damage on avoidance acquisition has attributed an associative role to this structure. Rather, the deficit in acquisition produced by cingulate cortical damage has been attributed to abnormality in one of two general nonassociative functions thought to be mediated by cingulate cortex in the normal subject.

One of these functions is emotionality. Thus, it has been suggested that subjects with cingulate lesions have difficulty in acquiring avoidance responses because they are deficient in the production of *fear*. Alternatively, it has been suggested that damaged subjects have *too much fear* (Lubar and Perachio, 1965). Yet another possibility that has been offered is that damaged subjects suffer an instrumental reinforcement deficit. They are unable to experience *relief* following successful instrumental performance (Coover *et al.*, 1974).

The second major category of general nonassociative deficit has been response modulation. In this instance, authors have attributed the deficit produced by cingulate cortical damage to factors such as excessive freezing (Thomas and Slotnick, 1962), absence of normal response facilitation (McCleary, 1966), and to a failure of mechanisms responsible for temporal integration of response sequences (Thomas *et al.*, 1968).

In reviewing the literature that gave rise to these hypotheses about the cingulate cortical deficit, it seemed to us that no single hypothesis is sufficient to account for the major findings. For example, attribution of the behavioral deficit to lessened emotionality, or fear, is contraindicated by findings demonstrating that lesioned subjects are able to acquire passive avoidance as readily as controls (McCleary, 1961; Lubar, 1964). Without added assumptions the lessened emotionality hypothesis would seem constrained to the expectation of deficient passive, as well as active avoidance learning. In addition, the idea that damage to cingulate cortex reduces emotionality is not consistent with findings indicating increases in indices of emotionality (excretion, vocalization) to be associated with such lesions (Lubar and Perachio, 1965).

The latter results raise the possibility that the avoidance deficit is produced by hyperfearfulness, and that intact cingulate cortex is a substrate of the inhibition of fearfulness. This is the hypothesis which was in fact invoked by Lubar and Perachio (1965) to account for the enhanced emotionality observed in their study, as well as the finding that only the acquisition in a two-way active avoidance task was impaired after cingulate lesions. Subjects in their study did not show a significant impairment in acquisition of one-way active avoidance. To incorporate this latter outcome with the enhanced fear hypothesis, Lubar and Perachio argued that the lesioned subjects were too fearful to reenter a compartment in which they had recently been shocked. It was assumed that they adopted a "freezing" strategy, instead. (Note that an advantage of the enhanced fear hypothesis is its compatibility with the normal passive avoidance learning shown by lesioned subjects, a finding which created problems for the lessened emotionality hypothesis.) It is also necessary to point out that the findings of Lubar and Perachio indicating that lesioned subjects manifest normal one-way avoidance learning, militate against the various response modulation arguments. If what is impaired following damage to cingulate cortex is merely deficient response facilitation as argued by McCleary (1961), or if lesioned subjects possess an excessive tendency to freeze, then behavior in the one-way avoidance task should show the same degree of impairment as that characterizing behavior in the two-way avoidance task.

Yet another observation argues against the response modulation hypotheses. It is the important demonstrations by Trafton and his colleagues (Trafton, 1967; Trafton *et al.*, 1969) that hungry rats with lesions in cingulate cortex were severely deficient in the acquisition of a conditioned emotional response (CER). If the animals in these experiments had been afflicted by excessive freezing behavior, or by deficient behavioral facilitation, they should have performed well in CER acquisition since the latter is a task which requires the withholding of behavioral responsiveness.

The results of Trafton in relation to performance of the CER also raise difficulties for the enhanced fear hypothesis of Lubar and Perachio (1965). It is difficult to see why subjects already primed by a cortical lesion to manifest fearfulness would fail to show a disruption of ongoing activity in response to the fear-inducing CS in this study.

The nonassociative accounts assert uniformly that lesioned subjects are afflicted with a generalized impairment in performance, not in learning capacity. As such, the impairments should be independent of the stage of training in which the lesion is made, and they should appear during tests of posttraining performance of the learned behavior. Contrary to this expectation, several studies have shown that rats and cats have little difficulty in reacquiring a cued active avoidance habit when cingulate lesions are induced during the retention interval (Moore, 1964; Slotnick, 1971; Eckersdorf, 1974). One of these studies (Eckersdorf, 1974) is especially noteworthy because it contrasted the behavior of cats lesioned during the retention interval with that of cats lesioned prior to acquisition. The results showed virtually normal savings in the attainment of criterion on the preoperatively acquired habit in cats lesioned after acquisition. However, the cats lesioned before acquisition "could not achieve criterion, remaining until the end of the experiment at a low level of reactivity" (Eckersdorf, 1974, p. 105).

Our conclusion is that no single nonassociative hypothesis provides an adequate interpretation of the full configuration of effects produced by cingulate cortical lesions. It is our suggestion that the difficulty with these hypotheses is that each omits inclusion of a fundamental associative process in defining the functional role of cingulate cortex. Let us examine now what may be achieved in attempting to interpret the results of the lesion experiments in light of the hypothesis which states that cingulate cortex mediates associative acquisition of the neuronal code for stimulus significance.

The electrophysiological data indicated that the neuronal activity in the deep laminae of cingulate cortex was associatively altered during conditioning so that a greater neuronal response occurred to the CS+, than to the CS−. The altered responsiveness was assumed to represent a neuronal code for stimulus significance, presumed to provide a basis for coordination of the avoidance response with occurrence of the CS+. In other words, our account views cingulate cortex as a substrate which mediates precise coordination of avoidance with specific, phasically presented cues.

Recall that lesions of cingulate cortex disrupt acquisition of avoidance in the two-way shuttle box apparatus, and acquisition of the CER. However, lesions do not interfere with acquisition of one-way active avoidance, nor do they affect acquisition of passive avoidance. It is the specificity of the disruption to the two-way shuttle and CER tasks which requires explanation.

By our account, the disruption of two-way avoidance and the CER would be linked to the fact that of all of the conditioning tasks under consideration, the two-way avoidance task and the CER task are the only ones in which the subject must use a discrete, unimodal, phasically presented CS as a cue for the behavioral response. In the other tasks (one-way avoidance and passive avoidance), it is likely that the stimuli which control the conditioned response are the redundant tonically acting contextual cues of the learning situation.

Our account states that the cue-specific discriminative neuronal activity that is rapidly acquired within cingulate cortex during avoidance acquisition is an important precursor of the rabbit's selective behavioral response to the CS+. Thus, we would propose that it is this discriminative function which is impaired in the lesioned subjects. When the task is such that behavior may be predicated on a multiplicity of redundant, tonically acting cues, then no advantage is conferred by intact cingulate cortex. Its discriminative function would not be expected to contribute importantly to behavioral acquisition in the latter variety of task.

We have seen that damage to cingulate cortex severely impairs acquisition of two-way active avoidance behavior, but lesions administered after acquisition do not greatly impair reacquisition of the behavior. The nonassociative hypotheses reviewed previously in this essay are without added assumptions unable to account for failure of cingulate cortical lesions to impair reacquisition. However, this finding is encompassed by our account in terms of the relegation process (see Section III,A,d). Thus, we view the cingulate cortical substrate as primarily involved in acquisition and specification of the code for significance (Section III,A, b). By the process of relegation the AV nucleus assumes the mediation of the significance code subservient to postacquisitional performance and retention of the behavioral discrimination. Thus, by our account damage to cingulate cortex induced after behavioral acquisition is well underway and does not affect retention because processes critical for retention are mediated by the AV nucleus.

   *b. Lesions of the AV Nucleus.* Unfortunately, few studies have examined the role of the AV nucleus in mediation of cued active avoidance behavior. Nevertheless, the work that has been carried out on this issue has supported the idea of a critical involvement of this structure in postacquisitional performance and retention of avoidance. Specifically, Rich and Thompson (1965) reported that rats with damage to the AV nucleus and adjacent areas of the thalamus showed severe impairment in performance of active avoidance behavior (a jump and wall-cling response to a light CS) which they had acquired prior to the lesion. In addition, involvement of the AV nucleus in mediation of retentive and memorial phenomena in humans is suggested by studies of human brain pathology, indicating that damage to the AV nucleus and neuro-anatomically related structures (e.g., mammillary bodies) is associated with phenomena of amnesia (see Section I). Thus, findings obtained from the literature on humans and animals are compatible with the retentive, memorial interpretation of the function of the AV nucleus. It may be that human patients with damage to these structures lack the ability to generate cue-specific significance codes which have become associatively linked to contents constituting the output of the memory system. In general, results from studies of the effects of brain damage on learning and performance are compatible with our view implicating cingulate cortex and the AV nucleus, respectively, in production of covert associative processes essential for acquisition and maintenance of learned behavior. We would point out that all of the evidence reviewed supporting an associative role for these limbic structures is at odds with the evolutionary divergence hypothesis.

## C. The Cingulate–AV Thalamic System May Not Be the Only System for Encoding of Stimulus Significance

   In setting forth our ideas on the behavioral relevance of activity in cingulate cortex and the AV nucleus we do not want to overstate our case by implying that the code for significance which develops in these structures constitutes a necessary condition for the acquisition of discriminative behavior. Several circumstances indicate that it would be inappropriate to adopt such a strong position. One of these is simply the existence of a considerable expanse of limbic cortical tissue in the anterior one-third of the hemispheric medial wall which on preliminary evidence from our laboratory seems to display electrophysiological response properties similar in certain ways to those reported here for the more posteriorly situated cingulate cortex. In addition, this anterior limbic cortical tissue would appear to have reciprocal neuroanatomical interconnection with the mediodorsal (MD) nucleus of the thalamus (e.g., Krettek and Price, 1977; Siegel *et al.*, 1977). Moreover, the MD nucleus has shown, like the AV nucleus, the late variety of neuronal discrimination in the small number of cases that we have examined to date. In other words, there exist two major areas of limbic cortex, one area (prefrontal cortex) comprising the anterior medial walls of the cerebral hemispheres, and the second area (cingulate cortex) comprising the posterior medial walls. Each of these communicates reciprocally with its own medially situated "nonspecific" thalamic nucleus. Because of their structural similarity, it seems reasonable to assume that these two thalamocortical configurations may have similar or related behavioral relevance. Moreover, each may provide a sufficient substrate for mediation of significance code in the behavioral task employed in our studies.

Of pertinance here is the recent study of Mishkin indicating that combined but not separate removal of hippocampal formation and amygdala yields severe memory impairment in monkeys (*Macaca mulatta*) (Mishkin, 1978). In interpreting these findings, Mishkin suggested that the amygdala is a component of one neuroanatomical subsystem and that the hippocampus is a component of a distinct subsystem. Each of these subsystems, he argued, may contribute a share of memory-related neural processing and joint action of both subsystems is critical for normal memorial functioning of the intact subject. It would be our suggestion that the two limbic corticothalamic configurations that we have just discussed may represent, respectively, the corticothalamic components of Mishkin's two subsystems. This possibility is suggested by the substantial afferents which reach the AV nucleus from hippocampus via the internal capsule (e.g., Meibach and Siegel, 1977a) and postcommissural fornix (e.g., Shipley and Sorensen, 1975; Poletti and Creswell, 1977; Sikes *et al.*, 1977; Nauta, 1956; Raisman *et al.*, 1965; Guillery, 1956), as well as major afferents which course to the MD nucleus from the amygdala in the rat (Siegel *et al.*, 1977).

In addition to the possibility that two limbic subsystems may participate jointly in mediating coding of significance one must recognize the further possibility that areas of cortex beyond the limbic medial wall also participate in the significance-coding process. This is suggested by findings indicating that neodecortication of rabbits (sparing prefrontal and cingulate cortices) nevertheless retarded the acquisition of classically conditioned discriminative eyeblink responses (Oakley and Russell, 1973, 1974a,b). The retardation was not pronounced, suggesting that participation of neocortex may have been tangential in this learning situation. In any case, findings suggesting a role in discriminative learning for cortical and thalamic areas other than cingulate cortex and the AV nucleus raise the possibility that *acquisition, specification, and relegation* of significance code may constitute a very general set of associative functions characterizing the entire corticothalamic axis of the mammalian brain.

D. BEHAVIORAL RELEVANCE OF CINGULATE CORTEX
   AND THE AV THALAMUS: EVIDENCE
   FROM REVERSAL TRAINING

Information of value in understanding the behavioral role of discriminative neuronal activity in cingulate cortex and in the AV nucleus is provided by the data obtained in our laboratory during reversal training.

One might easily suppose that reversal would be a replay of acquisition. Under this view neurons of the deep laminae of cingulate cortex would be expected to acquire a new neuronal discrimination (one appropriate to the reversal problem) in the early stages of reversal training. Later in reversal a neuronal discrimination should appear in the AV nucleus.

What actually happens is indicated in Figs. 15, 16, 17, and 18, which show the data collected from the cingulate cortex, in the form of average $z$-scores and average $T$-scores to CS+ and CS− in four stages of reversal training. Data of the deep laminae of cingulate cortex are shown separately from the data of the superficial laminae. The primary finding here is the absence of neuronal reversal in cingulate cortex in any stage of reversal training. Instead, neurons of the deep cingulate cortex manifested the original discrimination in the first session of reversal training. In other words, the CS+ of original training evoked a greater neuronal response than the original CS− in this session. In subsequent sessions there was a falling away of the original neuronal discrimination, but there were no signs of neuronal reversal (i.e., a significantly greater response to the CS+ relative to CS− in reversal training) at any stage of behavioral reversal.

Inspection of Figs. 15 through 18 reveals that the neuronal retention of the original habit was present in both deep and superficial laminae of

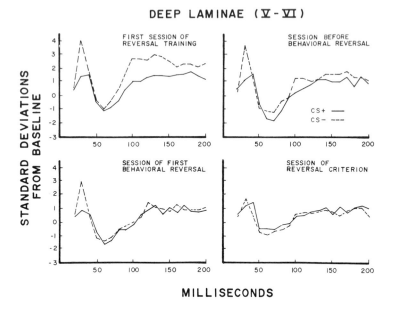

FIG. 15. Average neuronal response in the deep laminae of cingulate cortex in the form of z-scores to CS+ and CS− for the initial 19 10-millisecond bins following tone-onset, in four stages of reversal training. The stages are first session of reversal (R1), session before the first significant behavioral reversal (BR), session of first significant behavioral reversal (FR), and session in which reversal criterion was met (RC). Ordinate and abscissa values are as described in the legend to Fig. 4. Reprinted with permission from Gabriel *et al.* (1980b).

cingulate cortex, during the first session of reversal training. Thus, in both neuroanatomical loci, the z-scores representing the neuronal response to the origical CS+ exceeded significantly the scores representing the response to the original CS−, in several bins. Nevertheless, the original habit effect was more pronounced in the deep cortical laminae than in the superficial laminae. Only five bin-differences were significant in the superficial laminae whereas eight were significant in the deep laminae. Also, the deep laminae showed significant original habit reten- tion at a short-latency (20–30 milliseconds) bin. This effect persisted through reversal training to the day of first significant behavioral rever- sal. Although the effect was also present in the superficial laminae in the first session of reversal training, it did not persist beyond the first ses- sion, in those laminae. Finally, there were only marginal signs of original habit retention in the superficial laminae during R1 when the neuronal

# DEEP LAMINAE ($\underline{V}-\underline{VI}$)

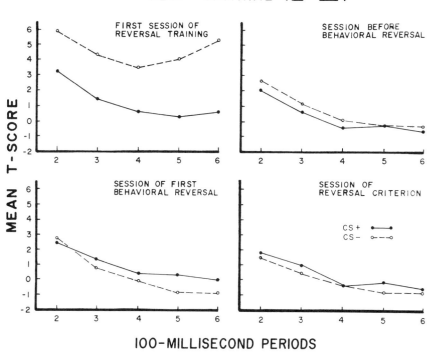

IOO-MILLISECOND PERIODS

Fig. 16. Average neuronal response of the deep laminae of cingulate cortex to CS+ and CS− for five consecutive periods of 100 milliseconds, in four stages of reversal training. The stages of reversal are defined in the caption of Fig. 15. The ordinate and abscissa values are as described in the legend to Fig. 5. Reprinted with permission from Gabriel *et al.* (1980b).

responses at the long latencies (100–600 milliseconds) were considered. However, the deep laminae manifested highly significant original habit retention in the first session of reversal training, at all latencies for which analysis was done.

To summarize, neurons of cingulate cortex manifested disrciminative neuronal activity appropriate to original acquisition, but they did not show discriminative activity appropriate to the reversal task. Instead, retention of the original discrimination was manifested during the first session of reversal training. This effect was greater in the deep laminae than in the superficial ones.

In stages of reversal training beyond the first session, retention of the original discrimination was not observed at any but the shortest latency

## SUPERFICIAL LAMINAE ( I - Ⅳ )

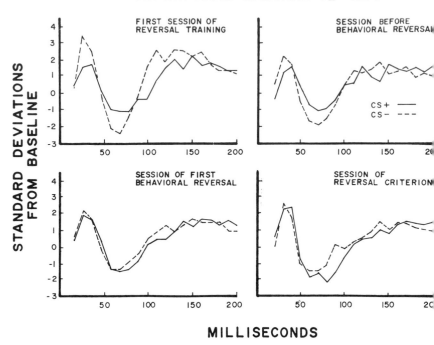

## MILLISECONDS

Fig. 17. Average neuronal response in the superficial laminae of cingulate cortex in the form of z-scores, to CS+ and CS− for the initial 19 10-millisecond bins following tone-onset, in four stages of reversal training. The stages of reversal are defined in the legend to Fig. 15. Ordinate and abscissa values are as described in the legend to Fig. 4. Reprinted with permission from Gabriel *et al.* (1980b).

of the evoked neuronal response and only in the deep laminae of cingulate cortex. However, the short-latency deep evoked response showed the retention effect throughout reversal training until and including the session of first significant behavioral reversal.

Recall that the predominant outcome obtained from the AV nucleus during original acquisition was a late-forming neuronal discrimination—an outcome also obtained from the superficial laminae of cingulate cortex. The question is what pattern of results was displayed by the AV nucleus during reversal training?

Data pertaining to this question are portrayed in Figs. 19 and 20, which show, respectively, the average results for the short- and long-latency neuronal responses of the AV nucleus in the four stages of reversal training. The results were clear. Significant neuronal discrimination appropriate to the reversal task occurred in the short-latency data and in

## SUPERFICIAL LAMINAE (I-Ⅳ)

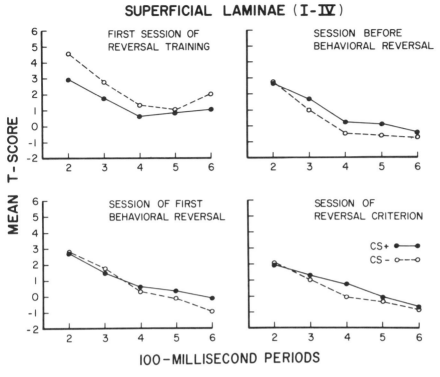

100-MILLISECOND PERIODS

FIG. 18. Average neuronal response of the superficial laminae of cingulate cortex to CS+ and CS− for five consecutive periods of 100 milliseconds, in four stages of reversal training. The stages of reversal are defined in the legend to Fig. 15. The ordinate and abscissa values are as described in the legend to Fig. 5. Reprinted with permission from Gabriel *et al.* (1980b).

the long-latency data during the day of the first significant behavioral reversal, and during the session in which the criterion of reversal was attained. Thus, unlike cingulate cortex, the neuronal discrimination formed in the AV nucleus during original acquisition underwent reversal. Furthermore, the relationship between neuronal discrimination in the AV nucleus, and behavioral discrimination, was unlike that displayed during acquisition. Whereas neuronal discrimination during acquisition formed after the session of first significant behavioral discrimination, neuronal reversal first occurred on the day of first significant behavioral reversal—simultaneously with the onset of behavioral reversal.

To recapitulate briefly, we have found that discriminative activity of cingulate cortex occurs shortly after the onset of training and is followed

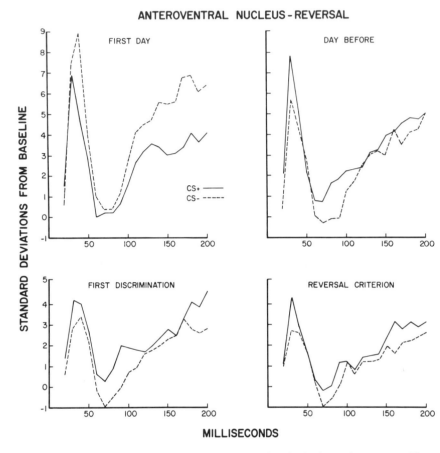

FIG. 19. Average neuronal response in the AV nucleus in the form of $z$-scores to CS+ and CS− for the initial 19 10-millisecond bins following tone-onset, in four stages of reversal training. The stages of reversal are defined in the legend to Fig. 15. Ordinate and abscissa values are as described in the legend to Fig. 4. Reprinted with permission from Gabriel *et al.* (1980b).

by discriminative activity in the AV nucleus, which first occurs after the task is well-learned. However, only the AV nucleus, not cingulate cortex, manifested discriminative activity appropriate to the reversal task. The only discriminative activity to occur in cortex during reversal training was that appropriate to original acquisition.

These results indicate that the processes which occurred within the cingulate cortex–AV nucleus system during reversal training were not a straightforward recapitulation of the acquisition processes. Neurons in

## ANTEROVENTRAL NUCLEUS - REVERSAL

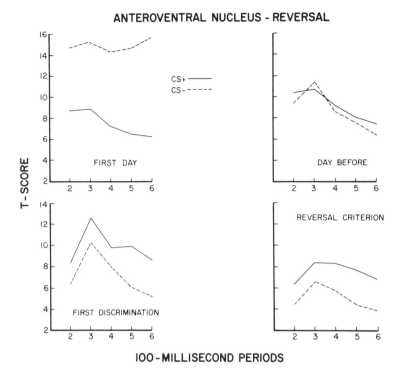

FIG. 20. Average neuronal response of the AV nucleus to CS+ and CS− for five consecutive periods of 100 milliseconds, in four stages of reversal training. The stages of reversal are defined in the legend to Fig. 15. The ordinate and abscissa values are as described in the legend to Fig. 5. Reprinted with permission from Gabriel et al. (1980b).

cingulate cortex and in the AV nucleus participated jointly in acquisition and in relegation of the code for stimulus significance. However, only neurons in the AV nucleus manifested reversal of the code. Evidently, the processing of coded signals remains in the domain of the AV nucleus, once relegation of coding to that region has taken place.

The findings indicating that the cingulate cortex shows a persistent retention of the original discrimination throughout the precriterial stages of reversal training suggest that cingulate cortical neuronal influences may not merely be withheld from participation in the reversal process. The cortical influences may in fact conflict with the reversal process, and thus retard its development. This conclusion receives support from studies of reversal in decorticate rabbits (e.g., Oakley and Russell, 1973) which indicate that the presence of neocortex is associated with retarded reversal learning, relative to reversal learning in subjects that underwent neodecortication during the period between original acquisition and reversal.[6]

Generally, the absence of direct one-to-one correspondence between discriminative behavioral responding and discriminative neuronal activity reinforces the contention stated previously in Section II,A that the neuronal activity is not *directly* tied either as cause or as effect to the behavioral response measured in our studies. This general finding is compatible with our view that the function in learned avoidance behavior of the cingulate cortex and of the AV nucleus involves primarily the processing of significant task-related stimuli, rather than direct control of behavioral output.

E. BEHAVIORAL RELEVANCE OF NEURONAL ACTIVITY
   IN CINGULATE CORTEX AND IN THE AV
   THALAMUS: EVIDENCE OBTAINED FROM
   MANIPULATION OF THE AMOUNT OF OVERTRAINING
   IN THE ORIGINAL DISCRIMINATION

Animals trained to a criterion of discrimination are retarded in the attainment of discrimination reversal, compared with animals given overtraining. In other words, training beyond criterion facilitates reversal (see reviews by Paul, 1965; Sperling, 1965; Lovejoy, 1965; Denny, 1970; Sutherland and Mackintosh, 1971; Mackintosh, 1974). This finding has come to be known as the overtraining reversal effect (ORE). Information pertaining to the issue of the behavioral relevance of the code for significance in cingulate cortex and in the AV nucleus is provided by consideration of the possible involvement of these processes in production of the ORE.

We manipulated the amount of overtraining for a subset of the rabbits in our studies of the neuronal correlates of discriminative avoidance learning. Specifically, a total of 36 rabbits were run under identical conditions of training except that 19 of them were begun in reversal in the session which followed completion of criterion, and 17 others were given either three or six sessions of acquisition training after criterion but prior to the initiation of reversal training. We refer here to sessions of training given after criterion as "overtraining." Since the amount of overtraining

[6]The fact that cingulate cortex was at l    t partially spared by the neodecortication procedures of these experiments provides fuɪ ɯer evidence beyond that cited previously (Section III,C) to indicate that noncingulate cortex plays a role similar to that of cingulate cortex in these behavioral situations.

(three or six sessions) did not produce significant effects on the data of reversal, we will confine our discussion to the two principal groups—the overtrained group and the nonovertrained group.

Figure 21 shows the mean number of sessi⌒ns required for the attainment of the criterion of behavioral reversal, for the overtrained rabbits, and for the nonovertrained rabbits. The difference was significant ($p <$ 0.05), indicating retarded behavioral reversal in the nonovertrained rabbits. Thus, the ORE was found to occur in our learning task.

Effects of the overtraining factor on neuronal activity in cingulate cortex are shown in Fig. 22. Here we see neuronal discrimination appropriate to original learning, in the initial, short-latency component of the cortical response. In the overtrained group, this original habit effect was present in the first session of reversal training, but it was absent from the day before first significant reversal, and from the day of first significant reversal. However, in nonovertrained subjects, the effect persisted throughout the day before and the day of significant behavioral reversal, as well as the day of reversal criterion. Analysis for cortical laminar differences showed that the persistent short-latency retention of the original neuronal discrimination took place entirely within the deep laminae of cingulate cortex. Retention of the original neuronal discrimination was manifested in the superficial laminae of the nonovertrained rabbits, in the first session of reversal training, but it did not appear in any of the subsequent stages of reversal. Persistent retention of

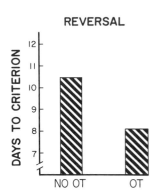

FIG. 21. Mean number of training sessions required to meet the criterion of reversal training in the nonovertrained (NO OT) rabbits ($N$ = 19) and in the overtrained (OT) rabbits ($N$ = 17).

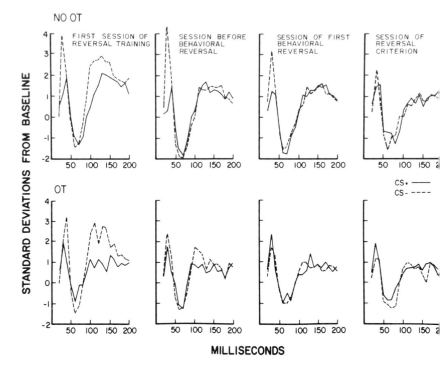

FIG. 22. Average neuronal response of cingulate cortex (all laminae) in the form of $z$-scores associated with CS + and CS −, for the initial 19 10-millisecond bins following tone-onset. Data are shown separately for overtrained (OT) and nonovertrained (NO OT) rabbits. The stages of reversal are defined in the legend to Fig. 15 and the ordinate and abscissa values are as described in the legend to Fig. 5. See Section III,E for a description of the effects of the overtraining manipulation on the neuronal response of the superficial and deep cortical laminae. Reprinted with permission from Orona *et al.* (1980).

the original neuronal discrimination did not occur within either deep or superficial laminae in the overtrained rabbits.

In addition to the more persistent neuronal discrimination appropriate to original learning in nonovertrained rabbits, there was a greater overall (nondiscriminative) cortical neuronal response in these subjects, relative to the overtrained subjects. In this instance, the effect of overtraining operated at both superficial and deep cortical laminae (Fig. 23).

The major idea that emerges in relation to the effects of overtraining is that the persistence of the original discrimination in neurons of the deep cortical laminae may have interfered with behavioral reversal. Also, the relatively high *overall* level of cingulate cortical neuronal reac-

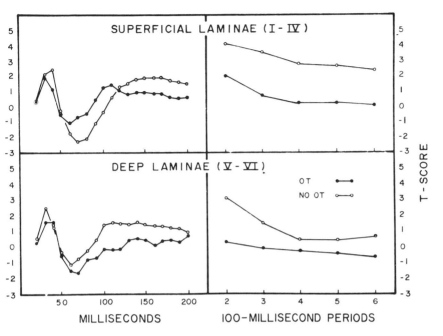

FIG. 23. Average neuronal response of nonovertrained (NO OT) subjects and over-trained (OT) subjects in superficial and deep cortical laminae, during reversal training. The data are collapsed over the four stages of reversal training. The left half of the figure presents the $z$-score results, and the right half presents the $T$-score results. Reprinted with permission from Orona *et al.* (1980).

tivity in nonovertrained rabbits during reversal training may have represented a relatively high weighting for the interfering cortical significance code. Thus, overtraining may facilitate reversal by lessening the normally interfering influence of significance code in cingulate cortex during reversal training.

This conclusion fits well with the data indicating that neodecortication of rabbits performed following original learning but prior to reversal training facilitated behavioral reversal (e.g., Oakley and Russell, 1973). It is interesting to note that the facilitation resulted primarily from a relative absence of response to the CS−, during reversal, in the neodecorticated rabbits. This feature of the behavioral data accords with our findings indicating a highly persistent short-latency cortical respon-siveness to the CS− during reversal, in our nonovertrained rabbits with cortices intact (Fig. 22).

## Overtraining and Neuronal Activity
## of the AV Nucleus

Recall that the AV nucleus was unlike cingulate cortex in that reversal of neuronal discrimination did occur in the AV nucleus. Unfortunately, the number of rabbits with electrodes in the AV nucleus was too small to permit demonstration of a behavioral ORE. Nevertheless, the results obtained from the AV nucleus were of interest.

The $z$-score data of the overtrained rabbits showed a large original habit effect in the first session of reversal training. Also, these data seemed to show reversal of neuronal discrimination in the session of first significant behavioral reversal, and in the criterial session (Fig. 24). The reversal effect did not appear to be as clear in the nonovertrained rabbits (Fig. 25) compared to the overtrained rabbits. It must be pointed out, however, that the interaction term of the analysis relevant to the inference that there was a difference in reversal between the overtrained and nonovertrained rabbits did not reach significance for $z$-scores or for $T$-scores. This may be attributed to the relatively small sample. Thus, it seems reasonable to suggest that with additional work, a more pro-

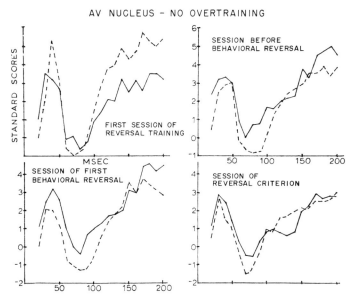

FIG. 24. Average neuronal response of the AV nucleus in four stages of reversal training for nonovertrained (NO OT) rabbits. The stages of reversal are as defined in Fig. 15 and the ordinate and abscissa values are as described in Fig. 5. Reprinted with permission from Orona et al. (1980).

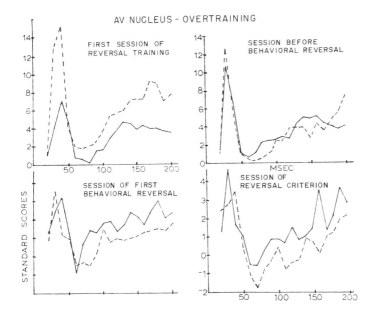

FIG. 25. Average neuronal response of the AV nucleus in four stages of reversal training, for overtrained (OT) rabbits. The stages of reversal are as defined in Fig. 15 and the ordinate and abscissa values are as described in Fig. 5. Reprinted with permission from Orona *et al.* (1980).

nounced reversal effect would be observed in the AV nucleus in overtrained as opposed to nonovertrained subjects.

An effect of overtraining which did attain statistical significance was the greater overall (nondiscriminative) short-latency neuronal response of neurons in the AV nucleus in overtrained rabbits, compared to the response of nonovertrained rabbits (Fig. 26). This effect is to be contrasted with the results obtained for cortical neurons, which showed greater overall reactivity in the nonovertrained as opposed to the overtrained group (Fig. 23). These results indicate that there is, with overtraining, a decreased reactivity of cingulate cortical neurons and an increased reactivity of neurons of the AV nucleus.

It is necessary to bear in mind that the inferences made here concerning the effects of overtraining on neuronal reactivity are derived from data obtained during reversal training. Thus, one should ask whether the inferred changes may be observed directly, during overtraining itself. Is there a decline over sessions of overtraining, in reactivity of cingulate cortical neurons, and is there an increase over sessions in the reactivity of neurons in the AV nucleus?

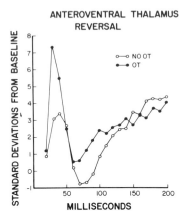

FIG. 26. Average neuronal response of the AV nucleus, in the form of $z$-scores, obtained during reversal training, for nonovertrained ($\bigcirc$) and overtrained ($\bullet$) rabbits. The data are collapsed over the four stages of reversal training. The ordinate and abscissa values are as defined in Fig. 5. This figure illustrates the greater overall reactivity during reversal training of AV nucleus neurons in overtrained as opposed to nonovertrained rabbits. Reprinted with permission from Orona *et al.* (1980).

We have already seen that a considerable number of electrode placements in cingulate cortex manifested acquisition followed by fading of the discriminative neuronal response, during the course of behavioral acquisition. It is possible that the reduced neuronal reactivity observed in cingulate cortex during reversal, following overtraining, is attributable to the greater opportunity for fading provided by overtraining. With greater opportunity for fading, one would expect a greater proportion of the neuronal records from overtrained rabbits to manifest low reactivity during reversal training relative to records of animals who experienced training to criterion only. This line of reasoning is supported by the observation that records classified by us as "faders" (see Section II,F,1) had significantly reduced overall response during reversal training, relative to records classified as "persisters." These results are in accord with the idea that cingulate cortical neurons which disengage from the significance coding process during acquisition remain disengaged during reversal training. By our account, such cortical neuronal disengagement results from inhibitory axonal feedback originating from neurons of the AV nucleus—neurons which have had their discriminative response relegated to them by cortical neurons of the deep laminae during prior stages of acquisition. All in all it seems reasonable to attribute the overtraining-related differences in cingulate cortical reactivity observed during reversal to overt changes in cortical reactivity that occurred during overtraining.

On the other hand we did not see changes during overtraining in reactivity of the AV nucleus—changes which could serve to account for the overtraining-related changes in reactivity of the AV nucleus observed in reversal. In other words, there was no evidence for progressively increasing neuronal reactivity in the AV nucleus during overtraining. This outcome suggests that the imputed changes remain latent during original training, and they become manifest only in situations such as reversal training, when processes of habit-revision are initiated.

## IV. Role of the Hippocampal Formation in the Encoding of Stimulus Significance

A. NEURONAL ACTIVITY OF THE
   HIPPOCAMPAL FORMATION

Reciprocal neuroanatomical pathways interconnect the cingulate cortex with structures of the hippocampal formation (e.g., Domesick, 1970; Meibach and Siegel, 1977b). Similarly, reciprocal pathways interconnect the hippocampal formation with the AV nucleus (Meibach and Seigel, 1977a; Lenn, 1978; Shipley and Sorensen, 1975; Sikes et al., 1977; Nauta, 1956; Raisman et al., 1965; Guillery, 1956). Given these neuroanatomical relationships, it would seem reasonable to assume that the hippocampal formation plays a role in acquisition, specification, and relegation of the code for stimulus significance.

Our initial studies have revealed a bursting pattern of neuronal spikes during trials of conditioning, within CA1 and the subicular region of the hippocampal formation (Gabriel and Saltwick, 1980). The number of spikes per burst ranged from five to thirty and the bursts occurred at a variable frequency ranging from 1 or 2 per second to as high as 10 per second. At the highest frequency the bursts were very "rhythmic," that is, a relatively constant interval of 100 milliseconds intervened between their onsets. The most striking observation was that the rhythmic high-frequency bursts consistently occurred just prior to the behavioral conditioned responses of the rabbits (see Fig. 27).

High-frequency bursts were seen at times when the rabbits did not respond behaviorally. An example is burst activity observed during pretraining to tones presented with randomly interspersed noncontingent footshocks (Fig. 28).

Also, bursts were sometimes seen in the initial seconds of tone presentations not followed by a behavioral response in the trained animals. The crucial point is, however, that despite occurrence of bursts unaccompanied by conditioned responses, *all instances* of conditioned responses were preceded by a series of high-frequency rhythmic bursts.

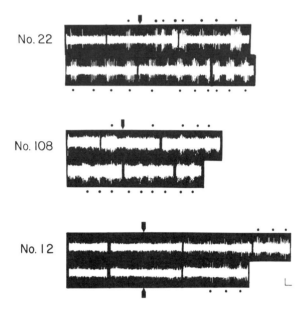

FIG. 27. Oscilloscope photographs of hippocampal multiple unit activity during the entire trials of conditioning are shown for three subjects. The onset of the CS is indicated by the pointers. A behavioral conditioned response occurred at the end of each trial. The horizontal calibration mark represents 50 milliseconds and the vertical mark represents 20 $\mu$V. A neuronal burst was defined as a cluster of at least three spikes. Dots were placed at each burst as an aid to visualization. Reprinted with permission from Gabriel and Saltwick (1980).

Other investigators have reported high-frequency (10–12 kHz) regular electroencephalographic (EEG) waves immediately preceding avoidance behavior of the rat (Vanderwolf *et al.*, 1973; Vanderwolf and Cooley, 1974; Whishaw and Nikkel, 1975). This EEG effect was recorded from the dorsal hippocampus, and was identified as the hippocampal "theta rhythm" (Greene and Arduini, 1954). Since the frequency of the neuronal bursts was very similar to the frequency of theta seen in these studies, and since both effects originated from similar regions of the hippocampal formation, it seemed reasonable to speculate that our hippocampal bursts may represent neuronal activity which is involved in the production of preavoidance theta.

Further evidence on this point is provided in Fig. 29, which shows a histogram produced by adding bursting spikes from consecutive trials of conditioning. The bursting spikes which contributed to Fig. 29 were those which just preceded the occurrence of the behavioral conditioned response averaged over a total of 32 trials. The histogram was produced

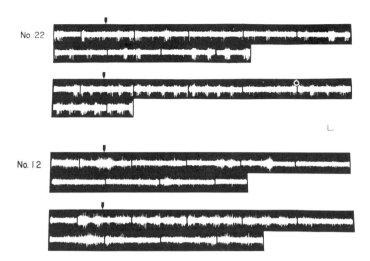

FIG. 28. Neuronal activity of the hippocampus to tones presented in pretraining is shown for two rabbits. Two tone presentations are shown for each rabbit. The pointers indicate tone-onset. The first series of tracings for each subject represents a tone which occurred just prior to a noncontingent shock, and at least three tones removed from the previous noncontingent shock. The second series of tracings for each subject represents the tone presentation which occurred just after the noncontingent shock. Calibration is given in the legend to Fig. 27.

by "averaging backward" from the response. The regular sinusoidal character of spike frequency is similar to the theta has been observed in several studies to precede avoidance responding (Vanderwolf *et al.,* 1973; Vanderwolf and Cooley, 1974; Whishaw and Nikkel, 1975). These observations support the idea that the neuronal bursts recorded from the CA1 and subicular region contribute to preavoidance theta.

There is currently considerable controversy surrounding the notion of the behavioral relevance of theta. Whereas certain investigators have maintained that theta is a phenomenon reflecting activities such as orienting, arousal, and other forms of information processing related to the assessment of external stimuli (e.g., Grastyan *et al.,* 1959; Bennett, 1975; Routtenberg, 1971), others have maintained that theta occurs in connection with a particular class of behaviors, termed "voluntary" (see Vanderwolf, 1971). The latter theory is supported by abundant evidence showing that theta occurs whenever rat subjects are engaged in behaviors such as walking, running, swimming, etc. (i.e., "voluntary behaviors"), but not in conjunction with motionlessness, or in conjunction with species typical behaviors such as grooming, eating, licking, or pelvic thrusting.

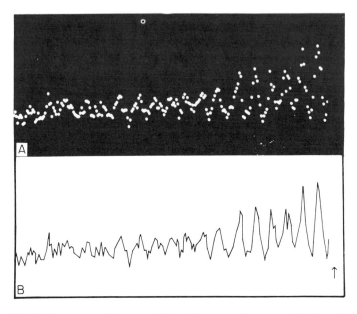

FIG. 29. (A) Preresponse histogram obtained by averaging neuronal spikes of the hippocampus that occurred just prior to the behavioral conditioned response in a trained subject. Thirty-two trials of conditioning were used to obtain the histogram. Each dot represents the frequency of spike in a 10-millisecond bin. The behavioral response occurrence is represented by the arrow at the left-most portion of the figure. Only large-amplitude spikes which showed the theta-like burst pattern contributed to the histogram. (B) The dots of (A) were connected to increase the visibility of the theta-like waveform of the spike histogram. Reprinted with permission from Gabriel and Saltwick (1980).

Data showing that theta consistently *precedes* the occurrence of learned avoidance responses is something of an embarrassment to this position, since presumably theta would not precede the behavioral activity (e.g., hurdle jumping, or wheel rotation) if that activity had never been subjected to the contingencies of the avoidance training situation. In fact, certain experiments have indicated specifically that in the rat, theta does *not* precede unconditioned wheel rotation (Whishaw and Vanderwolf, 1973) or initiation of other unconditional movements (Vanderwolf, 1975). The implication is that the theta effect which precedes conditioned avoidance behavior is acquired as a result of exposure to the conditioning situation.

To examine this issue, we carried out an analysis designed to detect change in theta-like neuronal activity as a function of stage of acquisition in our avoidance task (Gabriel and Saltwick, 1980).

The results of this analysis are presented in Fig. 30 which shows the

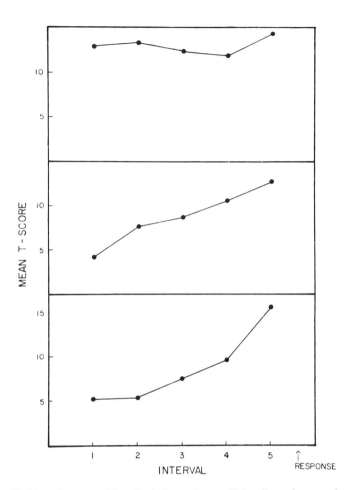

FIG. 30. Mean frequency ($N = 4$) relative to the pre-CS baseline, of neuronal spikes in five consecutive intervals prior to the behavioral conditioned response, in three stages of acquisition (early acquisition, top; at cirterion, middle; and during postcriterial performance, bottom). Each interval (abscissa mark) had a duration of 200 milliseconds. The occurrence of the behavioral response is indicated by the arrow at the right of the figure. Only theta-like bursting spikes of the hippocampus contributed to the analysis. The three curves are based on preresponse neuronal histograms obtained by "averaging backward" from the behavioral conditioned response. Each subject contributed the same number of response occurrences at each stage of training. The figure shows that the very "earliest" behavioral conditioned responses were not preceded by a build-up of theta-like neuronal bursts, but a build-up did precede responses that occurred in the middle and late stages of conditioning. Reprinted with permission from Gabriel and Saltwick (1980).

average frequency of neuronal spikes in five consecutive intervals (200 milliseconds each) prior to the occurrence of the locomotory avoidance response. Each of the graphs represents data of one of three stages of avoidance learning (early acquisition, criterion attainment, and postcriterial performance). Average results obtained from four rabbits are shown. Each rabbit provided a single neuronal record with a clear burst pattern of the kind shown in Fig. 28. Only the theta-like bursting spikes contributed to the analysis. The same number of trials (with conditioned responses) were involved in construction of each graph. Analysis of variance yielded a significant effect for the interaction of stage of training and interval, and subsequent tests showed that there was a significant build-up in theta-like neuronal activity prior to avoidance responses in the trained subject (second and third stages of training) but no such build-up occurred in the first stage of training, in connection with the initial-most avoidance responses. Instead, theta-like bursts were present at a high level throughout the entire CS-response interval, early in training. This "omnipresent" theta-like activity is similar in character to that which occurs during pretraining with to-be-conditioned tones and noncontingent footshock, as shown in Fig. 28.

These results indicate that theta-like unit activity of the hippocampal formation undergoes change during avoidance learning. The theta-like bursts were not temporally organized with respect to behavioral output early in training. Rather, they seemed to occur in a stationary fashion throughout the entire conditioning trial. Later in training, the bursts came to signal the occurrence of the behavioral response, as the animal gained experience with the CS–UCS contingencies of the task. Speaking anthropomorphically, it seemed as though the burst build-up that occurred in the trained subject reflected the subject's expectancy of shock, or his intention to perform the avoidance response.

It would be inaccurate to convey the impression that the theta-like burst phenomenon just reported represents the predominant form of hippocampal activity recorded in our studies. In fact, we have seen the burst effect in a small number of electrode placements relative to the total number of placements studied to date within the hippocampal formation.

Recently a preliminary analysis of the nonbursting hippocampal records has been completed (Saltwick and Gabriel, 1980). This analysis showed that for several of the records, there was substantial excitatory neuronal activity to both CS+ and to CS− in pretraining, in the first session of acquisition and in the first session of reversal training. However, no response, or an inhibitory response occurred during the intermediate and final sessions in each problem. These results suggest that processing of task stimuli by certain nonbursting hippocampal neurons occurs at the onset of new problems, but not during within-problem performance of an established habit.

Given our findings on hippocampal activity, what may be said about the relationship of the hippocampal formation with the other structures (cingulate cortex and AV nucleus) that we have studied, and with which the hippocampal formation is interconnected? What role is played by the hippocampal formation in manufacture and use of neuronal codes for stimulus significance?

In setting out to discuss these issues, we would like to assure the reader that it is not our intention to present yet another theory of hippocampal functioning. Rather, we will attempt to subject ideas that have been presented before to the constraints imposed by our own findings. The hope is that our findings will provide bases for selective reinforcement of extant proposals about the hippocampus. In discussing these issues we will use the general terms "cortex" and "thalamus" rather than cingulate cortex and AV nucleus, in view of the likelihood (Section III,C) that other cortical and thalamic centers manifest neuronal phenomena similar to those that we have observed in cingulate cortex and in the AV nucleus.

## B. Basic Functions of the Hippocampal Formation

### 1. Overview of the Hypothesis

In describing our view of hippocampal functioning, it is necessary first to elaborate briefly our basic assumptions about the behavioral role of the significance codes in cortex and thalamus. It is our view that the learned behavioral response is "primed" or made ready for elicitation, when trained subjects are placed into the learning situation. The neural mechanisms responsible for priming of the learned behavior are *not* the limbic structures discussed here (cingulate cortex and the AV nucleus). However, we propose that the firing of neurons in deep cingulate cortex, and in the AV nucleus, is *projected to* the centers for response priming. Neural input to the priming centers from cingulate cortex and the AV nucleus is in our view the trigger or "releaser" of the primed behavior. Thus, activation of deep cingulate and/or AV nucleus neurons, by whatever means (e.g., presentation of a CS + ; electrical brain stimulation) would be expected in our view to provoke behavioral output, provided that priming of the behavior has taken place. The major emphasis of the experimental work described in this article concerns the idea that through associative neural mechanisms, formerly neutral, external stimuli acquire control of the neuronal activity of cingulate cortex and AV nucleus. It is for this reason that conditional stimuli come to serve as external "releasers" of the primed behavioral response.

A fundamental role of the hippocampal formation in our view is to exercise modulatory control of the significance codes of cingulate cortex and the AV nucleus. When the hippocampal formation is in an active state, signified by the absence of pronounced high-frequency (10 per second) theta rhythm, then the flow of significance code from cingulate cortex and/or the AV nucleus is suppressed and the release of primed behavior is rendered unlikely. However, when the hippocampal formation is in an inactive state, signified by the presence of high-frequency theta rhythm, then hippocampal suppression of the significance code is withdrawn, and free flow of the code to the response priming center is permitted, triggering release of the primed behavior. By this view the hippocampal formation acts as a valve, governing the flow of behavior-triggering significance code from cingulate cortex and the AV nucleus, to the priming center.

These ideas define our conception of the output, or the "executive" functioning of the hippocampal formation. The question now becomes, what are the influences which govern the valve-like control that the hippocampal formation exerts over the code for significance? How does the hippocampal formation "know" when to suppress the flow of code to the priming center, and how does it know when to allow the flow to occur freely?

To answer these questions, we offer the suggestion that there are constructed within the tissues of the hippocampal formation neural models of the positive and the negative cues which operate in the learning situation. These models include a representation of the contingencies that each cue has with biologically significant events (i.e., reinforcements) that occur in the situation. The models are constructed on the basis of code inputs fed to the hippocampal formation from cingulate cortex and from other cortical and subcortical regions (e.g., entorhinal cortex, medial septal region) which send afferents to the hippocampal formation. After the models are constructed, then code inputs along these afferent pathways are compared to the existing models. If a positive cue is presented to the subject, there is a match with the hippocampal model of the positive cue. As a result of the match, the hippocampal formation "responds" by producing high-frequency theta rhythm. The result is that code for significance is fed to the priming center and the primed behavior is released. In this case, the "response" of the hippocampal formation is self-inactivation. If a negative cue is presented, there is a match with the hippocampal model of the negative cue, and the result is activation of the hippocampal formation. The activated hippocampal formation suppresses the flow of significance code to the priming center, and the behavioral response is withheld. In many learning situations, such as conditioned avoidance, the tonically acting background cues of the experimental environment serve as the negative cue, maintaining the hippocampal formation in a state of tonic activation, and thereby tonically holding in check output of primed behavior. In instances of this kind, occurrence of the positive cue produces phasic hippocampal inactivation and consequent behavioral release. This mode of action ensures precise temporal coordination of the behavioral response with occurrence of the critical positive cue.

We have seen that the neuronal code for significance which forms in the deep laminae of cingulate cortex in the early stages of discriminative conditioning is a rather generalized code. Both CS+ and CS− elicit excitation of the cortical response (Section III, A,b and c). For this reason we presume that cortical encoding of stimulus significance fosters generalized behavioral responding. The studies of Oakley and Russell cited previously (pp. 165, 171) provide empirical support for this assumption. Our hypothesis presumes in addition, that in contrast to the generalized nature of the cortical influence, the hippocampal models of cues and contingencies represent a more precise, less generalized, form of stimulus encoding. Thus a major feature of the adaptive relevance of the hippocampal formation lies in its ability to detect a negative cue, and to suppress the flow of code to the priming center, even though cortex may simultaneously produce a considerable generalized excitatory neuronal response to the negative cue. Thus, the hippocampal formation provides a mechanism for preventing the occurrence of falsely positive behavior to negative cues—behavior which would otherwise take place due to the influence of the generalized cortical code.

If the stimulus contingencies operating in a given learning situation are changed as in reversal shift, or an extinction paradigm, mismatch with existing hippocampal models is rapidly detected and hippocampal activation results. In consequence, cortical and thalamic codes for preshift stimulus significance, and behavioral responding in accordance with the preshift contingencies, are suppressed. This suppression is the first step leading to the construction of new codes for significance, and new hippocampal models appropriate to the postshift problem.

A final provision of our hypothesis is the idea that behavior-predictive, theta-like neuronal activity projected from the hippocampal formation to the AV nucleus during early training trials is one of two major inputs to the AV nucleus necessary for the construction of the relegated code for significance which develops in the AV nucleus at a late stage of training (Section III,A,d). The other input to the AV nucleus which contributes to code relegation is the short-latency discriminative activity projected to the AV nucleus from the deep cingulate laminae. Thus, in addition to hippocampal modulation of the flow of significance code from cortex and thalamus to the response priming center, our account assumes that the hippocampal formation is involved in construction of the late relegated code in the AV nucleus.

These assumptions are elaborated and supporting data are cited in subsequent paragraphs.

## 2. Modelling of Cues and Contingencies

The theta-like neuronal bursts recorded during trials of conditioning (Section IV,A) seemed to us to be very important in formulating fundamental assumptions about behavioral relevance of the late relegated code in the AV nucleus. In particular it seemed interesting that the build-up in rhythmic bursts was a delayed effect which started well after CS-onset and progressed to maximum prior to output of behavior. This behaviorally oriented pattern of neuronal activity should be contrasted with the temporal pattern of the differential neuronal responses of cortex and thalamus. In the latter cases the differential activity was time-locked to the *onset* of the stimuli and it occurred at short latency.

The differences between cortical and thalamic significance code on the one hand, and the hippocampal response on the other suggested to us that the hippocampal formation may be a "downstream" processor of cortical and thalamic code. In other words, the hippocampal formation may receive input of significance code from cortex and thalamus. In addition, the input may be "recognized" by hippocampal tissues, and depending on the nature of the code that is fed in, the hippocampal formation may produce various "responses" (e.g., either a build-up in theta-like activity or no build-up).

The recent findings of Berger and Thompson are compatible with these ideas. These studies show a dramatic increase in UCS-elicited discharge of hippocampal neurons after just a few pairings of the CS with the UCS during Pavlovian conditioning of the rabbit nictitating membrane response (NMR). In addition, hippocampal neurons showed early development of a preresponse discharge having a time course and amplitude highly correlated with the conditioned NMR, but which preceded the NMR by a few milliseconds. Changes of this kind did not occur in animals receiving unpaired presentations of CS and UCS (Berger et al., 1976; Berger and Thompson, 1977, 1978).

The acquired preresponse discharge has in our view an import similar to our own observation of build-up in theta-like neuronal activity. Both findings suggest that the hippocampal formation recognizes CS-driven significance code inputs and "responds" on the basis of the nature of the code. In addition, the specificity of this effect to CS–UCS pairing, and the very rapid increase in UCS-elicited discharge which immediately follows pairing, implicate the hippocampal formation in detection and processing of associative relationships (contingencies) among stimuli.

Based on the findings from our laboratory and from the Thompson laboratory we would propose that the hippocampal formation is able shortly after the onset of training to construct neuronal models of the cues and contingencies operating in a learning task. Once the models are constructed, hippocampal formation "recognizes" code input that it receives from cortex and/or from thalamus, by virtue of its conformity or lack thereof, with the model. Depending on the nature of the input the hippocampal formation programs various outputs that it has at its disposal. The modelling processes discussed here represent fundamental kernal processes underlying the behavioral relevance of the hippocampal formation.

It should be mentioned that the importance of the hippocampal formation for detection of altered contingencies is supported by two sources of information additional to the ideas mentioned. One is the work of Ranck (1973, 1975) demonstrating activity of hippocampal neurons which was specific to the detection of altered stimulus–reward contingencies, such as failure of rats to find a drinking spout in the expected location, following performance of a previously learned approach response to that location (Ranck, 1975, p. 224). The second source is the large body of literature indicating that failure to alter behavior appropriately when stimulus-reinforcement contingencies are altered is one of the most consistently reported results of hippocampal damage (see reviews by Douglas and Pribram, 1966; Douglas, 1967, 1972; Altman et al., 1973; Kimble, 1968; Nadel et al., 1975). Both items of data are consistent with the idea that the hippocampal formation is a region critical for encoding or "modelling" of stimulus–reinforcement contingencies. Specific instances relevant to this point, from the literature on hippocampal damage, are considered in Section IV,C,1.

### 3. Nature of Stored Code and the Role of Contextual Stimuli

It is our tentative working hypothesis that neuronal models of cues and contingencies constructed in the hippocampal formation during acquisition, and the encoding of cue-significance in cortex and thalamus are real engrammic modifications of neural tissues. They represent storage of information concerning the nature of the critical stimuli operating in a given task. The changes represent stored information in the sense that by virtue of their presence certain stimuli have *potential* to elicit unique forms of activity (i.e., code for stimulus significance) in the neural tissues that they occupy. Nevertheless, the existence of the engrammic modifications of tissue does not guarantee that unique neural activity will occur when the appropriate stimuli occur. Rather, the stimuli will not trigger the neuronal codes unless the subject is located in the training environment. Thus, in our view, engrams mediating neuronal response to significant cues for many different learning situations are laid down in the hippocampal formation, as well as in cortex and thalamus, during the lifetime of a typical mammal. However, these engrams for the most part lie dormant, until the subject confronts the environmental context for which a given set of engrams is appropriate. Once a given context is confronted, the detailed pattern of auditory, visual, tactile, olfactory (etc.) stimuli produced by that environment is conveyed to cortex, thalamus, and to the hippocampal formation. The specific configuration of sensory inputs activates the specific set of engrams appropriate to the situation. Thus, engrams representing the hippocampal models and the engrams for cortical and subcortical significance code are made ready for use by contextual inputs. Discussion of the implications of contextual control for electrophysiological analysis of neural substrates of learning is provided by Gabriel (1976) and by Disterhoft (1978).

It should be pointed out that the distinction between contextual stimuli and cue stimuli is not an absolute one. Rather, the occurrence of cues and contingencies represents an important component of the experimental context. For this reason the activation of engrams stored in cortex, thalamus, and in the hippocampal formation in trained subjects depends not only on the presence of appropriate background stimuli. It also depends on occurrence of cues and contingencies. We would propose that the phenomenon of "warm-up" seen in most learning situations is at least in part the result of engram activation contributed by the initial occurrences of the cues and contingencies in a given situation.

It is also likely that occurrences of the cues and contingencies are especially effective, relative to background contextual stimuli, in calling forth the hippocampal cue models, since cues and contingencies represent the special provinces of the hippocampal formation. We propose that alteration of background stimuli should not harm greatly the activation of hippocampal engrams provided that the altered stimuli are accompanied by occurrences of the original cues and contingencies. In contrast, occurrences of cues and contingencies should be of little value in calling forth cortical and thalamic engrams, if the background stimuli have been altered. In other words, background stimuli are more effective for evoking cortical and thalamic engrams, relative to cues and contingencies; however, cues and contingencies are more effective for evoking hippocampal engrams.

Evidence supporting these assumptions is provided by data recently reported by Winocur and Olds (1978). This study involved performance by rats in a Y-maze with simultaneously presented visual pattern stimuli (horizontal versus vertical stripes) as cues. In experiment 1, lesioned animals acquired the discriminative response as rapidly as controls. However, alteration of the contextual cues of the experimental environment (e.g., backgound illumination, maze color, clothing of the experimenter, etc.) produced in lesioned subjects a severe disruption in retention assessed in terms of reacquisition performance.

The disruption was not due in this study to the novelty per se of the altered environment. Subjects in a second experiment showed similar disruption even though they were familiarized with the altered environment prior to testing.

In experiment 3 lesioned subjects showed a very severe disruption when they were required to reverse the original visual pattern discrimination with continuing presence of the contextual stimuli from original learning. However, lesioned subjects were only mildly retarded relative to controls, when reversal took place in conjunction with alteration of background contextual stimuli.

Of particular interest in these data was the different way in which altering the contextual stimuli affected transfer performance of lesioned subjects when the transfer task involved reversal, and when it involved continuing performance of the original discrimination. Contextual alteration disrupted ongoing performance of the original discrimination by lesioned subjects, but such alteration proved helpful to lesioned subjects when they were required to *reverse* the original discrimination. Thus, changes in context are damaging to animals lacking hippocampi because they disrupt performance even when the significance of critical cues does not change. When the hippocampal formation is intact changes in context have a minimal effect on discriminative behavior. The hippocampus in some way permits the animal to prescind from contextual changes and to focus on the critical discriminanda. The conclusion that is suggested is that although the hippocampal formation makes use of background contextual cues, its essential function concerns the management of the discriminanda. With hippocampi intact, effective use of the discriminanda can take place despite change in background context.

This outcome is due in part, we believe, to the ability of cue and contingency occurrences to activate the hippocampal models of these events. Such activation occurs even if there has been a shift in the background contextual stimuli, provided that the preshift cues and contingencies continue to operate after the shift. Once the hippocampal models for the cues and contingencies have been activated, then postshift reestablishment of relegated thalamic significance code appropriate to the cues can take place. Reestablishment of the thalamic code is what is needed for reestablishment of appropriate discriminative behavior. We suggest that the reestablishment of thalamic code occurs by virtue of the constructive, relegatory influence of the hippocampal formation on thalamic code for significance (Section IV,B,5).

The findings indicating that change in background cues severely disrupted ongoing performance of the original discrimination in subjects with hippocampal lesions may be viewed as compatible with our assumption that cortical and thalamic engrams (and the significance code which these engrams mediate) are critically dependent on the presence of the background contextual stimuli. Without these stimuli there is no agency to call forth the engrams and the consequent significant code appropriate to the contingencies. Of course, we have just seen that there is missing as well, the constructive role of the hippocampal formation in reestablishing the thalamic code.

The critical dependence of cortical and thalamic engrams on background contextual stimuli is also illustrated by the finding that lesioned subjects were actually *aided* by a change in background stimuli, when the change was accompanied by reversal of the preshift stimulus contingencies. It is our assumption here that the background cues were ineffective in activating the cortical and thalamic engrams appropriate to the original contingencies. Thus, new engrams, and new significance code, appropriate to the reversal problem could be formed in cortex and thalamus without competition from inappropriate preshift codes. The severest disruption occurred when lesioned subjects were required to reverse with presence of preshift contextual stimuli.

These indications that cortical significance codes are "context-bound" accord nicely with the findings of Oakley and Russell (1973, 1974) who have demonstrated that neodecortication induced between acquisition and reversal facilitated discriminative reversal. Also, the context-bound nature of cortical significance codes is indicated by our own findings (Section III,D) that cingulate cortex manifests persistence of the original neuronal discrimination, with gradual reduction of that discrimination, but no reversal, during the course of reversal training.

Contextual stimuli are not only important for the activation of cortical, thalamic, and hippocampal engrams. In addition, the contextual stimuli are essential for the response priming effect discussed in Section IV,B,1. Specifically, we assume that the contextual stimuli acquire, through associative conditioning, the ability to call forth or to prime neural representations of the behavior or set of behaviors appropriate to a given learning task. Once primed, the appropriate behavioral representations are held in a mode of readiness, awaiting input of cortical and/or thalamic significance code necessary for behavioral elicitation. This idea is similar to the hypothetical mechanism of priming described by Lashley in his well-known essay on the problem of serial order in behavior (Lashley, 1951). We offer the suggestion that the caudate nucleus and other striatal structures may be important substrates of such priming, by virtue of the involvement of these structures in motor control, and by virtue of the widespread cortical and thalamic projections to these structures (e.g., Webster, 1965).

Evidence for the importance of response priming is provided by the phenomenon of pseudoconditioning, which refers to the observation that any phasically presented novel stimulus will elicit a behavioral response if there have been several prior elicitations of the response by presentation of a UCS in the experimental situation (see Kimble, 1961, p. 60–64). Our assumption here is that background stimuli of the experimental situation acquire the ability to prime the behavior elicited by the UCS, by virtue of the repeated "pairing" of those stimuli with the UCS. Once primed, any novel stimulus will trigger elicitation of response, because novel stimuli are effective in evoking neuronal activity of cingulate cortex and the AV nucleus (Gabriel and Saltwick, 1977), and such activity is in our view the necessary condition for eliciting primed behavior (see Section IV,B,1).

Finally, we would like to stress the point that priming of responses, and activation of cortical and thalamic significance codes, depend upon the *associative* conditioning of these activities to contextual stimuli of the experimental environment. This idea receives support from past studies demonstrating that extended exposure of trained subjects to the experimental environment prior to extinction testing abolishes the performance of conditioned responses during the test (Gabriel, 1970, 1972). Our interpretation of this outcome is that exposure to the apparatus produces extinction of the associative linkages between the apparatus stimuli and response priming, and between the apparatus stimuli and activation of cortical and thalamic engrams for significance codes. Thus, critical mediational mechanisms of the nervous system are lost due to apparatus exposure. The result is that presentation of the CS is without behavioral effect.

## 4. Behavioral Relevance of Hippocampal Models
of Cues and Contingencies

In our own studies, increased cue-evoked neuronal activity (i.e., neuronal excitation) in cingulate cortex and in the AV nucleus was associated with performance of the behavioral response. Lesser neuronal activation or absence of activation was generally associated with absence of response. Given these relationships we have adopted the view that the cortical and thalamic significance codes observed in our studies represent neuronal influences which trigger or facilitate active behavioral output. That is, the cortical and thalamic events are behavior-inducing neuronal events; these regions represent a neural "go" system.

One of the chief functions of the hippocampal formation involves its action as a counterweight to the cortical and thalamic go system. Thus, presuming that a hippocampal cue-model has been constructed, when a positive cue (e.g., CS + ) is presented, the hippocampal formation enters the theta mode, which represents a state of hippocampal inactivity (see Grastyan *et al.*, 1959). With inactivation of the hippocampal formation, full expression of cortical and thalamic significance code is permitted. When a negative cue is presented, the hippocampal formation sends off neural output which suppresses significance code in cortex and in thalamus.

By this view two opposing systems are operating, one (the cortical and thalamic system) fostering active behavioral responding, by virtue of significance code, and the second (the hippocampal system) fostering suppression of significance code. In this sense, our view is similar to the view of cingulate cortical and hippocampal function espoused in the theoretical accounts of McCleary (1966) and Altman *et al.* (1973). Nevertheless, the present account places emphasis on limbic substrates as essential for the behavioral expression of associative stimulus significance. In contrast, the accounts of McCleary and of Altman *et al.* view the limbic structures as essential for nonassociative modulation of behavior.

To summarize briefly, we have said that the hippocampal formation constructs neuronal models of experimental cues and contingencies. Once the models exist the hippocampal formation responds in a unique way to cue presentation; when a positive cue occurs the hippocampal formation is inactivated. The inactivation is signified by the occurrence of 10 per second theta rhythm. When a negative cue occurs the hippocampal formation is activated and it suppresses the cortical and thalamic significance code. Hippocampal activation is signified by absence of 10 per second theta. Contextual stimuli activate engrams for these functions in cortex, thalamus, and hippocampal formation when subjects are placed into the experimental environment. Background stimuli are of prime effectiveness for activating cortical and thalamic engrams, whereas occurrences of cues and contingencies are most effective for activating hippocampal engrams.

## 5. Hippocampal Participation in Production of Relegated Neuronal Code for Significance of Cues

Our results showed that neurons in the deep laminae of cingulate cortex acquired a discriminative response to the cues (CS + and CS − ) used for avoidance acquisition. The discriminative effect, proposed by us to represent neuronal code for stimulus significance, was acquired in the very early stages of acquisition, and in certain placements it showed a tendency toward reduction in later stages. Of particular importance for the present analysis was the finding that the discriminative activity appropriate to original learning persisted through the precriterial stages of reversal training. Thus, there were sessions in reversal in which the rabbits responded with discriminative behavior appropriate to the reversal problem, while cingulate cortex manifested neuronal discrimination appropriate to original acquisition. Discriminative neuronal activity appropriate to original acquisition showed greater persistence through reversal in subjects that did not receive overtraining in the original task, relative to overtrained subjects. We inferred from these results a possible role of cingulate cortex in mediating the behavioral ORE. The idea is that the highly persistent "old habit" effect in cingulate cortex is responsible for retardation of behavioral reversal seen in nonovertrained subjects.

A more general viewpoint to emerge from these data is the idea that cortex is involved in the initial significance coding of stimuli which serve to cue behavior in learning situations. Once cortical processing has established the identity of the significant stimuli, there is cortical disengagement from active task processing and the job of producing a unique neuronal response to such stimuli is relegated to thalamus, as indicated by the late-developing neuronal discrimination seen in the AV nucleus in our studies.

One of several aspects of the adaptive value of the late-formed thalamic code (see Section III,A,d) may involve a kind of "automatic pilot" notion. Thus, production of neuronal code for significance at the thalamic level allows disengagement of cortex from active stimulus coding in the task. Such disengagement would free cortex for subsequent discriminative problems that may occur. It would thereby allow a more flexible behavioral adaptation to revision of the original problem, as indicated by our own studies of the ORE (Section III,E).

An important point concerns the finding that the code for significance seen in the deep laminae of cingulate cortex was a rather generalized code. Thus, in the very initial-most stage of acquisition both CS+ and CS− evoked ample associative cortical neuronal responses. Progress in acquisition was accompanied by a gradual drop in the cortical response to the CS−, with little change in the response to CS+. On the other hand, the discriminative neuronal effect which developed in the AV nucleus was not at all generalized. Instead, advent of discriminative activity in the AV nucleus was characterized by a sharp step-up in the neuronal response evoked by the CS+, with no change in the response evoked by the CS−. This sharp discriminative effect was first observed in association with the advent of the first criterial-level performance of the behavioral discrimination. These results suggest that an aspect of the adaptive value of the relegated code is its role in promoting ample behavioral discrimination, by virtue of the clear-cut neuronal discrimination that occurs. More generally these results suggest that the relegated neuronal code observed in the AV nucleus reflects a *"significance extraction"* process (Section III,A,d).

If the relegated thalamic code underlies the substantial behavioral discrimination that one observes during performance at criterion, it is reasonable to propose that the generalized prerelegatory cortical code for significance may not be adequate to support ample behavioral discrimination. This idea follows from the observation that cortical encoding parallels initial behavioral discrimination and that it shows fading when behavioral discrimination is at maximum. Thus, the chief function of cortex is problem solution, i.e., identification and specification of the important task stimuli. Mediation of ample criterial-level behavioral discrimination is the province of the extracted thalamic code. This general idea will carry throughout our discussion.

In tying in these ideas with the functional role of the hippocampal formation we should report that rhythmic theta-like neuronal bursts increasing to 10 per second just prior to avoidance responses were observed in 3 of 13 electrode placements in the AV nucleus (see Fig. 31). Because we observed similar theta-like neuronal burst activity in CA1 and the subicular areas of the hippocampal formation, and because axonal projection from these areas has been shown to terminate within the AV nucleus, it seems reasonable to suppose that the theta-like neuronal bursting that occurs in the AV nucleus may represent activity being projected to that region from the CA1 and the subicular areas of the hippocampal formation. If this is so, then we know that the AV nucleus receives at least two distinct varieties of neuronal input during

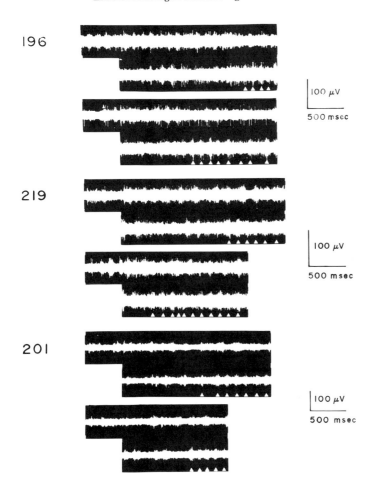

196

219

201

|00 μV

500 msec

|00 μV

500 msec

|00 μV

500 msec

FIG. 31. Oscilloscope photographs of multiple-unit activity of the AV nucleus during entire trials of conditioning are shown for three rabbits (196, 219, and 201). Two trials are shown for each rabbit. Each trial is comprised of two traces, an upper trace and a lower (indented) one. Time of CS onset on the upper trace is indicated by the left edge of the indented (lower) trace. Activity pictured above and to the left of the indented trace is pre-CS activity. A behavioral response occurred at the end (right-most point) of each trial. Calibrations for voltage and time are given at the right, for each subject. The purpose of the figure is to indicate that theta-like neuronal bursts occur prior to the avoidance response in the AV nucleus, as well as in the CA1-subicular region of the hippocampal formation (see Section IV,A and Fig. 27). Reprinted with permission from Lambert et al. (1980).

discriminative avoidance conditioning. One of these is the relatively short-latency discriminative neuronal activity that is time-locked to the onsets of the CS. This activity is projected to the AV nucleus over the corticothalamic pathway which originates in laminae V and VI of cingulate cortex. The second variety of activity which is fed to the AV nucleus is the behavior-related theta-like neuronal bursting from CA1 and from the subicular region of the hippocampal formation. It is worthwhile to consider that these two inputs to the AV nucleus may be instrumental in constructing the neuronal discrimination which forms within the AV nucleus, in the late stages of discriminative acquisition. In other words, we would propose that one of the functions of the hippocampal formation is its instrumentality in construction of the late relegated thalamic code for significance of stimuli.

We have suggested (Section III,A,d) that the late advent of relegated code in the AV nucleus may signify the switching-in of a stimulus analyzer indicating a focusing by the subject upon the relevant cues operating in a given task.

Isaacson (1974) has reviewed work by Kimble (e.g., Kimble, 1963) involving study of simultaneous and successive brightness discrimination by rats in Y-mazes. These studies demonstrated that training in a successive discrimination problem transferred positively to a simultaneous problem. Detailed analysis of the protocols of individual rats suggested that rats trained on the successive problem performed well in the simultaneous problem because they adopted a brightness hypothesis at the outset, suggesting that an analyzer for brightness had been switched-in during original training. Rats with hippocampal lesions did not benefit from prior training in the successive problem, and detailed analysis of their behavior suggested that they adopted a positional hypothesis—behavior typical of animals starting out on their first problem. If one is willing to grant a correspondence between late developing relegated code in thalamus, and switching-in, these results may be viewed as compatible with our contention that the hippocampal formation contributes to code relegation.

We have seen that advent of relegated code in thalamus is associated with advent of ample behavioral discrimination. If the relegated code is an important causal mediator of the clear cut behavioral discrimination seen during criterion attainment, and if as we suggest here, the hippocampal formation contributes to relegation of neuronal code, then it follows that hippocampal processing should contribute importantly to the efficiency of discriminative behavioral acquisition.

That it does so has been well-documented in a review by Fish (1975), indicating lesion-related impairment in acquisition for each of five commonly employed discriminative procedures (visual pattern discrimination, simultaneous and successive brightness discrimination, successive auditory discrimination, and position discrimination).

It is not the case that impairments occurred in every study employing one of these procedures. However, a substantial proportion of the studies with each procedure yielded impairment. Moreover, Fish's review indicated that one could distinguish commonalities among studies yielding impairment, and among those not yielding impairment—commonalities which provided insight into factors responsible for the impairment.

For example, studies reporting impaired acquisition of positional discrimination were those which adopted relatively stringent criteria for acquisition (e.g., Means et al., 1972), whereas studies reporting no impairment employed lenient criteria (e.g., Kimble and Kimble, 1965). We interpret these data as indicating a hippocampal involvement in relegation of significance code essential for attainment of the stringent criteria. A further presumption would be that performance at the lenient criteria was mediated by cortical encoding mechanisms, in the absence of the ample relegated code of thalamus.

The idea of a hippocampal role in relegation of significance code must be qualified by observations indicating the critical importance of the hippocampal formation only for tasks in which the subject is required to use discrete, isolated cues that are imbedded in a context of other non-cue stimuli. Evidence to be discussed (Section IV,C,2) suggests that the importance of the hippocampal contribution to relegation is diminished in certain situations, such as when many stimulus elements serve redundantly as cues for the behavior or when task discriminanda are very salient permitting little opportunity for confusion or interference. In such situations we would propose that the significance of the redundant cueing stimuli is encoded in thalamus at the outset of training, with little or no prerelegatory encoding by cortex, and no substantial role of the hippocampal formation in the relegation process. This restriction of hippocampal influence to tasks involving discrete nonredundant cues is reminiscent of the restriction of effects of cingulate damage to tasks with discrete unimodal stimuli as CSs for avoidance (Section III,B, a). The implication is that cortex and hippocampal formation are jointly involved in the initial stages of stimulus encoding for tasks with discrete cues. However, neither cortex nor hippocampus participates uniquely when task cues are redundant or very salient.

To summarize, we have proposed that there are two basic processes underlying the behavioral relevance of the hippocampal formation. One of these involves modelling of cues and contingencies, and consequent control of significance code in cortex and in thalamus. The second is a contribution of the hippocampal formation in relegation of the neuronal code for stimulus significance. In the following sections we will attempt to indicate how these ideas may be used to account for changes in behavior known to result from hippocampal lesions.

## C. APPLICATION OF THE ACCOUNT TO STUDIES OF THE BEHAVIORAL EFFECTS OF HIPPOCAMPAL LESIONS

### 1. Studies Involving Transfer of Training

Our results suggested that with training beyond criterion, there is a gradual diminution in the weighting of cortical significance code, and a gradual increase in the weighting of thalamic code, in the governance of behavioral responding (see Section III,E). Thus, there would eventually occur in many tasks a stage at which the cortex has disengaged from the processing of task stimuli. When disengagement has taken place, significance coding of cues occurs largely in thalamus. The major observation indicating disengagement of cortex as well as continuing relevance of thalamus is our finding indicating that the predominant discriminative activity seen in cortex during reversal training was that appropriate to original learning, whereas thalamus showed discriminative activity appropriate to acquisition and to reversal. The concept of cortical disengagement suggests that cortex is specialized for identification of relevant stimuli, but not as much for behavioral expression of stimulus significance. The latter job is carried out primarily in thalamic substrates.

The persistence in cortex of the residual discriminative neuronal response appropriate to original learning not only suggested a disengagement of cortex from task processing, it also raised the possibility that the residual activity in cortex would interfere with behavioral reversal. This suggestion was supported by our finding that overtraining in the original task reduced the persistence of old habit activity in cortex and facilitated behavioral reversal. The suggestion also receives support by the data of Oakley and Russell (1973, 1974) indicating that neodecortication of rabbits after acquisition but before reversal facilitated behavioral reversal.

We would like to propose here relevance of these findings to a major facet of hippocampal functioning. We have argued that relegation of significance code to thalamus results from joint action of inputs from cortex and from hippocampal formation. Thus by our account cortex and hippocampal formation are the two structures responsible for construction of relegated significance code in thalamus. Given that the cortex gradually relinquishes control of stimulus processing during acquisition, the hippocampal formation is the only remaining structure that is likely to be involved in interaction with thalamus, to bring about changes in stimulus processing and in behavior, should there be alteration of task contingencies. Even for tasks in which the hippocampal formation plays little or no role in acquisition, it may nevertheless become importantly engaged during transfer of training.

Thus we would suggest a 2-fold role of the hippocampal formation during transfer of training. First, inappropriate residual significance code operating in cortex is suppressed by the hippocampal formation. In addition, relegated code in thalamus is suppressed, and new code is formed in thalamus by virtue of interaction of thalamic structures with the hippocampal formation.

Suppression is the result of altering cues and/or task contingencies. Thus if a positive cue (e.g., CS + ) is made negative by removing its usual consequence (e.g., the UCS) the hippocampal formation will rapidly detect the change, because of mismatch of the input with the original model. Suppression of ongoing cortical and thalamic coding is a direct result of mismatch detection. A new model of the positive cue will be formed rapidly in the hippocampal formation so that before long, presentation of the formerly positive cue will elicit suppression of cortical and thalamic excitatory code, rather than hippocampal inactivation.

Hippocampal involvement in reconstruction of code appropriate to the postshift task is viewed as a process similar to hippocampal involvement in relegation of code during original training.

Contribution to relegation on the one hand, and suppression and revision of excitatory code on the other represent two proposed hippocampal functions which involve hippocampothalamic communication. We have tentatively identified the first of these putative neuronal functions with the rhythmic theta-like bursts which our studies have suggested are sent from CA1 and from the subicular complex, to the AV nucleus.

We have not observed any unique form of neuronal activity common to the hippocampal formation and the AV nucleus, which might subserve the second form of hippocampothalamic communication (suppression of excitatory relegated code in the AV nucleus). However, excitatory neuronal responses to CS+ and CS− of nonbursting hippocampal neurons occur at the outset of training, and at the outset of reversal training. These excitatory effects manifested transition to no effect, or to an inhibitory effect in the intermediate and final stages in each problem (Section IV,B,1). It is possible that the excitatory effects seen at the outset of acquisition and reversal reflected issuance by the hippocampal formation of a "command" to "clear" or "initialize" the substrates in cortex and in thalamus, so as to prepare for the incorporation of new codes within these substrates. Again, the occasion for this hippocampal effect is the advent of new cueing stimuli and/or contingencies, leading to rapid reformulation of the hippocampal cue models. Once reformulation is underway formerly positive, presently negative cues suppress the original excitatory cortical and thalamic codes. Formerly negative presently positive cues inactivate the hippocampal formation itself, allowing full expression of excitatory codes.

The viewpoint presented here suggests that it is absence of the ability to suppress obsolete cortical and thalamic significance code in hippocampectomized animals which creates the often-reported deficit in transfer tasks such as reversal learning (e.g., Winocur and Olds, 1978, exp. 3), certain passive avoidance tasks involving inhibition of previously acquired approach behavior (e.g., Wishart and Mogenson, 1970), extinction of the straight alley approach response (e.g., Jarrard *et al.*, 1964), acquisition involving differential reinforcement for low rates of response (DRL: e.g., Schmaltz and Isaacson, 1966), blocking (Solomon, 1977; Rickert *et al.*, 1978), and latent inhibition (Solomon and Moore, 1975).

We have already applied our account to the deficit in reversal training, produced by hippocampal lesions (Section IV,B,3). Let us now consider certain other transfer paradigms.

Lesioned subjects are notoriously deficient in their ability to inhibit previously acquired approach responses. By our account, the positive "cue" modelled by the hippocampal formation during original learning is the entire experimental context and the cue-consequence relation modelled is the contingency between contextual stimuli and reward. Replacement of reward by nonreward or by punishment produces mismatch of inputs with the existing hippocampal models, consequent suppression of cortical and thalamic codes and rapid reformulation of new codes and models. In lesioned subjects there is no suppression and the contextual stimuli continue to elicit codes which drive approach behavior.

Our studies have indicated that the significance code seen early in training in the deep laminae of cingulate cortex is a generalized code. Both CS+ and CS− elicit associatively acquired neuronal responses in this substrate. A critical premise of our account is that construction of a hippocampal model of cues and contingencies and subsequent relegation of significance code to thalamus are sequential processes which supplement the generalized cortical code by providing more precise, less generalized neuronal representation of the critical stimuli. In other words, model construction and relegation represent processes of *significance extraction* (Section III,A,d) which occur during learning, and which underlie the improvement during training in the discriminative behavior of normal subjects.

These ideas provide background relevant to one of the interesting effects of hippocampal damage—elimination of the phenomenon of blocking.

In the blocking paradigm subjects are first given paired presentations of a CS [CS(A)] and a UCS, followed by compound conditioning with CS(A), and a second CS [CS(B)]. Finally, each component of the compound is tested separately to determine its associative strength. The results indicate that only CS(A) elicits the CR in normal subjects, but considerable associative strength is manifested by both stimuli in lesioned subjects.

We would suggest that CS(B) acquires ability to elicit the cortical code during the compound conditioning phase of the blocking paradigm. However, CS(B) is excluded from the hippocampal model of positive cues, by virtue of its redundancy with CS(A). Thus, when CS(B) is presented to a normal subject in the test it is "classified" as a negative cue by the hippocampal formation. Consequent hippocampal outputs suppress the cortical code elicited by CS(B) and no behavioral output occurs. In lesioned subjects the cortical code is not suppressed and CS(B) elicits a behavioral response. These assumptions do not explain the mechanisms whereby the hippocampal formation classifies CS(B) as a negative cue, but they do indicate how the lesion-produced elimination of the blocking effect is compatible with the general idea of hippocampal supplementation or "sharpening" of the cortical code.

The idea that hippocampal processing sharpens to the generalized cortical code is supported by results of Solomon and Moore (1975), demonstrating that rabbits with hippocampal lesions manifest flattened gradients of stimulus generalization relative to controls following conditioning of the rabbit NMR. In our view the flat gradients in lesioned subjects represent the product of generalized cortical significance coding alone, whereas the sharper gradients in normal animals reflect the more precise modelling of cue stimuli, contributed by hippocampal processing.

In the latent inhibition paradigm a model of the prospective CS is constructed within the hippocampal formation during "CS-alone" presentations. The contingency in this situation is in fact a cue-no consequence relationship, since the CS is paired with no UCS. Thus the hippocampal model formed during CS-alone training is a negative cue model, which fosters output of hippocampal suppression directed toward the cortical and thalamic substrates of the significance code. At the outset of acquisition training there is a brief period during which this suppressive influence retards the formation of the code essential to performance of the behavioral CR. This produces the retardation defining the latent inhibition effect. That the retardation is a relatively minimal and transient effect is testimony to hippocampal flexibility defined in terms of the potential for rapid replacement of the negative-cue model with a positive-cue model. In lesioned subjects there is no retardation of significance coding and acquisition takes place at a normal pace. That is, there is no latent inhibition effect.

### 2. Hippocampal Lesions and Behavioral Acquisition

We have been considering the role of the hippocampal formation in relation to transfer of training paradigms. Nevertheless, it is clear that hippocampal lesions alter behavioral acquisition in several learning situations. Discussions of hippocampal function must deal with the role of the hippocampal formation in acquisition, and in particular, such discussions must deal pointedly with demonstrations indicating that hippocampal damage disrupts acquisition in certain tasks, leaving acquisition in other tasks unaffected.

Of relevance to this point is the observation that the distinction between acquisition and transfer may have validity only at the procedural level. At a more fundamental level virtually all of the behavioral paradigms used for study of hippocampal function are in fact transfer paradigms.

The validity of this assertion is evident in relation to operant paradigms such as DRL, and for many "passive avoidance" paradigms. Subjects trained in DRL, for example, almost without exception have been given "pretraining" on a CRF schedule, and subjects trained in passive avoidance in many studies received prior approach training. [It is interesting to note that hippocampal lesions reliably retard "acquisition" in both situations, *unless* special pains are taken to avoid pretraining of subjects. This point has received documentation by Isaacson (1974) in relation to the DRL task and for passive avoidance by Black *et al.* (1977).]

The sense in which certain other paradigms involve transfer of training is more subtle. Nevertheless it becomes apparent by considering that after the initial trial in any multitrial learning task it is necessary to evaluate the "transfer" of past trials to the current trial. Thus, for example, all alley entries in a complex maze but the first may be viewed as transfer tests.

These ideas provide the background for considering hippocampal functioning in original acquisition. The basic principle here is that the hippocampal formation performs exactly the same functions in acquisition as in transfer of training. Thus, there will be an essential contribution of the hippocampal formation to acquisition for tasks in which current performance involves suppression of excitatory significance code in cortex and in thalamus. The question then becomes, what are the situations in which suppression is likely to be required?

We would expect the contribution of the hippocampal formation to behavioral acquisition to be critical in situations in which there is need to suppress generalized cortical significance code elicited by negative cues. Situations likely to require suppression of code elicited by such stimuli are those situations in which subjects are required to predicate their behavioral responses upon the occurrence of nonsalient, isolated, positive stimuli imbedded in a context of other stimuli having negative or neutral behavioral significance.

Stated another way, when tasks require subjects to respond to specific, isolated, nonsalient cues, problems may be created by virtue of the tendency for negative cues present in the situation to elicit generalized significance code in cortex. When this happens the subject is likely to emit falsely positive behavioral responses. However, the hippocampal formation by virtue of its precise cue-model suppresses the excitatory code when negative cues are presented.

We would stress again the idea that the hippocampal function in acquisition is identical to the function proposed previously in relation to transfer tasks. In both cases, hippocampal action is expected to aid performance when deleterious effects of excitatory significance codes operate. The excitatory codes requiring suppression in the case of transfer tasks are the established cortical and thalamic codes appropriate to original learning. Potentially interfering codes requiring suppression in the acquisition tasks are the generalized cortical responses evoked by negative cues in early stages of training, prior to the development of maximally differential cortical codes, and prior to advent of the clearly differential relegated code of thalamus.

There is an important connection between the idea of relegation and hippocampal involvement in behavioral acquisition.

Prior to relegation all that is available to control behavioral response is the generalized cortical significance code. The more precise hippocampal model of task stimuli represents an important supplement to cortical significance codes in this phase of acquisition. However, after relegation has taken place there is available the highly precise relegated code in thalamus, characterized by ample neuronal response to positive cues, and no response to negative cues (Section III,A,d).

We propose that prior to relegation the precise hippocampal model is of great value in terms of its ability to mediate suppression of the cortical code when negative cues occur. After relegation, the precise hippocampal model does not play as vital a role, because appropriate discriminative responding without falsely positive behavior is mediated by the precise relegated code in thalamus.

It is important to bear in mind that there is overlap of cortical and thalamic significance codes. Typically the cortical code is formed in advance of the thalamic code during the course of acquisition, but the cortical code does not cease to operate as soon as the thalamic code develops. Instead, our results suggest that there is a period of training during which codes operate in both structures with progressive increase in the weighting of the thalamic code and progressive decrease in the weighting of the cortical code (Section III,E). Thus, the suppressive control exerted by the hippocampal formation may be of continuing value after relegation, as a counterweight to the generalized cortical code, during the period of overlap.

There is one final point of importance in considering the contributions of the hippocampal formation to behavioral acquisition. It is the idea that in addition to its role in mediating suppression of the generalized excitatory code, the hippocampal formation may play a direct role in bringing about relegation of significance codes as manifested in the AV nucleus (see Section IV,B,5). In our view a hippocampal contribution to relegation of codes in original learning is likely to be of value in promoting behavioral acquisition, again, in situations in which the stimuli whose codes are to be relegated are isolated, nonsalient ones.

When is the hippocampal contribution to acquisition unimportant?

Clearly our view expects no lesion-related deficit in situations that do not require suppression of an excitatory cortical significance code. In fact, need for code suppression and lesion-produced deficit are both absent for several learning situations, including single-stimulus acquisition by rabbits of the conditioned NMR, acquisition of approach in the straight alley, and acquisition of operant behavior on a continuous reinforcement (CRF) schedule. In each case subjects have no way to damage their performance scores by overresponding. Thus, the excitatory codes in cortex and thalamus are unmitigated goods in these tasks.

Even when some suppression of the excitatory code may be required, there is a reduced likelihood of falsely positive behavior due to a generalized cortical code, provided that the cues that operate are salient and/or redundant. This is so because negative cues are less likely to evoke the generalized excitatory code to the extent that they are distinct from positive cues. Moreover, by our account the significance of salient and/or redundant stimuli is encoded in thalamus at the outset of training, with little or no prerelegatory phase involving exclusively cortical encoding.

Thus, when task stimuli are salient and/or redundant, there is little or no hippocampal contribution to acquisition. This is so because the hippocampal formation is not needed either for suppressing the generalized cortical code, or for constructing the relegated subcortical code.

If cue salience and redundancy are the factors which determine the importance of the hippocampal contribution in acquisition, then manipulation of salience and redundancy should affect the probability of observing an acquisition deficit in lesioned subjects. This prediction fares well in terms of studies of maze learning (e.g., Winocur and Breckenridge, 1973), single alternation learning (e.g., Stevens and Cowey, 1972), positional discrimination learning (e.g., Lash, 1964), and go, no-go operant discrimination learning (e.g., Freeman, 1978). In each study cited addition of redundant, relevant stimuli employable as cues for behavior eliminated lesion-produced deficit in acquisition. In addition, the principle receives support from between-experiment comparisons in relation to passive avoidance behavior. Thus, in a recent review Black *et al.* (1977) point out that a lesion-related deficit in passive avoidance acquisition occurs only in situations that require subjects to use cues distant from the source of punishment. In tasks yielding no deficit, "salient cues were available and could be perceived from all parts of the apparatus" (p. 1211).

Behavioral acquisition of simultaneous pattern discrimination, and simultaneous brightness discrimination are unaffected by hippocampal damage. Yet, it may seem arbitrary and gratuitous to assume that such tasks represent easy problems with unconfusable discriminanda, or problems in which neuronal stimulus codes undergo immediate relegation.

In this regard it should be mentioned that not all visual discrimination problems are normally learned by animals with damaged hippocampi. Thus, Isaacson's review indicates that tasks learned normally typically involve use of the Y-maze or the T-maze, as in the study of Winocur and Olds (1978) previously discussed (Section IV,B,3). Hippocampal lesions retard acquisition in tasks such as successive discrimination (e.g., Kimble, 1963) and operant learning situations in which a light cue signals availability of reinforcement (Woodruff and Isaacson, 1972). Following arguments presented by Moore (1979), it is worthwhile to consider that the insensitivity of the simultaneous tasks to hippocampal lesions may be attributable to the fact that the discriminanda in these tasks not only provide subjects with information about correct choice, they also provide information about the locus of reward, by virtue of the proximity of cues with the postchoice alleys of the maze. It may be that by adopting the relatively simple strategy "approach the positive cue" lesioned subjects are able to perform adequately in the simultaneous problems, despite deficient suppression of the excitatory code by the negative cue. Even though the negative cue is present, simultaneous presence of the positive cue may preempt the subject's approach behavior in simultaneous discrimination tasks. We offer the additional suggestion that this simple "sign tracking" strategy (Hearst and Jenkins, 1974) may be employable on the basis of the kind of neuronal encoding that we have seen in the AV nucleus, involving ample neuronal response to the positive cue and no response to the negative cue. Successive discrimination tasks may create problems for lesioned subjects because of the requirement that they suppress falsely positive behavior at times when there is no salient, directional positive cue present to preempt their approach response.

In support, we would point out that in one of the rare studies reporting a lesion-related deficit in Y-maze pattern discrimination (Niki, 1962), the discriminanda were not adjacent. Under such circumstances viewing the negative cue could take place without simultaneous influence of the positive cue. This circumstance would reduce the probability of preemption of approach behavior by the positive cue.

Among the most dramatic deficits in acquisition occur when lesioned animals are required to perform in the radial maze (see Olton *et al.*, 1978; Jarrard, 1978). In this task the subject is placed on a central platform from which it has access to a series (usually 8) of alleyways projecting outwardly in spokelike fashion. Typically, goal areas at the end of each alley are baited and optimal performance involves collection of reward in each alley, without reentry of any of the alleys.

A unique feature of the radial maze task is the way in which behaviorally significant stimuli alter their significance as the subject performs. Thus, all stimuli are positive cues at the outset of a maze trial, presuming that the subject has learned that all alleys have been baited. As soon as a given alley is chosen the pattern of extramaze and intramaze cues associated with that choice undergoes transition from the status of a positive cue to the status of a negative cue. That is, the subject must withold entry on subsequent confrontations of the once-chosen alley. It is very likely that the generalized cortical significance code is of little value in this situation because of the high confusability of the stimuli. Moreover, the discriminability of cues mediating specific alley choices in this task cannot be enhanced by repeated performance, and by relegation, because no single stimulus confronted by a given subject possesses cue value which endures from trial to trial. Thus, at the end of a given trial all patterns have become negative cues, but at the onset of the next trial all patterns become, once again, positive cues.

This situation places a heavy load on hippocampal precision, speed, and flexibility of encoding: highly confusable patterns of stimuli associated with each chosen alley must be encoded by the hippocampal mechanism as negative cues so that the excitatory cortical significance code may be suppressed should these patterns be confronted a second time; at the end of each trial all codes must be abandoned, and new codes must be reformulated during the course of each trial; finally, the within-trial encoding cannot profit by formation of nongeneralized (relegated) code. Given these requirements it is understandable by our account that hippocampal damage is disruptive to normal performance in the radial maze.

Our point that relegation is of no value in the temporary coding that must underly radial maze performance is not intended to rule out the possibility that relegation may aid other sorts of coding processes important for radial maze performance.

In this connection, a recent experiment by Jarrard (1978) suggests that relegation may indeed play a role. Gross hippocampal lesions disrupted maze performance when subjects were lesioned before acquisition, and when they were lesioned after acquisition. However, when lesions were restricted to CA1 and the subicular complex, only postoperative acquisition was affected. Subjects trained preoperatively showed normal performance after surgery.

These results are compatible with the idea that significance codes for the radial maze may be relegated to subcortical structures during acquisition and that once relegation occurs, lesions of CA1 and the subicular complex do not degrade performance.

We have already argued that codes for cues inhibiting reentry during a given trial cannot undergo relegation to thalamic centers. Thus, it becomes interesting to inquire into the nature of the significance codes which do undergo relegation in this task. They must be codes for stimuli whose significance endures from trial to trial.

It may be worth considering that the extramaze stimuli confronted by the animal as it adopts various bodily orientations in the maze may possess such enduring cue value. Perhaps the subject learns to associate certain of these cues (such as the window shade or the door knob) with a particular set of alley choices. Acquisition of distinctive neuronal codes for such cues may help the subject to organize and to separate the full set of alley choices into a series of subsets, each controlled by a different extramaze cue. With this arrangement, choices within each subset may be run off without interference from choices in other subsets. This kind of organizing function for extramaze stimuli would be expected to carry over from trial to trial. It would also be expected to decrease the processing load placed upon the hippocampal formation in relation to inhibition of reentry. If extramaze stimuli are in fact used in the fashion suggested, it becomes possible to imagine how relegation and consequent amplification of significance codes associated with extramaze stimuli may be of substantial benefit in radial maze performance.

A final point of interest concerns again the lesion in Jarrard's study which interfered with acquisition but not with performance of the acquired habit. We interpreted this outcome to indicate that the damaged region is essential for relegation of significance codes to the AV nucleus. We would point out that the locus of the lesion included the subicular complex, a site of origin of postcommissural projections to the AV nucleus—projections which seem to convey theta-like preresponse discharge from the subicular complex to the AV nucleus (Section IV,B, 5). These observations are compatible with our suggestion that theta-like influences projected from subicular complex to the AV nucleus may aid in construction of late relegated code in the AV nucleus.

Firing patterns of hippocampal neurons seem to be correlated with occupation by subjects of specific locations in an experimental environment (e.g., Ranck, 1973). On this basis it has been suggested that hippocampal neurons perform a place coding function. This and other arguments have led to the formulation of a compelling hypothesis stating that the hippocampal formation is the neural locus for construction of environmental (spatial) maps, which in turn make possible problem solution on the basis of spatial strategies (see O'Keefe and Nadel, 1978).

Our own account is in fundamental agreement with the spatial mapping idea, insofar as both viewpoints impute to the hippocampal formation a role in the precise and rapid encoding of nonsalient, nonredundant properties of the experimental environment. Nevertheless, we are not convinced that hippocampal functioning contributes only to the elaboration of spatial strategies in task solution. In support we would cite the build-up in theta-like discharge which precedes the occurrence of the avoidance response (Section IV,A) as evidence that the hippocampal formation participates in coding processes relevant to temporal properties of the critical CS-UCS relationship. A similar conclusion follows from the studies of Berger and Thompson demonstrating that the discharge of hippocampal neurons which precedes the conditioned NMR by a few milliseconds, also shows a temporal pattern nearly identical to the time course of the NMR (Section IV,B,2). Berger and Thompson concluded from these results that hippocampal neuronal response represents a temporal "model" of the conditioned NMR.

In addition there are many behaviors such as NMR conditioning itself and DRL acquisition which are dramatically affected by hippocampal damage yet which seem completely divorced from the concept of a spatial strategy.

By our view "place coding" manifested by hippocampal neurons represents a subclass of significance coding. Stimuli associated with particular locations, as well as stimuli totally lacking in spatial connotation, may come to be modelled through operation of the associative mechanisms of the hippocampal formation. The reader is referred to recent reviews by Solomon and by Moore (Solomon, 1979; Moore, 1979) for detailed documentation of the involvement of the hippocampal formation in nonspatial processing.

Data obtained from study of performance in situations other than the radial maze may be viewed as compatible with the idea that the hippocampal formation is importantly involved in enabling subjects to use nonsalient nonredundant cues to suppress excitatory cortical significance code and thereby to stop behavior.

For example, Isaacson (1974, pp. 165–167) has reviewed literature compatible with the idea that distractability, and the impaired spontaneous alternation behavior seen in lesioned subjects may result from failure of these subjects to encode the inhibitory significance of incidental stimuli in the experimental environment.

Micco and Schwartz (1971) trained rats to run in a wheel to avoid unsignaled footshock. Following this all subjects received trials of discriminative Pavlovian fear conditioning in which a tone and a light served as CS+ and CS− and footshock served as UCS. After discriminative conditioning, the CSs were presented separately to the subjects during performance in the unsignaled shock-avoidance situation. Normals showed increase in wheel running to the CS+ and decrease to the CS−. Hippocampals also increased running to the CS+, but there was no attenuation of running to the CS−. These results may be interpreted to reflect a failure of suppression of cortical and thalamic significance codes driven by the tonically acting contextual stimuli of the wheel-running apparatus.

The idea that intact hippocampal functioning is critical for inhibitory stimulus control of behavior is contraindicated by the conclusion of Solomon and Moore (1975) to the effect that the hippocampal formation is not necessary for the development of conditioned inhibition during discriminative Pavlovian conditioning of the rabbit NMR. In elaborating this idea Solomon (1979) and Moore (1979) have argued that the hippocampal formation is involved in "tuning out" irrelevant cues, but that other brain substrates mediate the distinctive phenomena defined as conditioned inhibition (see Rescorla, 1969).

The work of Solomon and Moore points up an important qualification which must be borne in mind in relation to our account. We have been using the term "negative stimulus" to refer to a broad class of stimuli, all of which are ineffective in evoking excitatory activation of neuronal activity in cortex and in thalamus. Included in this class are stimuli which are negatively correlated with reinforcement, stimuli which are uncorrelated with reinforcement, and stimuli which are correlated with reinforcement, but redundantly so, as in the case of CS(B) in the blocking paradigm (Section IV,C,1). In each case, there is a failure to elicit cortical code due to hippocampal categorization of these cues as negative. What is important is to recognize that by our account the hippocampal formation, cortex, and thalamus are involved exclusively with the production and suppression of neuronal *excitations* which directly induce active behavioral responding. The process referred to in our account of hippocampal suppression of cortical and thalamic code for significance is compatible in all respects with Solomon's and Moore's idea of tuning out. Our account does not preclude the possibility that other substrates of the brain exist which are specialized for active inhibitory control of behavior. Indeed, the existence of such substrates is supported by the work of Mis (Mis, 1977).

We have considered a number of experimental situations in which behavioral impairment may be accounted for in terms of the inappropriate operation of the excitatory cortical and thalamic significance code. In these situations lesioned subjects lack hippocampal suppression of the excitatory code. The suppression in intact subjects is based on the existence of a hippocampal model for the negative cue.

The reader may wonder about the utility of the model for the positive cue, whose construction we have also imputed to the hippocampal formation. What are the observations which give rise to the idea of positive cue modelling? What is gained by our assumption that the hippocampal formation undergoes self-suppression when a modelled positive cue is actually presented?

Relevant to these questions are the results of Blanchard and his colleagues (Blanchard and Blanchard, 1969; Blanchard *et al.*, 1970) indicating that the tonically acting contextual cues in the experimental situation (apparatus cues) induce "freezing" after rat subjects have experienced shock during avoidance training. These experiments demonstrated additionally that acquired freezing controlled by apparatus stimuli was countered by an opposite behavioral tendency (running) controlled by the specific shock-signaling cue. In subjects with hippocampi intact the freezing response controlled by the apparatus stimuli interfered with successful performance of running to the shock-predictive CS. However, there was an absence of apparatus-related freezing in subjects with hippocampal lesions, and a consequent facilitation of avoidance responses to the specific cue. These data suggest that in active avoidance tasks the apparatus stimuli may function as a negative cue, whereas the specific CS may serve as a positive cue. Because the apparatus stimuli are present tonically there would be tonic hippocampal suppression of the excitatory cortical and thalamic code. In this situation the CS must serve to remove the tonic suppression so that the excitatory code may trigger active avoidance.

These assumptions provide an account of the commonly reported facilitation produced by hippocampal lesions, of active avoidance acquisition in the two-way shuttle-box situation (see the reviews by Isaacson, 1974; Black *et al.*, 1977). The idea here is that in normal subjects, the suppressive conrol exerted by the stimuli of the to-be-entered shuttle-box compartment blocks entry and thereby retards acquisition. In lesioned subjects this suppressive influence is absent and the excitatory control mediated via CS driven significance codes in cortex and in the AV nucleus operate unopposed to promote frequent and successful avoidance.

These assumptions may be used to provide an account of our own findings on the relation between avoidance performance in the wheel apparatus and the rhythmic theta-like neuronal bursts of rabbit CA1 and subicular complex (Section IV,A).

Of prime importance here is the observation that the rabbits perform relatively little locomotory behavior during the intertrial interval in our task. Moreover, locomotion does not typically occur in the trained animal following onset of the CS+, until more than 70% of the CS–UCS interval has elapsed (see Fig. 1). In Pavlovian terms, the animal is said to be undergoing inhibition of delay, during the initial 70% of the interval. Speaking anthropomorphically, the animal seems to withhold committment to response until the last instant.

During the final 30% of the CS–UCS interval there is a volley of rhythmic 10 per second theta-like neuronal bursts, followed by the locomotory avoidance response. Thus, occurrence of the behavior is preceded by 10 per second theta-like activity and the absence of behavior is associated with the absence of 10 per second theta-like activity, in the trained animal.

We suggest that the absence of 10 per second activity and the relative behavioral immobility that accompanies that absence reflect the operation of contextually driven, hippocampally mediated suppression of the excitatory code for significance.

The contextually driven inhibitory effect holds movement in check until exactly the right circumstance (presentation of the CS+) occurs. When this happens input to the hippocampal formation, in the form of the significance code from cingulate cortex and/or from the AV nucleus, provides a match with the existing hippocampal model of the CS+, and thereby serves to remove the hippocampal suppression of excitatory code for significance. The result is that primed behavior is released. The net effect is that output of behavior is precisely coordinated with critical stimulating circumstances. These ideas provide a basis for our assumption that hippocampal models are constructed for positive cues as well as for negative cues.

### D. NEUROPATHOLOGY OF LEARNING AND MEMORY IN HUMANS

#### 1. A Word on the Comparability of Human and Animal Performance

A basic premise of our account is that associative evoked activity in cortex and in thalamus serves as a "go" signal which fosters active behavioral responding. We have assumed that the behavior measured in our experiment is in some sense primed and held in an output mode, awaiting a signal for elicitation, in the trained animal (see Section IV,B, 1).

A problem arises in applying these ideas to human learning situations, because the tests of learning and memory which appear to reflect sensitively amnesia resulting from limbic system damage in humans are typically tests of paired associate learning or free recall, involving many stimuli and many responses. These tasks tap stimulus and response selection processes not tapped by the relatively simple conditioning paradigm which gave rise to our formulation. The question is, how may limbic significance coding processes operate in situations involving multiple stimuli and multiple responses?

One way to approach this issue would be to assume that all selection occurs at the level of significance code itself. In other words, we could argue that a qualitatively unique form of neuronal response develops in the limbic structures to each stimulus and that each unique code through S-R association elicits the appropriate response. This view places all of the burden of response selection upon the stimulus encoding properties of the limbic structures.

We do not believe that this idea represents a tenable approach to the problem, for it does not allow the stimulus properties of response items to contribute to acquisition and retention, a contribution known to occur on other grounds (e.g., Underwood *et al.*, 1959; Paivio *et al.*; 1968; Noble and McNeely, 1957). In addition, our own data do not lend themselves to the idea because of the requirement for assuming that encoding occurs in terms of qualitative differences in neuronal firing patterns that occur to different stimuli. Our data suggest that it is not the qualitative properties of the neuronal response which encodes significance but rather the quantity of firing. Large magnitude neuronal responses in the cingulate cortex and the AV nucleus are predictive of behavioral output whereas smaller responses or nonresponse are not. The suggestion is that a primed response will be triggered if a threshold of limbic neuronal activity is exceeded.

To incorporate into these ideas both the human and the animal situations one could assume that there is response priming (Sections IV,B,1, 3,4) in both situations and that each primed response sends a unique neuronal code for its identity to the limbic structures.

In the case of discriminative performance by the rabbit, there is only one response, and its identity code becomes a constant contextual input to the cingulate cortex and the AV nucleus. This input, identifying the response to these limbic structures is a must if the CS+ is to elicit a large neuronal effect in the limbic neurons. When the response code is coming in, the CS+ will work and the consequent large neuronal response in the limbic structures will serve to release the primed behavior. The main point is that conjoint input of the neuronal codes identifying stimuli *and* responses is essential for elicitation of significance code in these structures.

In the human case one could assume, using the paired-associate paradigm as a model, that all responses on the list are primed in an output mode and unique identity codes for each are sent sequentially to the cingulate cortex and the AV nucleus. In this instance the neurons in these structures receive conjoint input consisting of identity codes for stimuli and for responses.

In a typical recall test the cingulate cortex and the AV nucleus would receive the neuronal identity code for a given stimulus upon presentation of the stimulus item. At the same time there would be a succession of inputs to the cingulate cortex and the AV nucleus of the identity codes for the various primed responses. The neurons in the cingulate cortex and the AV nucleus would fire when the incoming response code corresponded to the response item that had been paired during learning with the currently operating stimulus code. In other words, neuronal activation of significance code in the cingulate cortex and the AV nucleus would occur when the stimulus code being sent to these structures represented a stimulu' item from the list, and when the response code being sent represented the response that was paired with that stimulus. Significance code triggered in the neurons in the cingulate cortex and the AV nucleus would elicit output of the response that was sending its identity code to these structures at that instant.

The hippocampal formation would have models of the S-R pairings appropriate to the list. Responses sending identity codes inappropriate to the stimulus item being presented would create mismatch with the hippocampal model, thereby eliciting code-suppression in cortex and thalamus. Thus, no response would occur.

These assumptions help in making a more direct application of our data from rabbits to the human learning case. The upshot of this formulation is that cingulate cortex and the AV nucleus provide a general facilitative form of neuronal activity, triggering primed responses when circumstances are appropriate. Stimulus and response information are both assessed in determining the appropriateness of circumstances. It is only the quantity of neuronal activity in these structures, not the quality, or pattern which has behavioral significance by this view.

## 2. Limbic Damage in Humans

Bilateral removal of the hippocampal formation by our account should deprive patients of capabilities for sharpening and extraction of generalized cortical significance code. On grounds of loss of sharpening, patients should be unable to form precise models of cues and contingencies. In addition, they should be unable to suppress generalized significance code elicited during acquisition by negative cues, and they should be unable to suppress codes appropriate to original learning, during tests involving transfer of training.

The process of relegation, in our account, confers temporal isolation of the significance code. Also, it represents switching-in of attention to stimulus dimensions of significance in a given learning situation (Section III,A,d). Finally, relegation underlies ample, criterial-level behavioral performance (Section III,A,d), characteristic of the highly trained individual. Absence of these functions in damaged humans should pro-

duce a deficient ability to retain information over relatively long intervals, deficient ability to focus attention on critical stimulus dimensions,
and an inability to manifest ample criterial-level memorial performance
after repeated exposure to stimuli and contingencies.

On the positive side, patients without hippocampi still have cortical
encoding mechanisms at their disposal. Thus, a rapid but generalized
form of encoding, only weakly in control of behavioral output should be
manifested by these patients.

The classic abnormality in hippocampectomized patients is the inability to show memory for events (such as a conversation) if there is a
disruption between the event and the occasion of recall. The disruption
need only be brief (such as going for a drink of water) to produce the
loss of memory. Information processing and very short-term memory
needed to sustain the patient's involvement during the original event appear to be intact.

The question of relevance here is, which of the abnormalities defined
in our account may be invoked to explain this classic amnesic syndrome?
It is not possible to single out any one of the several deficiencies suggested by our account. However, discriminative insufficiency due to inability to suppress generalized cortical code, inability to switch-in or attend to relevant stimulus dimensions, and absence of the (relegated)
neural code needed for clear-cut discriminative behavior may all contribute a share in production of the classic syndrome.

Compatible with the idea of cortical mnemonic processing in amnesic
patients is the general finding that memories *are* indeed formed in the
amnesic patients (see review by Weiskrantz, 1978). Nevertheless, several
studies indicate that special pains must be taken, such as provision of
"recall cues" about material to be remembered, in order to demonstrate
retention by amnesics in paradigms such as paired associate learning or
free recall (Warrington and Weiskrantz, 1968, 1971, 1974). This outcome is generally in accord with our idea of the remoteness of cortical
encoding from behavioral expression.

Also, highly abnormal, dogged persistence by amnesics in inappropriate recall of originally learned material has been shown for situations in which similar recall cues were employed in original learning and
in subsequent tests (Warrington and Weiskrantz, 1974; Winocur and
Weiskrantz, 1976). This effect is reminiscent of the "context bound"
features of cortical activity (Section IV,B,3), such as persistence in
cingulate cortex during reversal training of neuronal activity appropriate
to original learning (Section III,D). It is also reminiscent of the per-

sistence of originally acquired responses of hippocampectomized animals, during transfer of training.

Patients suffering Korsakoff's syndrome frequently display amnesia, with correlated damage to certain midline diencephalic structures (mammillary bodies, MD nucleus, fornix, AV nucleus, Section I). By our account, such patients should be capable of forming precise models of cues and contingencies, unlike the bilaterally hippocampectomized patients. However, diencephalic patients should be as deficient as the hippocampectomized patients in producing the precise and long-enduring relegated codes formed in the thalamic substrates.

To our knowledge, there is no evidence clearly in support of these assertions. Human amnesia associated with damage to midline diencephalic structures and amnesia associated with hippocampal damage seem to be indistinguishable. On the other hand, it would be inappropriate to accede to the impression of similarity of these groups in the absence of substantial experimental work directed explicitly at comparing them. In addition, one must allow that the diencephalic limbic structures may act with the hippocampal formation as one functional system (see Brion, 1969). Thus, whereas certain diencephalic structures (e.g., the AV nucleus, the MD nucleus) may serve as substrates for ample relegated code for significance, other diencephalic structures (e.g., fornix, mammillary bodies) often damaged in Korsakoff patients, may be essential to normal expression of the exclusively hippocampal processes of cue-modelling and code suppression that operate prior to relegation.

To summarize briefly, the fundamental proposition to emerge from our work is the idea that the behavior of anmesic human patients with limbic damage represents behavior mediated by a cortical mnemonic system. The cortical system lacks the functions of significance extraction in the form of construction of precise neural models for cues and contingencies, and in the form of relegated code associated with hippocampal and thalamic substrates, respectively. The cortical mechanism also lacks the attentional benefits of the switching-in process, and the advantages for endurance of memory afforded by the temporal isolation of the thalamic substrates.

These ideas suggest that consideration be given to a reorientation of the debate centering on whether human limbic amnesia is due to deficient storage or to deficient retrieval. The cortical mechanism which in our view mediates learning and memory in amnesics stores information and it retrieves information. Rather than questioning whether storage or retrieval is affected, it may turn out to be more productive to ask what are the neurophysiological mechanisms of storage and retrieval that operate in the cortical system, and what are the mechanisms of sharpening and relegation carried out by hippocampal and thalamic substrates?

One final point. Our electrophysiological studies have indicated a clear importance of animal limbic structures in mediation of animal learning and memory. We hope in addition that in deriving from our animal data inferences concerning human learning and memory, we have in some measure lessened the impact of the evolutionary divergence hypothesis, and broadened the base of support for use of animal models as an approach to the understanding of these processes.

## V. Summary

Our studies have shown that associative (discriminative) neuronal activity is acquired in cingulate cortex and in the anteroventral (AV) nucleus during the course of acquisition of discriminative avoidance behavior. The discriminative neuronal activity occurred in the form of a greater neuronal response to the CS+, than to the CS−.

The fundamental assertion that we advanced in relation to this finding is that the discriminative activity represents an acquired neuronal code for the significance of the conditional stimuli (CS+ and CS−). The neuronal code for significance is viewed here as discriminative neuronal activity essential for the rabbit's ability to use the CSs as cues for discriminative behavior.

The data indicated that the neuronal code for significance is established in three consecutive stages. The first two of these, labeled by us as *acquisition* and *specification* of the neuronal code, are processes reflected by activity in cingulate cortex.

*Acquisition* of the code denotes the increased neuronal response which occurs in the first session of avoidance training, relative to pretraining with tones and noncontingent footshock. The increased response is not discriminative within the modality of the CS (i.e., it occurs both to CS+ and CS−). However, we have adopted the working hypothesis that the increased response is specific to the modality of the CS. Thus, we predict that it would not occur to stimuli outside of the CS modality, should such stimuli be interspersed among the CSs during the initial trials of conditioning. Finally, our studies have indicated that acquisition of the code is specific to the deep laminae of cingulate cortex. It does not occur in superficial laminae or in the AV nucleus.

With continuation of training the CS+ retains its capacity to elicit the acquired neuronal code but the CS— shows a progressive loss of that capacity. This is the phenomenon denoted by our concept of *specification*. It is by way of *specification* that the acquired code for significance is made unique to a single stimulus (the CS+) within the modality of the CS. (It should be noted that *specification* occurs in parallel with the onset of behavioral discrimination in the course of training. This fact is important because it is requisite to our assertion that the discriminative neuronal activity is a causal precursor of behavioral discrimination.)

The third and final process whereby the neuronal code for significance is established is *relegation*, a term used to denote the development of discriminative neuronal activity in the AV nucleus, in a late stage of acquisition, during performance of ample behavioral discrimination. Through *relegation* the neuronal code which is acquired and specified in the deep laminae of cingulate cortex is transferred to neurons of the AV nucleus. These neurons now produce the significance code, freeing cingulate cortex to process other new incoming discriminative problems. Properties of the late developing relegated code suggest that it may play an important role in mediating ample criterial level behavioral performance, long-term retention of the behavioral discrimination, and focusing of attention on the CS.

Our data indicate that discriminative neuronal activity develops in the late stage of behavioral acquisition, in the superficial laminae of cingulate cortex, as well as in the AV nucleus. The late developing activity in the superficial laminae is presumed to represent the relegated discrimination in the AV nucleus fed back to the superficial laminae via the thalamocortical pathway. We suggest here that the feedback signal informs cingulate cortex that *relegation* of the code for significance has taken place. This information promotes disengagement of the cingulate cortex from direct participation in the significance coding process. Thus, as mentioned previously, cingulate cortex is freed to engage new problems. Given disengagement, production of the significance code for the current problem is handled at the level of the AV nucleus.

Studies of the behavioral effects of lesions indicate that cingulate cortex is an important neural substrate for acquisition of aversively motivated behavior, but not for retention of the behavior. Lesions in the AV nucleus have been shown to disrupt retention. These findings are in fundamental agreement with the inferences derived from our data implicating cingulate cortex in *acquisition* and *specification* of significance code, and envisioning the AV nucleus as a substrate for relegated significance code.

Of major influence in the development of our concept of significance code are findings from studies of brain damage in animals indicating that lesions in cingulate cortex disrupt acquisition of aversively motivated behavior only when subjects are required to respond to a discrete, unimodal, phasically presented cue. Disruption does not occur if the task employed is one-way active avoidance, or passive avoidance—tasks which involve use of the tonic multimodal stimulus context as the "cue" for the behavior. These findings coupled with our data on neuronal discrimination suggest that what is conferred by intact cingulate cortex is the ability to use a discrete unimodal stimulus as a cue for avoidance behavior. It is precisely this function that we maintain is conferred by code for significance of conditional stimuli.

The convergence of ideas developed from the two diverse methodologies, involving induced brain damage on the one hand, and neuronal recording on the other, illustrates the complementary nature of these two approaches.

The idea that subordination of cingulate cortex to the AV nucleus in processing of task stimuli occurs after relegation was supported by the results obtained during reversal training. Specifically the results indicated that reversal of neuronal discrimination occurred in the AV nucleus, but not in cingulate cortex. Viewed in the context of our current framework we interpret this outcome to indicate that cingulate cortex does not reinitiate acquisition and specification of the significance code for reversal. Rather, once relegation of the significance coding process to AV nucleus has taken place, further modification of the code, such as its reversal, is carried out in terms of interactions between the AV nucleus and the hippocampal formation.

This is not to imply that cingulate cortex manifests a passive noninvolvement in the reversal process. In fact neurons of the deep laminae showed a pronounced retention of the originally acquired neuronal discrimination which persisted throughout a considerable extent of reversal training. The persistence was greater in nonovertrained rabbits than in overtrained rabbits. In addition, the overall (nondiscriminative) reactivity of neurons in all laminae of cingulate cortex was greater throughout reversal training in nonovertrained rabbits, compared to overtrained rabbits. Conversely, reactivity of neurons in the AV nucleus during reversal was enhanced by overtraining. These differences occurred in conjunction with the behavioral ORE. That is, nonovertrained rabbits required a significantly greater number of training sessions than that required by overtrained rabbits, to meet the criterion of reversal.

We interpreted these results to indicate that the significance code appropriate to original training, which persisted in the deep cingulate laminae throughout reversal in nonovertrained rabbits, interfered with the attainment of behavioral reversal in these animals. Moreover, the greater reactivity of deep cingulate neurons during reversal in nonovertrained as opposed to overtrained rabbits may have represented a greater overall weighting for the interfering cortical activity. Thus, our results suggested that the behavioral ORE occurs because of greater persistence in cortex of residual discriminative neuronal activity appropriate to original learning, for nonovertrained subjects compared to overtrained subjects.

The hippocampal formation is reciprocally interconnected with cingulate cortex and with the AV nucleus. This fact coupled with observations of hippocampal neuronal activity made in our laboratory and in other laboratories led us to a formulation about the behavioral relevance of the hippocampal formation. This formulation involved the following propositions: (a) Significance code in cingulate cortex and in the AV nucleus triggers the output of primed behavioral responses; these structures are part of a neural "go" system. (b) The hippocampal formation receives significance code from cingulate cortex and from the AV nucleus as a major source of input—i.e., the hippocampal formation is a "downstream" processor of significance code. (c) The hippocampal formation uses generalized significance code from cortex at the outset of training, to construct more precise less generalized neuronal models of the positive and negative cues, and of the contingencies of the cues with their consequences. (d) Model construction in the hippocampal formation occurs very rapidly at the outset of training, and reconstruction of the models occurs rapidly, following experimental shift in cues and/or their contingencies. (e) Activity projected from the hippocampal formation serves to suppress facilitative significance code in cingulate cortex and in AV nucleus. Such suppressive output serves to inhibit the output of primed behavioral responses. (f) Once cue-models are constructed, occurrence of a positive cue blocks the suppressive hippocampal output, allowing cortical and thalamic significance code to trigger the output of primed responses. (g) Occurrence of a negative cue promotes suppressive hippocampal output and prevents behavioral response. (h) Theta-like neuronal activity projected from the hippocampal formation to the AV nucleus contributes to construction of relegated code for significance in that structure, for problems in which the subject is required to predicate behavioral responding on the occurrence of discrete, isolated nonsalient cues.

These propositions were used along with our observations on neuronal activity in cingulate cortex and the AV nucleus, to provide an interpretation of some of the well-established consequences of limbic system damage for performance in learning and memory tasks. The totality of our work suggests that cingulate cortex, hippocampal formation, and the AV nucleus act in a coordinated fashion to bring about initial encoding and subsequent extraction of stimulus significance, during learning in animals and in humans.

## References

Adams, R. D. (1969). The anatomy of memory mechanisms in the human brain. *In* "The Pathology of Memory" (G. A. Talland and N. C. Waugh, eds.), pp. 91–106. Academic Press, New York.

Altman, J., Brunner, R. L., and Bayer, S. A. (1973). The hippocampus and behavioral maturation. *Behavioral Biology* **8**, 557–596.

Angelergues, R. (1969). Memory disorders in neurological disease. *In* "Handbook of Clinical Neurology" (P. J. Vinken and G. W. Bruyn, eds.), "Disorders of Higher Nervous Activity," Vol. 3. American Elsevier, New York.

Barbizet, J. (1963). Defect of memorizing of hippocampal–mammillary origin: A review. *Journal of Neurology, Neurosurgery and Psychiatry* **26**, 127–135.

Bennett, T. L. (1975). The electrical activity of the hippocampus and processes of attention. *In* "The Hippocampus." Vol. II: "Neurophysiology and Behavior" (R. L. Isaacson and K. H. Pribram, eds.), pp. 71–97. Plenum, New York.

Berger, T. W., and Thompson, R. F. (1977). Limbic system interrelations: Functional division among hippocampal–septal connections. *Science* **197**, 587–589.

Berger T. W. and Thompson, R. F. (1978). Neuronal plasticity in the limbic system during classical conditioning of the rabbit nictitating membrane response. I. The hippocampus. *Brain Research* **145**, 323–346.

Berger, T. W., Alger, B., and Thompson, R. F. (1976). Neuronal substrates of classical conditioning in the hippocampus. *Science* **192**, 483–485.

Berger, T. W., Milner, T. A., Swanson, G. W., Lynch, G. S., and Thompson, R. F. (1979). Reciprocal anatomical connections between cingulate-retrosplenial cortex and anteroventral thalamus in the rabbit studied with horseradish peroxidase. *Society for Neuroscience, Abstract Bulletin,* #888, p. 270.

Black, A. H., Nadel, L., and O'Keefe, J. O. (1977). Hippocampal function in avoidance learning and punishment. *Psychological Bulletin* **84**, 1107–1129.

Blanchard, R. J., and Blanchard, C. D. (1969). Passive and active reactions to fear-eliciting stimuli. *Journal of Comparative and Physiological Psychology* **18**, 129–135.

Blanchard, R. J., Blanchard, C. D., and Fial, R. A. (1970). Hippocampal lesions in rats and their effect on activity, avoidance, and aggression. *Journal of Comparative and Physiological Psychology* **71**, 92–102.

Brion, S. (1969). Korsakoff's syndrome: Clinico-anatomical and physiopathological conditions. In "The Pathology of Memory" (G. A. Talland and N. C. Waugh, eds.), pp. 28–40. Academic Press, New York.

Brogden, W. J., and Culler, F. A. (1936). A device for motor conditioning of small animals. *Science* **83**, 269.

Buchwald, J. S., and Brown, K. A. (1973). Subcortical mechanisms of behavioral plasticity. *In* "Efferent Organization and the Integration of Behavior" (J. D. Maser, ed.), pp. 100–136. Academic Press, New York.

Carey, R. J., Fitzpatrick, D., and Diamond, I. J. (1979). Thalamic projections to layer I of striate cortex shown by retrograde transport of horseradish peroxidase. *Science* **203**, 556–559.

Coover, G., Ursin, H., and Levine, S. (1974). Corticosterone levels during avoidance learning in rats with cingulate lesions suggest an instrumental reinforcement deficit. *Journal of Comparative and Physiological Psychology* **87**, 970–977.

Correll, R. E., and Scoville, W. B. (1967). Significance of delay in performance of monkeys with medial temporal lobe resections. *Experimental Brain Research* **4**, 85–96.

Denny, M. R. (1970). Elicitation theory applied to an analysis of the overlearning reversal effect. *In* "Current Issues in Animal Learning" (J. H. Reynierse, ed.), pp. 175–194. Academic Press, New York.

Dickinson, A. (1974). Response supression and facilitation by aversive stimuli following septal lesions in rats: A review and model. *Physiological Psychology* **2**, 444–456.

Disterhoft, J. (1977). Short latency discriminative unit responses: One way to search for the engram. *Physiological Psychology* **7**, 498–500.

Disterhoft, J., and Segal, M. (1978). Neuron activity in rat hippocampus and motor cortex during discrimination reversal. *Brain Research Bulletin* **3**, 583–588.

Domesick, V. B. (1969). Projections from cingulate cortex in the rat. *Brain Research* **12**, 296–320.

Domesick, V. B. (1970). The fasciculus cinguli in the rat. *Brain Research* **20**, 19–32.

Domesick, V. B. (1972). Thalamic relationships of the medial cortex in the rat. *Brain, Behavior and Evolution* **6**, 141–169.

Douglas, R. J. (1967). The hippocampus and behavior. *Psychological Bulletin* **67**, 416–422.

Douglas, R. J. (1972). Pavlovian conditioning and the brain. *In* "Inhibition and Learning" In (R.A. Boakes and M. S. Halliday, eds.), pp. 529–565. Academic Press, New York.

Douglas, R. J., and Pribram, K. H. (1966). Learning and limbic lesions. *Neuropsychologia* **4**, 197–220.

Eckersdorf, B. (1974). The effects of lesions in the posterior part of the gyrus cinguli on the conditioned defensive response of active avoidance in cats. *Acta Physiological Polonica* **2**, 105–114.

Fish, B. S. (1975). Unpublished review of studies and effects of hippocampal lesions on acquisition and performance of discriminative behavior.

Foster, K., Orona, I., Lambert, R. W., and Gabriel, M. (1980). Unit activity of the deep and superficial laminae of rabbit cingulate-retrosplenial cortex, and the anteroventral nucleus of thalamus, during discriminative avoidance conditioning and overtraining. *Journal of Comparative and Physiological Psychology* (in press).

Freeman, F. G. (1978). Cue utilization and hippocampal lesions in rats. *Physiological Psychology* **6**, 275–278.

Gabriel, M. (1970). Intersession exposure of rabbits to the conditioning apparatus, avoidance extinction and intertrial behavior. *Journal of Comparative and Physiological Psychology* **72**, 244–249.

Gabriel, M. (1972). Incubation of avoidance produced by generalization to stimuli of the conditioning apparatus. *Topics in Learning and Performance* (R. F. Thompson and J. V. Voss, eds.), pp. 50–84. Academic Press, New York.

Gabriel, M. (1976). Short latency discriminative unit reaction: Engram or bias? *Physiological Psychology* **4**, 275–280.

Gabriel, M., and Saltwick, S. E. (1977). Effects of unpaired footshock on rabbit limbic and auditory neuronal responses to tone stimuli. *Physiology and Behavior* **19**, 29–34.

Gabriel, M., and Saltwick, S. E. (1980). Rhythmic, theta-like unit activity of the hippocampal formation during acquisition and performance of avoidance behavior in rabbits. *Physiology & Behavior* (in press).

Gabriel, M., Wheeler, W., and Thompson, R. F. (1973a). Multiple-unit activity of the rabbit cerebral cortex in single-session avoidance conditioning. *Physiological Psychology* **1**, 45–55.

Gabriel, M., Wheeler, W., and Thompson, R. F. (1973b). Multiple-unit activity of the rabbit cerebral cortex during stimulus generalization of avoidance behavior. *Physiological Psychology* **1**, 313–320.

Gabriel, M., Miller, J. D., and Saltwick, S. E. (1976). Multiple-unit activity of the rabbit medial geniculate nucleus during conditioning, extinction and reversal. *Physiological Psychology* **4**, 124–134.

Gabriel, M., Saltwick, S. E., and Miller, J. D. (1977a). Unit activity of anterior cingulate cortex in differential conditioning and reversal. *Bulletin of the Psychonomic Society* **9**, 207–210.

Gabriel, M., Miller, J. D., and Saltwick, S. E. (1977b). Unit activity in cingulate cortex and anteroventral thalamus of the rabbit during differential conditioning and reversal. *Journal of Comparative and Physiological Psychology* **91**, 423–433.

Gabriel, M., Foster, K., and Orona, E. (1980a). Unit activity in limbic cortex and anteroventral thalamus during acquisition and overtraining of discriminative avoidance behavior in rabbits. *In* "Neural Mechanisms of Goal-Directed Behavior and Learning" (R. F. Thompson, L. H. Hicks, and V. B. Shvyrkov, eds.), Academic Press, New York (in press).

Gabriel, M., Orona, E., Lambert, R. W., and Foster, K. (1980b). Neuronal activity of deep and superficial laminae of cingulate cortex and the anteroventral thalamus during reversal of discriminative avoidance behavior in rabbits. Submitted.

Gabriel, M., Orona, E., Foster, F., and Lambert, R. W. (1980c). Neural bases of the over-training reversal effect. Submitted.

Gabriel, M., Foster, K., and Orona, E. (1980d). Interaction of superficial and deep laminae of cingulate cortex with anteroventral nucleus of thalamus during behavioral learning. *Science* (in press).

Gaffan, D. (1974). Recognition impaired and association intact in the memory of monkeys after transection of the fornix. *Journal of Comparative and Physiological Psychology* **86**, 1100–1109.

Grastyan, E., Lissak, K., Madarasz, I., and Donhoffer, H. (1959). Hippocampal electrical activity during the development of conditioned reflexes. *Electroencephalography and Clinical Neurophysiology* **11**, 409–430.

Green, J. D., and Arduini, A. (1954). Hippocampal electrical activity in arousal. *Journal of Neurophysiology* **17**, 533–557.

Guillery, R. W. (1956). Degeneration in the post-commissural fornix and the mamillary peduncle of the rat. *Journal of Anatomy* **90**, 350–368.

Harper, R. M. (1973). Relationships of neuronal activity to EEG waves during sleep and wakefulness. *In* "Brain Unit Activity and Behavior" (M. I. Phillips, ed.), pp. 130–154. Thomas, Springfield, Illinois.

Hearst, E., and Jenkins, H. M. (1974). "Sign-tracking: The Stimulus–Reinforcer Relation and Directed Action." Psychonomic Society, Austin, Texas.

Hoffman, H. S. (1966). The analysis of discriminated avoidance. In "Operant Behavior: Areas of Research and Application" (W. K. Honig, ed.), Appleton-Century-Crofts, pp. 499–530. New York.

Horel, J. A. (1978). The neuroanatomy of amnesia: A critique of the hippocampal memory hypothesis. Brain 10, 403–445.

Isaacson, R. (1974). "The Limbic System." Plenum, New York.

Iversen, S. D. (1973). Brain lesions and memory in animals. In "The Physiological Basis of Memory" (J. A. Deutsch, ed.), pp. 305–356. Academic Press, New York.

Jarrard, L. E. (1975). Role of interference in retention by rats with hippocampal lesions. Journal of Comparative and Physiological Psychology 89, 400–408.

Jarrard, L. E. (1978). Selective hippocampal lesions: Differential effects on performance by rats of a spatial task with preoperative versus postoperative training. Journal of Comparative and Physiological Psychology 92, 1119–1127.

Jarrard, L. E., Isaacson, R. L., (1965). Hippocampal ablation in rats: Effects of intertrial interval. Nature (London) 207, 117–124.

Jarrard, L. E., Isaacson, R. L., and Wickelgren, W. O. (1964). Effects of hippocampal ablation and intertrial interval on acquisition and extinction of a runway response. Journal of Comparative and Physiological Psychology 57, 442–445.

Kahn, E. A., and Crosby, E. C. (1972). Korsakoff's syndrome associated with surgical lesions involving the mammillary bodies. Neurology 22, 117–124.

Kappers, C. U., Ariens, (1909). The phylogenesis of the paleocortex and archicortex compared with the evolution of the visual neocortex. Archives of Neurology and Psychiatry 4, 161–193.

Kesner, R. P., and Wilburn, M. W. (1974). A review of electrical stimulation of the brain in context of learning and retention. Behavioral Biology 10, 249–293.

Kimble, D. P. (1963). The effects of bilateral hippocampal lesions in rats. Journal of Comparative and Physiological Psychology 56, 273–283.

Kimble, D. P. (1968). The hippocampus and internal inhibition. Psychological Bulletin 70, 285–295.

Kimble, D. P., and Dannen, E. (1977). Persistent spatial maze learning deficits in hippocampal-lesioned rats across a 7-week postoperative period. Physiological Psychology 5, 409–413.

Kimble, D. P., and Gostnell, D. (1968). Role of cingulate cortex in shock avoidance behavior of rats. Journal of Comparative and Physiological Psychology 65, 290–294.

Kimble, D. P., and Kimble, R. J. (1965). Hippocampectomy and response perseveration in the rat. Journal of Comparative and Physiological Psychology 60, 474–476.

Kimble, D. P., and Pribram, K. H. (1963). Hippocampectomy and behavior sequences. Science 139, 401–407.

Kimble, G. (1961). "Hilgard and Marquis' Conditioning and Learning." Appleton-Century-Crofts, New York.

Krettek, J. E., and Price, J. L. (1977). The cortical projections of the mediodorsal nucleus and adjacent thalamic nuclei in the rat. Journal of Comparative Neurology 2, 157–192.

Lambert, R. W., Foster, K., Orona, E., and Gabriel, M. (1980). Rhythmic theta-like unit activity recorded from the rabbit anteroventral nucleus of the thalamus during performance of conditioned avoidance responses. In preparation.

Lash, L. (1964). Response discriminability and the hippocampus. Journal of Comparative and Physiological Psychology 57, 251–256.

Lashley, K. S. (1951). The problem of serial ordering in behavior. In "Cerebral Mechanisms of Behavior" (L. A. Jeffress, ed.), pp. 112–136. Wiley, New York.

Lenn, N. J. (1978). Fornix afferents to the anteroventral thalamic nucleus: An EM study in the rat. *Brain Research Bulletin* **3**, 589–593.

Linesman, M. A., and Olds, J. (1973). Activity changes in rat hypothalamic, preoptic area and striatum associated with Pavlovian conditioning. *Journal of Neurophysiology* **36**, 1038–1050.

Lovejoy, E. (1966). Analysis of the overlearning reversal effect. *Psychological Review* **73**, 87–103.

Lubar, J. F. (1964). Effect of medial cortical lesions on the avoidance behavior of the cat. *Journal of Comparative and Physiological Psychology* **58**, 38–46.

Lubar, J. F., and Perachio, A. A. (1965). One-way and two-way learning and transfer of an active avoidance response in normal and cingulectomized cats. *Journal of Comparative and Physiological Psychology* **60**, 46–52.

Mackintosh, N. J. (1974). "The Psychology of Animal Learning." Academic Press, New York.

McCleary, R. A. (1961). Response specificity in the behavioral effects of limbic system lesions in the cat. *Journal of Comparative and Physiological Psychology* **54**, 605–613.

McCleary, R. A. (1966). Response-modulating functions of the limbic system: Initiation and suppression. *In* "Progress in Physiological Psychology" (E. Stellar and J. M. Sprague, eds.), Vol. 1, pp. 209–272. Academic Press, New York.

Malamud, M., and Skillicorn, S. A. (1956). Relationship between the Wernicke and the Korsakoff syndrome. *AMA Archives of Neurology and Psychiatry* **76**, 585–596.

Means, L. W., Walker, D. W., and Isaacson, R. L. (1970). Facilitated single alternation go, no–go acquisition following hippocampectomy in the rat. *Journal of Comparative and Physiological Psychology* **72**, 278–285.

Means, L. W., Leander, J. D., and Isaacson, R. L. (1971). The effect of hippocampectomy on alternation behavior and response to novelty. *Physiology and Behavior* **6**, 17–22.

Means, L. W., Woodruff, M. L., and Isaacson, R. L. (1972). The effect of a twenty-four hour intertrial interval on the acquisition of a spatial discrimination by hippocampally damaged rats. *Physiology and Behavior* **8**, 457–462.

Meibach, R. C., and Siegel, A. (1977a). Thalamic projections of the hippocampal formation: Evidence for an alternate pathway involving the internal capsule. *Brain Research* **134**, 1–12.

Meibach, R. C., and Siegel, A. (1977b). Subicular projections to the posterior cingulate cortex in rats. *Experimental Neurology* **57**, 264–274.

Micco, D. J., and Schwartz, M. (1971). Effects of hippocampal lesions upon the development of Pavlovian internal inhibition. *Journal of Comparative and Physiological Psychology* **76**, 371–377.

Milner, B. (1970). Memory and the medial temporal regions of the brain. *In* "The Biology of Memory" (K. H. Pribram and D. E. Broadbent, eds.), pp. 29–50. Academic Press, New York.

Milner, B. (1972). Disorders of learning and memory after temporal lobe lesions in man. *Clinical Neurosurgery* **19**, 421–446.

Mis, F. W. (1977). A midbrain–brain stem circuit for conditioned inhibition of the nictitating membrane response in the rabbit (*Oryctolagus cuniculus*). *Journal of Comparative and Physiological Psychology* **91**, 975–988.

Mishkin, M. (1978). Memory in monkeys severely impaired by combined but not by separate removal of amygdala and hippocampus. *Nature (London)* **273**, 297–298.

Mishkin, M., and Pribram, K. H. (1954). Visual discrimination performance following partial ablation of the temporal lobes. I. Ventral vs. lateral. *Journal of Comparative and Physiological Psychology* **47**, 14–20.

Moore, J. W. (1979). Information processing in space-time by the hippocampus. *Physiological Psychology* **7**, 224–232.

Moore, R. Y. (1964). Effects of some rhinencephalic lesions on conditioned avoidance behavior in cats. *Journal of Comparative and Physiological Psychology* **57**, 65–71.

Nadel, L., O'Keefe, J., and Black, A. (1975). Slam on brakes: A critique of Altman, Brunner, and Bayer's response-inhibition model of hippocampal function. *Behavioral Biology* **14**, 151–162.

Nauta, W. J. H. (1956). An experimental study of the fornix system in the rat. *Journal of Comparative Neurology* **104**, 247–272.

Niki, H. (1962). The effects of hippocampal ablation on the behavior in the rat. *Japanese Psychological Research* **4**, 139–153.

Noble, C. E., and McNeely, D. A. (1957). The role of meaningfulness (m) in paired-associate verbal learning. *Journal of Experimental Psychology* **53**, 16–22.

Oakley, D. A., and Russell, I. S. (1973). Differentiation and reversal of conditioning in decorticate rabbits. *IRCS Journal, Medical Sciences* (73-11) 46-13-1.

Oakley, D. A., and Russell, I. S. (1974a). Differential and reversal conditioning in partially neodecorticate rabbits. *Physiology and Behavior* **13**, 221–230.

Oakley, D. A., and Russell, I. S. (1974b). Pavlovian discrimination learning in decorticate and hemidecorticate rabbits. *IRCS Journal, Medical Sciences* **2**, 1065.

O'Keefe, J. O., and Nadel, L. (1978). "The Hippocampus as a Cognitive Map." Oxford University Press, Oxford.

Olds, J., Disterhoft, J., Segal, M., Kornblith, L. D., and Hirsh, R. (1972). Learning centers of rat brain mapped by measuring latencies of conditioned unit responses. *Journal of Neurophysiology* **35**, 202–219.

Olton, D. S., Walker, J. A., and Gage, F. H. (1978). Hippocampal connections and spatial discrimination. *Brain Research* **139**, 295–308.

Orbach, J., and Fantz, R. L. (1958). Differential effects of temporal neo-cortical resections on overtrained and nonovertrained visual habits in monkeys. *Journal of Comparative and Physiological Psychology* **51**, 126–129.

Orona, E., Foster, K., Lambert, R. W., and Gabriel, M. (1980). Contribution of rabbit cingulate-retrosplenial cortex and anteroventral nucleus of thalamus to the overtraining reversal effect. In preparation.

Paivio, A., Smythe, P. C., and Yuille, J. C. (1968). Imagery versus meaningfulness of nouns in paired associated learning. *Canadian Journal of Psychology,* **22**, 427–441.

Paul, C. (1965). Effects of overlearning upon single habit reversal in rats. *Psychological Bulletin* **63**, 65–72.

Penfield, W., and Milner, B. (1958). Memory deficit produced by bilateral lesions in the hippocampal zone. *AMA Archives of Neurology and Psychiatry* **79**, 475–497.

Poletti, C. E., and Creswell, G. (1977). Fornix system efferent projections in the squirrel monkey: An experimental degeneration study. *Journal of Comparative Neurology* **175**, 101–128.

Pribram, K. H., and Weiskrantz, L. (1957). A comparison of the effects of medial and lateral cerebral resection on conditioned avoidance behavior of monkeys. *Journal of Comparative and Physiological Psychology* **50**, 74–80.

Raisman, G., Cowan, W. M., and Powell, T. P. S. (1965). An experimental analysis of the efferent projection of the hippocampus. *Brain* **89**, 83–108.

Ranck, J. B. Jr. (1973). Studies on single neurons in dorsal hippocampal formation and septum in unrestrained rats: I. Behavioral correlates and firing repertoires. *Experimental Neurology* **41**, 461–531.

Ranck, J. B. (1975). Behavioral correlates and firing repertoires of neurons in dorsal hippocampal formation and septum of unrestrained rats. *In* "The Hippocampus" (R. L. Isaacson and K. H. Pribram, eds.), vol. 2, pp. 207–246. Plenum, New York.

Ranson, S. W., and Clark, S. L. (1959). "The Anatomy of the Nervous System: Its Development and Function," 10th ed., p. 351. Saunders, Philadelphia.

Rescorla, R. A. (1967). Pavlovian conditioning and its proper control procedures. *Psychological Review* **74**, 71–80.

Rescorla, R. A. (1969). Pavlovian conditioned inhibition. *Psychological Bulletin* **72**, 77–94.

Rich, I., and Thompson, R. (1965). Role of the hippocampo-septal system, thalamus, and hypothalamus in avoidance conditioning. *Journal of Comparative and Physiological Psychology* **59**, 66–72.

Rickert, E. J., Bennett, T. L., Lane, P., and French, J. (1978). Hippocampectomy and the attenuation of blocking. *Behavioral Biology* **2**, 147–160.

Rose, J. E., and Woolsey, C. N. (1948). Structure and relations of limbic cortex and anterior thalamic nuclei in rabbit and cat. *Journal of Comparative Neurology* **89**, 279–340.

Rose, M. (1933). Zytoarchitektonischer Atlas der Grosshirnrinde des Kaninchens. *Journal für Psychologie und Neurologie* **43**, 353–440.

Routtenberg, A. (1971). Stimulus processing and response execution: A neurobehavioral theory. *Physiology and Behavior* **6**, 589–596.

Saltwick, S. E., and Gabriel, M. (1980). Relationships of non-bursting neuronal activity of the hippocampal formation to acquisition and performance of discriminative avoidance behavior in rabbits. In preparation (1966).

Schmaltz, L. W., and Isaacson, R. L. (1966). The effects of preliminary training conditions upon DRL performance in the hippocampectomized rat. *Physiology and Behavior* **1**, 175–182.

Schmaltz, L. W., and Theios, J. (1972). Acquisition and extinction of a classically conditioned response in hippocampectomized rabbits (*Oryctolagus cuniculus*). *Journal of Comparative and Physiological Psychology* **79**, 328–333.

Schreiner, L., and Kling, A. (1953). Behavioral changes following rhinencephalic injury in the cat. *Journal of Neurophysiology* **16**, 59–65.

Scoville, W. B. (1954). The limbic lobe in man. *Journal of Neurosurgery* **11**, 64–66.

Scoville, W. B., and Milner, B. (1957). Loss of recent memory after bilateral hippocampal lesions. *Journal of Neurology, Neurosurgery and Psychiatry* **20**, 11–21.

Segal, M. (1973). Flow of conditioned responses in limbic telencephalic system of the rat. *Journal of Neurophysiology* **36**, 840–854.

Segal, M., and Olds, J. (1972). Behavior of units in hippocampal circuit of rat during learning. *Journal of Neurophysiology* **35**, 680–690.

Shiffrin, R. M., and Schneider, W. (1977). Controlled and automatic human information processing: II. Perceptual learning, automatic attending, and a general theory. *Psychological Review* **84**, 127–190.

Shipley, M. T., and Sorensen, L. F. (1975). On the laminar organization of the anterior thalamus projections to the presubiculum in the guinea pig. *Brain Research* **86**, 473–477.

Shvyrkov, V. B., and Aleksandrov, Yu. I. (1973). Cortical neurons, the treatment of information, and the behavioral act. *Doklady Akademii Nauk SSSR* **212**, 1021–1024.

Siegel, A., Fukushima, T., Meibach, R., Burke, L., Edinger, H., and Weiner, S. (1977). The origin of the afferent supply to the mediodorsal thalamic nucleus: Enhancement of HRP transport by selective lesions. *Brain Research* **135**, 11–23.

Sikes, R. W., Chronister, R. B., and White, L. E., Jr. (1977). Origin of the direct hippocampus-anterior thalamic bundle in the rat: A combined horseradish peroxidase-Golgi analysis. *Experimental Neurology* **57**, 379–395.

Slotnick, B. M. (1971). Visual discrimination and avoidance behavior in rats with cingulate cortical lesions. *Neuropsychologia* **9**, 61–66.

Solomon, P. R. (1977). Role of the hippocampus in blocking and conditional inhibition of the rabbit's nictitating membrane response. *Journal of Comparative and Physiological Psychology* **91**, 407–417.

Solomon, P. R. (1979). Temporal versus spatial information processing theories of the hippocampal function. *Psychological Bulletin* **6**, 1272–1279.

Solomon, P. R., and Moore, J. W. (1975). Latent inhibition and stimulus generalization of the classically conditioned nictitating membrane response in rabbits (*Oryctolagus cuniculus*) following dorsal hippocampal ablations. *Journal of Comparative and Physiological Psychology* **89**, 1203.

Sperling, S. E. (1965). Reversal learning and resistance to extinction: A review of the rat literature. *Psychological Bulletin* **63**, 281–297.

Stevens, R., and Cowey, A. (1972). Enhanced alternation learning in hippocampal rats by means of added light cues. *Brain Research* **46**, 1–22.

Sutherland, N. S., and Mackintosh, N. J. (1971). "Mechanisms of Animal Discrimination Learning." Academic Press, New York.

Sweet, W. H., Talland, G. A., and Ervin, F. R. (1959). Loss of recent memory following section of the fornix. *Transactions of the American Neurological Association* **84**, 76–82.

Thomas, G. J., and Otis, L. S. (1958). Effects of rhinencephalic lesions on conditioning of an avoidance response in the rat. *Journal of Comparative and Physiological Psychology* **51**, 130–134.

Thomas, G. J., and Slotnick, B. M. (1962). Effects of lesions in the cingulum on maze learning and avoidance conditioning in the rat. *Journal of Comparative and Physiological Psychology* **55**, 1085–1091.

Thomas, G. J., Hostetter, G., and Barker, D. J. (1968). Behavioral functions of the limbic system. *In* "Progress in Physiological Psychology" (E. Stellar and J. M. Sprague, eds.), Vol 2, pp. 230–311. Academic Press, New York.

Thompson, R. F., and Kramer, R. F. (1965). Role of association cortex in sensory preconditioning. *Journal of Comparative and Physiological Psychology* **60**, 186–191.

Thompson, R. F., and Shaw, J. A. (1965). Behavioral correlates of evoked activity recorded from associative areas of the cerebral cortex. *Journal of Comparative and Physiological Psychology* **60**, 329–339.

Thompson, R. F., and Smith, H. E. (1967). Effects of association area lesions on auditory frequency discrimination in cat. *Psychonomic Science* **8**, 123–124.

Thompson, R. F., Johnson, R. H., and Hoopes, J. J. (1963). Organization of auditory, somatic sensory, and visual projection to association fields of cerebral cortex in the cat. *Journal of Neurophysiology* **26**, 343–364.

Trafton, C. L. (1967). Effects of lesions in the septal area and cingulate cortical areas on conditioned suppression of activity and avoidance behavior in rats. *Journal of Comparative and Physiological Psychology* **63**, 191–197.

Trafton, C. L., Filbey, R. A., and Johnson, R. W. (1969). Avoidance behavior in rats as a function of the size and location of anterior cingulate cortex lesions. *Psychonomic Science* **14**, 100–102.

Underwood, B. J., Runquist, W. N., and Schulz, R. W. (1959). Response learning in paired-associate lists as a function of intralist similarity. *Journal of Experimental Psychology* **58**, 70–78.

Ursin, H., Linck, P., and McCleary, R. A. (1969). Spatial differentiation of avoidance deficit following septal and cingulate lesions. *Journal of Comparative and Physiological Psychology* **68**, 74–79.

Vanderwolf, C. H. (1971). Limbic-diencephalic mechanisms of voluntary movement. *Psychological Review* **78**, 83–113.

Vanderwolf, C. H. (1975). Neocortical and hippocampal activation in relation to behavior. *Journal of Comparative and Physiological Psychology* **88**, 300–323.

Vanderwolf, C. H., and Cooley, R. K. (1974). Hippocampal electrical activity during long-continued avoidance performances: Effects of fatigue. *Physiology and Behavior* **13**, 819-823.

Vanderwolf, C. H., Bland, B. H., and Whishaw, I. Q. (1973). Diencephalic, hippocampal and neocortical mechanisms in voluntary movement. *In* "Efferent Organization and the Integration of Behavior" (J. D. Maser, Ed.), pp. 229-262. Academic Press, New York.

Victor, M., Adams, R. D., and Collins, G. H. (1971). "The Wernicke-Korsakoff Syndrome." David, Philadelphia.

Vinogradova, O. S. (1970). Registration of information and the limbic system. *In* "Short-Term Changes in Neural Activity and Behavior" (G. Horn and R. A. Hinde, eds.), pp. 95-141. Cambridge University Press, Cambridge.

Walker, H. M., and Lev, J. (1953). "Statistical Inference." Holt, New York.

Warrington, E. K., and Weiskrantz, L. (1968). A new method of testing long-term retention with special reference to amnesic patients. *Nature (London)* **217**, 972-974.

Warrington, E. K., and Weiskrantz, L. (1971). Organizational aspects of memory in amnesic patients. *Neuropsychologia* **9**, 67-73.

Warrington, E. K., and Weiskrantz, L. (1973). An analysis of short-term and long-term memory defects in man. *In* "The Physiological Basis of Memory" (J. A. Deutsch, ed.), pp. 365-395. Academic Press, New York.

Warrington, E. K., and Weiskrantz L. (1974). The effect of prior learning on subsequent retention in amnesic patients. *Neuropsychologia* **12**, 419-428.

Webster, K. E. (1965). The cortico-striatal projection in the cat. *Journal of Anatomy* **99**, 329-337.

Weiskrantz, L. (1978). A comparison of hippocampal pathology in man and other animals. *In* "Functions of the Septo-Hippocampal System," pp. 373-387. Ciba Foundation Symposium 58 (new series), Exerpta Medica, Elsevier, North-Holland, Amsterdam.

Whishaw, I. Q., and Vanderwolf, C. H. (1973). Hippocampal EEG and behavior: Changes in amplitude and frequency of theta (Theta rhythm) associated with the spontaneous and learned movement patterns of rats and cats. *Behavioral Biology* **8**, 461-484.

Whishaw, I. Q., and Nikkel, R. W. (1975). Anterior hypothalamic electrical stimulation and hippocampal EEG in the rat: Suppressed EEG, locomotion, self-stimulation and inhibition of shock avoidance. *Behavioral Biology* **13**, 1-20.

Winer, B. J. (1962). "Statistical Principles in Experimental Design." McGraw-Hill, New York.

Winocur, G. (1979). The effects of interference on discrimination learning and recall by rats with hippocampal lesions. *Physiology and Behavior* (in press).

Winocur, G., and Black, A. H. (1978). Cue induced recall of a passive avoidance response by rats with hippocampal lesions. *Physiology and Behavior* **21**, 39-44.

Winocur, G., and Breckenridge, C. B. (1973). Cue dependent behavior of hippocampally damaged rats in a complex maze. *Jouranl of Comparative and Physiological Psychology* **82**, 512-522.

Winocur, G., and Olds, J. (1978). Effects of context manipulation on memory and reversal learning in rats with hippocampal lesions. *Journal of Comparative and Physiological Psychology* **92**, 312-321.

Winocur, G., and Weiskrantz, L. A. (1976). Investigation of paired associate learning in amnesic patients. *Neuropsychologia* **14**, 97-100.

Wishart, T., and Mogenson, G. (1970). Effect of lesions of the hippocampus and septum before and after passive avoidance training. *Physiology and Behavior* **5**, 31-34.

Woodruff, M. L., and Isaacson, R. L. (1972). Discrimination learning in animals with lesions in hippocampus. *Behavioral Biology* **7**, 489-501.

PROGRESS IN PSYCHOBIOLOGY AND PHYSIOLOGICAL PSYCHOLOGY, VOL. 9

# Neural Mechanisms in Taste Aversion Learning

## John H. Ashe

*Department of Physiology*
*University of California at San Francisco*
*San Francisco, California*

### and

## Marvin Nachman

*Department of Psychology*
*University of California at Riverside*
*Riverside, California*

## I. Introduction

It is well established that if an animal experiences a change in internal state after consumption of a distinctly flavored food that animal will avoid future ingestion of that food. The prototypical paradigm to demonstrate food aversion learning consists of allowing an animal a brief period of ingestion of a novel food (CS) that is followed by the administration of a substance which alters the internal state (UCS) and usually produces behavioral signs of gastrointestinal distress. Although, the paradigm resembles traditional classical conditioning, taste aversion learning differs from it in two important ways. In contrast to the relatively brief optimum CS–UCS intervals (milliseconds to seconds) that will support the acquisition of most classically conditioned

233

Copyright © 1980 by Academic Press, Inc.
All rights of reproduction in any form reserved.
ISBN 0–12–542109–5

behaviors, a robust food aversion can be acquired when the interval between ingestion and change in internal state extends over several hours
(Etscorn and Stephens, 1973; Nachman, 1970a; Revusky, 1968; Smith
and Roll, 1967). In addition, food-related stimuli are apparently selectively associated with internally rather than externally initiated consequences (Garcia and Koelling, 1966). These major parametric deviations
suggest that biologically significant associations are formed much more
readily than biologically arbitrary associations (Seligman, 1970) and as
such may be particularly important for insight into the essential nature
of the neural associative process.

Because of the unique parametric properties of food aversion learning, a fundamental concern of many contempory psychologists has been
expressed in the question of whether a unitary process and set of principles underlies associative learning (Krane and Wagner, 1975; Revusky
and Garcia, 1970; Seligman, 1970; Testa, 1974). Numerous articles and
a recent symposium (Barker *et al.*, 1977) have been devoted to a review
of the theoretical aspects of taste aversion learning. In contrast,
the present article is a discussion of the neural mechanisms involved in
taste aversion learning with consideration of such issues as the identification of anatomical loci, the characteristics of those neural systems that
comprise the functional components of taste aversion learning, and the
identification of enduring cellular events that may be necessary for learning with long CS–UCS intervals.

As a consequence of the long-delay phenomenon, food aversion learning offers a unique model for the study of central associative
mechanisms, because these processes can be modulated by treatments interposed in the CS–UCS interval. However, some features of food aversion learning have presented particular difficulties for the study of
neural mechanisms, precluding, for example, the extensive use of intracellular or extracellular recording techniques to identify correlates of
the formation of long-delay associations. The problem lies in the difficulty of establishing experimental control of stimulus onset and other
parameters of both the CS and UCS. These difficulties have hampered
the rigorous investigation of the temporal characteristics and interrelationships of neural loci in the acquisition of learned taste aversions.
Accordingly, the bulk of research concerning the neurobiological
substrates of learned food aversions has utilized ablation and stimulation techniques. However, it should be recognized that these techniques,
though useful in suggesting the presence or absence of involvement of
certain loci in particular functions, cannot provide conclusive evidence
of integrative mechanisms.

## II. The Nature of the Conditioned Stimulus

It is clear that gustatory stimuli, in contrast to the appearance, texture, or location of the food, are the most sensitive stimuli for the acquisition of food aversions (for review see Nachman *et al.,* 1977a). Indeed, the most remarkable feature of taste aversion learning is the fact that the learning is specific to gustatory stimuli, i.e., robust, one-trial acquisition with an extended CS-UCS interval is obtained only when gustatory stimuli are used. As demonstrated in the pioneering study of Garcia and Koelling (1966), an animal somehow learns with remarkable ease and strength to avoid a particular taste when that taste is followed by sickness or some other internal consequence, but does not learn a similar aversion to visual, cutaneous, or auditory stimuli. Thus, it is appropriate to examine the nature of the specific neuronal events evoked by gustatory stimuli that are requisite for the acquisition of a learned taste aversion. A major question with which we are confronted is how can gustatory input persist in a potentially associable state such that when visceral events arise sometime later, an association can be established? Likewise, why is it that such an association cannot be established with visual, cutaneous, or auditory stimuli? One might suppose that a gross difference between the morphology or physiology of the primary gustatory system and the other primary sensory modalities could account for this dichotomy. However, no such obvious difference has yet been described.

### A. THE ANATOMICAL HYPOTHESIS

In a particularly important discussion, Garcia and Ervin (1968) hypothesized that the neural mechanisms underlying gustatory-visceral associations are anatomically distinct from those subserving telereceptive-cutaneous associations. The conceptual basis of this argument rests upon the observations and suggestions of C. Judson Herrick (1948) who described a gustatory-visceral integrative region in the brainstem of the tiger salamander which is coupled to visceral motor mechanisms, and a separate integrative region receptive to exteroceptive-cutaneous stimuli and coupled to somatic motor mechanisms. According to Garcia and Ervin, the direct convergence of primary gustatory and visceral afferents, but not telereceptive or cutaneous afferents, at the nucleus of the solitary tract is considered to be of particular, but undefined, importance.

In mammals, the rostral nucleus of the solitary tract receives primary gustatory afferents which enter the brain via the facial and glossopharyngeal nerves (Brodal, 1969). Secondary afferents emerge from the nucleus of the solitary tract, course ipsilaterally to the dorsal pontine taste area, and subsequent tertiary afferents ascend in the central tegmental tract to distribute bilaterally in the medial aspect of the thalamic ventrobasal complex, hypothalamus, and amygdala (Norgren, 1976; Norgren and Leonard, 1973). Thalamic gustatory projections to the neocortex terminate in a well-defined region just dorsal to the rhinal sulcus (Norgren and Wolf, 1975).

In addition to the gustatory afferent projection to the solitary tract, general visceral afferents also terminate within the nucleus of the solitary tract (Brodal, 1969). There is also evidence of a close anatomical relationship between the nucleus of the solitary tract and the area postrema, a chemoreceptive zone which may also be receptive to visceral input. Available anatomical evidence indicates that the area postrema is in both afferent and efferent connection with the solitary nucleus (Morest, 1960, 1967).

In view of the hypothesis that anatomical convergence at the solitary nucleus may be of importance for the establishment of gustatory-visceral associations, it is noteworthy that somatosensory projections from the tongue also project directly to the solitary nucleus. Following section of the trigeminal (maxillary and mandibular divisions) and facial nerve, extensive preterminal degeneration has been noted in the solitary nucleus (Torvik, 1956). Furthermore, Blomquest and Antem (1965) stimulated the glossopharyngeal, chorda tympani, and lingual nerves and recorded evoked multiple-unit discharge at the solitary nucleus. Short-latency (2-4 msec) responses were noted upon stimulation of any of the three nerves, and the response field of the lingual nerve was found to overlap the response fields of the glossopharyngeal and chorda tympani nerves. Likewise, single-unit studies provide evidence that afferents that convey chemical, mechanical, and thermal information from the tongue converge upon single cells of the rostral solitary nucleus (Makous *et al.,* 1963).

Activation of the somatosensory afferents from the tongue has been shown to be an adequate CS for the acquisition of long-delay learning with a visceral UCS. Nachman (1970a) demonstrated that a change in the temperature of distilled water was a sufficient CS when followed by LiCl. Learning was established in one trial and with a CS–UCS interval of 15 minutes. Similarly, it has been demonstrated (Nachman *et al.,* 1977b), that rats can acquire CS–UCS learned aversions when the CS is the pattern of tongue-tactile stimulation that is required by the nature of the drinking task. Using somatosensory discriminations such as lapping versus licking and licking from a spout with a large versus a small opening, it has been possible to form aversions with CS–UCS intervals as long as 1 hour. However, it should be noted that the magnitude of the aversion, number of trials necessary for acquisition, and length of the associative CS–UCS interval found with orosomatic stimuli are not comparable to those found when gustatory stimuli are used.

Certainly, one is impressed by the fact that two quite separate inputs, gustatory and visceral, converge at the primary synaptic level and that these two modalities provide the most effective stimuli for taste aversion learning. Indeed, as previously indicated, the convergence of the CS and UCS at the nucleus of the solitary tract is the critical aspect of Garcia and Ervin's (1968) conceptualization of the underlying basis of taste aversion learning. However, it is important to examine more closely the meaning and implications of anatomic convergence, as well as its relationship to the equally important temporal convergence that is necessary for learning to occur.

Related lines of inquiry have also suggested that cells upon which the CS and UCS converge are more likely to exhibit conditioned changes than cells responsive to only one of the conditioning sensory modalities (O'Brien and Fox, 1969; Yoshii and Ogura, 1960). However, while convergence of CS–UCS input at some neural level is probably a necessary factor for the acquisition of classically conditioned neuronal responses (Brauth and Olds, 1977; Oleson *et al.*, 1975), the functional significance of converging input remains to be elucidated. With regard to taste aversion learning in particular, several obvious, but important, questions concerning the convergence hypothesis remain unanswered. Do gustatory and visceral afferents converge directly upon the same postsynaptic neuron within the solitary nucleus, or are more extensive intranuclear connections necessary? Assuming direct convergence, are there differences in the regional distribution of synapses upon the soma-dendritic surface depending upon the type of afferent input? And a related question can be asked: assuming either direct or indirect convergence via intrinsic neurons, are there differences in the characteristics of the postsynaptic response which are dependent upon the type of afferent input? For example, synaptic potentials with durations lasting minutes provide a mechanism for long-term temporal summation which could contribute to the long CS–UCS interval in taste aversion learning. The proximity of such synapses to the impulse-generating region of the cell may also be of importance in determining the effectiveness and duration of temporal summation. Hence, we are still confronted with the task of identifying the physiological substrata (which may or may not be secondary to anatomical convergence) that account for the extended CS–UCS interval that will support the acquisition of a learned taste aversion. Thus, while it is likely that a spatial and temporal convergence of CS and UCS afferents is a necessary factor for the development of conditioned neuronal responses, there is no evidence to indicate that anatomical convergence per se is sufficient for the acquisition of a taste aversion with a long CS–UCS interval. That is, the knowledge that gustatory and visceral afferents converge on the same nucleus does not satisfactorily account for interactive effects since the gustatory CS and visceral UCS may be arriving several hours apart. Nor is there any compelling reason to assume a single physiological process as the basis of the pronounced length of the CS–UCS interval. It is at least as likely that several physiological responses interact to result in the prolonged CS–UCS interval observable by behavioral testing.

## B. POSSIBLE PHYSIOLOGICAL MECHANISMS

The long-lasting effects produced by gustatory stimuli cannot be attributed solely to a lingering peripheral aftertaste (Rozin, 1969), but must be due to some type of central mediating state that accounts for the animal's ability to associate the CS and UCS over a long interval. Conceivably, the synaptic drive of primary synapses could be optimum for the induction of long-lasting cellular events capable of bridging the CS–UCS interval. If so, this may be reflected in neuronal discharge rate. For example, Perrotto and Scott (1976) report that LiCl perfused over the tongues of rats evokes an average discharge of 53 spikes/second at the solitary nucleus but only 13 spikes/second at the pontine taste area. Similar findings were reported for a wide variety of chemical stimuli applied to the tongue. It is possible that the time course of excitability is proportional to the magnitude of evoked discharge rate, and this in turn may determine to some extent the length of the CS–UCS interval. That is, it may be that gustatory input produces long-lasting activity of neurons of the solitary nucleus which in turn mediates the length of the associative gradient. Studies which examine the time course of excitability at the nucleus of the solitary tract are nonexistent, but related evidence indicates that this approach may prove to be particularly fruitful. For example, electrical stimulation of the rabbit abducens nucleus, if delivered within a defined period following an acoustic stimulus, results in an augmented evoked nictitating membrane response with a magnitude that is dependent on the interval between the two stimuli (Young et al., 1976). Furthermore, the interstimulus interval functions for the augmented reflex excitability of abducens motoneurons and the interstimulus interval functions for tone-air puff conditioning of the nictitating membrane show a close correspondence (Thompson, 1976). Thompson (1976) has suggested that similar alterations in neuronal excitability of certain brain systems may mediate the long interstimulus interval seen in taste aversion learning. It is also possible that the long interstimulus interval is a by-product of the fact that the central effect of the CS is highly repetitive and prolonged neuronal activation that is induced by the animal's lapping at a fluid for a period of several minutes. Consistent with these notions are the findings that for a constant level of taste aversion the duration (or amount) of CS access and the concentration of the CS bear an inverse relationship to each other (Barker, 1976). Likewise, the length of the CS–UCS interval that will support conditioning can be extended by increasing the concentration of the CS (Braun and Rosenthal, 1976).

It should be noted that hypotheses which require a prolonged central aftereffect of the gustatory CS, regardless of their form, do not explain why a UCS such as peripheral electrical stimulation is not associated with a gustatory CS. One would expect that paradigms using a gustatory CS and a shock UCS separated by a long CS–UCS interval or an audiovisual CS paired with a sickness UCS at a short CS–UCS interval would also be equally effective. The evidence indicates that this is not the case. Therefore, the specificity of the stimuli that can be associated may very well be the result of anatomical segregation of associative mechanisms. In support of the suggestion that telereceptive–somatosensory and gustatory–visceral associations are mediated by different anatomical subtrates (Garcia and Ervin, 1968), it has been found that large lesions of the hippocampus, lateral septum, or lesions limited to the posteroventral hippocampus produce deficits in CER or passive avoidance but not in gustatory aversion (McGowan *et al.*, 1972; Miller *et al.*, 1975). However, the converse, that is, a lesion which disrupts the learning mechanisms for acquisition of taste aversions but not CER or passive avoidance has not been demonstrated.

## 1. Susceptability of the CS Trace to Disruption

The durability of the central representation of the CS experience has been investigated by application of electroconvulsive shock treatment (ECS). Nachman (1970b) reports that ECS (50 mA for 200 msec) interpolated in the CS–UCS interval has only a limited effect on the acquisition of a taste aversion. ECS given immediately after 30 seconds of saccharin ingestion had no detrimental effect on learning a taste aversion, suggesting that the enduring effects of the 30-second CS are not mediated by processes known to be altered by ECS-induced seizures. On the other hand, Kral (1971) allowed a 10-minute period of ingestion and applied ECS (60 mA for 700 msec) at various times within a 4-hour CS–UCS interval and found that ECS disrupted acquisition regardless of the time within the CS–UCS interval that it was given. At this time the reason for these apparently discrepant findings remains to be resolved, and it is difficult to reach any firm conclusion regarding the efficacy of ECS in disrupting the enduring activity consequent to the CS. As has been shown with other paradigms (McGaugh and Gold, 1974), the relative effectiveness of ECS may be dependent upon the particular parameters of the electric current used and the strength of the original learning.

Buresová and Bures (1973) have found that cortical spreading depression (CSD) can have a time-dependent effect on the central after-effect of the CS. The efficacy of the gustatory stimulus as a CS is blocked if given during the period of CSD. In contrast, if CSD is initiated within the CS–UCS interval typical taste aversions are acquired, although it appears that CSD attenuates the duration of the possible CS–UCS interval (Buresová and Bures, 1974). These findings with CSD have been interpreted as indicating that the acquisition of a taste aversion requires the initial participation of the cortex for processing the memory of the indifferent gustatory experience, but that the actual physiological associative events are to be found at subcortical regions. Similar interpretations have been derived from comparable experiments using general anesthesia (Buresová and Bures, 1977). It is not yet clear what events underlie the effect of CSD in attenuating the CS–UCS interval, or how these events underlie the effect of CSD in attenuating the CS–UCS interval, or how these events differ from the effect of general anesthesia which has been reported to prolong the CS–UCS interval (Rozin and Ree, 1972). Nonetheless, it appears that the associative mechanisms and those mechanisms subserving the length of the CS–UCS interval can be uncoupled by CSD. It could be that the CS–UCS interval is determined predominately by functions intrinsic to cortical tissue. Or it could be that subcortical mechanisms are fundamental, but that subcortical neuronal activity is disrupted by CSD (Bures *et al.*, 1961). Additional evidence suggestive of the separate functioning of associative mechanisms and those mechanisms determining the extent of the CS–UCS interval comes from the study of immature rats. It has been reported that immature rats (23 days old) can readily acquire a learned taste aversion, but only with short CS–UCS intervals (Baker *et al.*, 1977). Baker *et al.* (1977) also found that immature rats differed from adults in lacking the usual neophobic response (Barnett, 1975) to novel gustatory stimuli. Whether the lack of long-delay learning and the lack of neophobia are functionally related or bear only a coincidental relation to each other remains to be clarified.

## 2. Possible Long-Lasting Synaptic Changes

To date the findings do not implicate a specific anatomical locus nor do they elucidate the mechanism by which anatomical convergence can give rise to the long CS–UCS interval. Enduring posttetanic potentiation, such as that reported for the hippocampus, is illustrative of the type of long-lasting neuronal event that is necessary to account for the temporal characteristics of learned taste aversions. Recent evidence indicates that the hippocampus has a remarkable capacity for long-lasting physiological plasticity (Alger and Teyler, 1976; Bliss and Gardner-Medwin, 1973; Bliss and Lømo, 1973; Deadwyler et al., 1976; Douglas and Goddard, 1975). In contrast to the effects of repetitive stimulation at the neuromuscular junction and spinal motoneurons which may last for a few hundreds of milliseconds to minutes (Eccles, 1964), the effect at certain synapses in the hippocampus has been found to persist for hours (Bliss and Gardner-Medwin, 1973; Bliss and Lømo, 1973) or days (Bliss and Gardner-Medwin, 1973; Douglas and Goddard, 1975). Indeed, potentiation has been reported to persist for several weeks in the chronic unanesthetized rabbit (Bliss and Gardner-Medwin, 1973). Gustatory stimuli may evoke qualitatively similar enduring changes at the solitary nucleus. If so, enduring increases in excitability may be the physiological mediator of the interstimulus interval in taste aversion learning.

Also, gustatory neurons may differ from other sensory neurons in ways that are more subtle than gross anatomical loci of terminating primary afferents and synaptic drive. For example, during the past few years evidence has pointed to an involvement of metabolic events in synaptically mediated modifications of neuronal excitability that are of long duration (Libet, 1979) and that may serve as a model for how anatomical convergence can be translated into cellular events capable of mediating the long CS–UCS interval. Electrical stimulation of the preganglionic nerve to the superior cervical ganglion of most mammals produces three distinct postsynaptic potentials: an EPSP that occurs after only a brief latent period (fast EPSP) and two long-latency synaptic potentials that differ qualitatively from the fast EPSP—the slow IPSP and slow EPSP (Libet, 1970). The fast EPSP is the direct result of the preganglionic release of acetylcholine acting upon nicotinic receptors of the postganglionic neuron. In contrast, the slow IPSP occurs as a result of the synaptic release of dopamine from ganglionic interneurons

(Libet and Owman, 1974), and the slow EPSP by the effect of preganglionically released acetylcholine acting at ganglion cell muscarinic sites. Utilizing this synaptic system, Libet and Tosaka (1970) have shown that brief perfusion of the *in vitro* superior cervical ganglion of the rabbit with small concentrations of dopamine, an intraganglionic neurotransmitter (Libet and Owman, 1974), results in the enhancement of the subsequent depolarizing response (slow EPSP) produced by the muscarinic agonist methacholine. The enhancement of the slow EPSP has been reported to last for several hours and is thought to be mediated by the intracellular production of cyclic adenosine 3,′5-monophosphate (cAMP). In addition, enhancement of the slow EPSP is susceptible to time-dependent blockade by cyclic guanosine 3,′5′-monophosphate (cGMP) which suggests that the cellular substrate of enduring facilitation undergoes a gradual change of state to a more stable form (Libet, et al., 1975). Hence, these data provide a model which is unique in demonstrating a biochemical interaction between qualitatively distinct postsynaptic processes in which an initial synaptic input enhances a second synaptic response that is separate in time and that utilizes a different neurotransmitter. Somewhat analogous modulating interactions between neurotransmitter systems also occur apparently in the central nervous system (Freedman *et al.,* 1977; Reader et al., 1977).

At present, there is no evidence that the intraneuronal events that occur in the superior cervical ganglion also occur in gustatory neurons, although this idea certainly merits investigation. The metabolic processes in the ganglion which produce synaptic plasticity with appropriately long temporal characteristics may serve as a significant model for long-delay taste aversion learning. The mechanisms elucidated in the superior cervical ganglion may also provide a basis for how anatomical convergence can be translated into physiological processes that can result in behavioral plasticity.

## III. The Nature of the Unconditioned Stimulus

A. The Range of Effective Unconditioned Stimuli

We have thus far emphasized the fact that certain unknown properties intrinsic to the neural representation of gustatory information are fundamental for the acquisition of a learned taste aversion. Of equal importance is the nature of the UCS. Garcia and Koelling (1966) have shown that gustatory stimuli can be readily associated with the internal consequences of X irradiation or LiCl injections, but not with noxious electrical stimulation of the paws. Yet, electrical stimulation of peripheral regions is the UCS of choice for learned associations using auditory/visual conditional stilmuli while internal consequences are generally ineffective. Evidently, not all UCS are adequate for the establishment of all types of aversive associations.

Ideally, for the neurobiological analysis of behavioral plasticity, one would like to specify the anatomical nature of the CS and UCS sensory input as well as the motor pathway subserving the response. While it is clear that the most effective CS pathway in food aversion learning is the gustatory pathway, the nature of both the UCS input and the motor output remains obscure. Taste aversions are readily acquired when the ingestion of a substance is followed by such diverse agents as scopolamine (Berger, 1972), LiCl (Nachman, 1963), apomorphine (Garcia *et al.*, 1966), α-methyl-*p*-tyrosine (Carey and Goodall, 1974), *d*-amphetamine (Cappell and LeBlanc, 1971), cyclophosphamide (Garcia, *et al.*, 1966), morphine (Cappell *et al.*, 1973), anesthetics (Brown and Glusman, 1971), and several common rodenticides (Nachman and Hartley, 1975), to list but a few. Similarly, a variety of treatments such as X irradiation (Garcia *et al.*, 1955), rotation (Braun and McIntosh, 1973; Hartley, 1977), and cortical spreading depression (Winn *et al.*, 1975) have been reported to be effective unconditioned stimuli.

The effectiveness of the UCS was originally attributed to induced gastrointestinal disturbance or illness (Garcia and Ervin, 1968). In part this was a result of the fact that the earliest unconditioned stimuli used were ionizing radiation and drugs such as apomorphine and cyclophosphamide which are known to produce nausea and gastrointestinal illness. Likewise, ionizing radiation is known to produce signs of gastric dysfunction which include diarrhea, nausea, emesis, and anorexia (Prosser *et al.*, 1947). Thus, it was not improbable that gastric disturbance was the functional UCS for producing learned taste aversions. However, this evidence was certainly not conclusive particularly since each of these treatments has other widespread effects and also because the correlation between the efficacy of a drug or treatment as a UCS and its effectiveness in producing gastric dysfunction is low. For example, Berger (1972) reported that learned aversions could be established with psychoactive drugs, such as amphetamine, scopolamine, and chlorpromazine, at dose levels that do not produce obvious signs of sickness. Similarly, LiCl has been found to be an effective UCS at low doses that apparently do not produce signs of gastrointestinal distress (Nachman and Ashe, 1973). Treatments such as ionizing radiation also appear to produce taste aversions at dose levels that are below the threshold for production of signs of gastric distress (Smith, 1971). In contrast, apomorphine appears to make animals exceedingly sick while producing a less pronounced learned aversion (Revusky and Garcia, 1970). On the other hand, Garcia and his associates (Coil *et al.*, 1978a) have recently shown that for animals that have already learned an aversion to saccharin, the degree of learned aversion can be attenuated by administration of an antiemetic drug. In this study saccharin aversion was induced by the use of the emetic LiCl as the unconditioned stimulus, and an antiemetic drug was given 30 minutes prior to the test for aversion. This finding of an attenuation of a learned aversion by an antiemetic was interpreted as indicating that the critical physiological effect of the UCS is nausea and that for aversions to occur nausea must be reestablished by the CS on test day.

Thus, while there is some evidence indicating that nausea may play a role in learned taste aversions when known emetic agents are used as unconditioned stimuli, the notion of induced nausea as a unifying principle or necessary condition is probably an oversimplification. The fact remains that pharmacological agents that contrast with LiCl in having no obvious emetic actions and are effective unconditioned stimuli; furthermore there is no indication that the effectiveness of these agents as unconditioned stimuli can be reduced by administration of antiemetics prior to testing.

B. Physiological Characteristics of the Unconditioned Stimulus

The very diversity of effective unconditioned stimuli has presented special problems for understanding the relevant physiological effects produced by these stimuli. A particularly perplexing finding is that both noxious and pleasurable drug states can be used as unconditioned stimuli for the production of learned taste aversions. For example, drugs such as morphine or amphetamine which animals will self-administer (Schuster and Thompson, 1969) are nevertheless effective unconditioned stimuli for taste aversion learning. These findings have led to the suggestion that all novel drug states are aversive (Amit and Baum, 1970) or that novel drug states are disruptive to normal physiological function and therefore aversive for the animal (Gamzu, 1977). Of course, these formulations do not account for why the animal will self-administer these drugs.

Another suggested explanation for the diversity of drugs that are effective unconditioned stimuli has been that many of the drug states produce a common stress response, perhaps reflected in an elevation of blood corticosterone concentration, and that this response is the underlying factor critical for taste aversion learning (Braveman, 1977). The principal evidence in support of this hypothesis is the observation that LiCl or morphine injections are accompanied by an elevation of blood corticosterone levels (A. L. Riley, unpublished observations discussed in detail in Braveman, 1977). Furthermore, Smotherman *et al.* (1976) report that pretreatment on the conditioning day with dexamethaxone, an inhibitor of ACTH release, attenuates LiCl-induced taste aversions. Also, presession injections of either ACTH or the ACTH analog $ACTH_{4-10}$ retard the extinction of a learned taste aversion (Rigter and Popping, 1976; Smotherman and Levine, 1978). But, because the peptide $ACTH_{4-10}$ is virtually devoid of adrenocorticotrophic activity while retaining its behavioral efficacy (de Wied, 1974) it appears that an ACTH-induced elevation of plasma corticosterone concentration is not a mandatory component of the ACTH effect on taste aversion extinction. More likely, the influence of ACTH and its analog $ACTH_{4-10}$ on taste aversions is the result of a postulated direct effect on the central nervous system (de Wied, 1974).

The possibility that stress is the common factor appears to be particularly unlikely in view of the fact that some well-known stress-inducing treatments are not effective as unconditioned stimuli. For example, Nachman (1970b) has shown that giving ECS, as an aversive treatment, does not result in the acquisition of learned taste aversions. Similarly, in earlier unpublished work, we attempted to test the stress hypothesis by using other nonchemical stressful treatments such as cold and restraint (treatments that would also be expected to elevate blood corticosterone levels) and have found them to be ineffective. Thus, elevation of plasma corticosterone levels may be a correlate of some effective unconditioned stimuli, but activation of the pituitary–adrenal system per se does may not appear to be sufficient for the learning of a taste aversion.

It has also been hypothesized that the effects of various unconditioned stimuli are mediated by some common substance such as histamine. It is known that one correlate of radiation treatment is an elevation of the blood histamine level, and Levy *et al.* (1974) found that the aversion-producing effect of radiation may be mediated via the histamine response. These investigators reported that either ionizing radiation or subcutaneously administered histamine diphosphate is an effective unconditioned stimulus for conditioning a saccharin aversion, and that an intraperitoneal injection of the antihistamine chlorpheniramine maleate prior to irradiation blocked the efficacy of radiation as a UCS. However, an elevation of blood histamine concentration cannot be a common factor for all effective unconditioned stimuli because Levy and her associates also found that antihistamine pretreatment had no effect on a learned taste aversion induced by LiCl.

In view of the diversity of drugs and toxic agents that are effective unconditioned stimuli for taste aversion acquisition (for a more extensive list see Riley and Baril, 1976), it is of particular interest to note that not all toxic agents function as UCSs. Nachman and Hartley (1975) examined the UCS properties of several toxic agents and found that cyanide and strychnine were relatively ineffective. These investigators concluded that the effects of different drugs may be mediated by different physiological systems in producing learned taste aversions. Similar findings for pyrrolopyrimidine, gallamine, malonate, and cyanide have recently been reported (Ionescu and Buresová, 1977). Continued investigation along these lines is needed. An understanding of the mechanism that allows some drugs to be effective UCSs but not others would be a very important advance in the understanding of the physiological/biochemical substrata of taste aversion learning. Also, the fact that potentially lethal substances such as cyanide and strychnine are relatively ineffective for conditioning aversions indicates that toxic action and novelty of drug state are insufficient explanations for the motivational properties of the UCS.

In summary, the difficulties in identifying the mechanisms that underlie the UCS effect have greatly hampered the analysis of the neural mechanisms of taste aversion learning. It appears that different drugs may work on different systems and possibly at different loci within a system to produce the same behavioral effect. It is clear from the work of Nachman and Hartley (1975) and Ionescu and Buresová (1977) that not just any alteration in internal state is sufficient to give rise to a functional UCS. Some drugs are effective in producing taste aversions while others are ineffective regardless of the magnitude of gross organismic effects. Moreover, when one examines the drugs that do produce taste aversions it is difficult to identify their common characteristic.

## C. Anatomical Locus of Action of the Unconditioned Stimulus

The behavioral and physiological effects of various drugs may be the direct result of the drug's action on the brain, peripheral neurons, or organs. The wide range of effective drugs and treatments has raised the question of what might be the nature and variety of the anatomical pathways that mediate the UCS consequences.

The viscera contains nociceptive and other receptors sensitive to chemical, mechanical, and thermal stimulation. The effects of these stimuli are conveyed centrally via the vagus and splanchnic nerves (Newman, 1974). A solution of $CuSO_4$ administered orally is a well-known emetic acting on the upper gastrointestinal tract (Wang and

Borison, 1952), and consistent with this fact is the demonstration by Coil *et al.* (1978b) that bilateral subdiaphragmatic vagotomy results in a suppression of conditioned taste aversions produced by $CuSO_4$. While the suppression is pronounced following intragastric administration of $CuSO_4$, there is only moderate to weak suppression following intraperitoneal or intravenous injections, respectively. On the other hand, similar experiments utilizing LiCl have yielded both positive (Greenberg *et al.*, 1977) and negative results (Martin *et al.*, 1978).

In 1949, Borison and Wang described an area at the dorsolateral border of the lateral reticular formation of the cat that when electrically stimulated elicited emesis. In addition, they described a "chemoreceptor trigger zone" for emesis located at the area postrema in the floor of the fourth ventricle near the obex (Wang and Borison, 1952). Lesions of the area postrema have been reported to have little effect on the vomiting reflex initiated by irritation of the gastrointestinal tract consequent to oral administration of peripheral acting chemicals such as $CuSO_4$, but do abolish the reflex to blood-borne emetics such as apomorphine (Wang and Borison, 1952). Apparently the primary locus of action for the emetic effect of orally administered $CuSO_4$ is the upper gastrointestinal tract, the effects of which are conveyed to the lateral reticular formation "vomiting center" by visceral afferent nerves. In contrast, apomorphine and intravenously administered $CuSO_4$ evidently have a direct effect on the area postrema. It is also noteworthy that the area postrema is in close anatomical and probably physiological communication with the nucleus of the solitary tract (Morest, 1960, 1967). As mentioned earlier, the area postrema has been of interest to those investigating the neural mechanisms of taste aversion learning because of its involvement in the physiological response to certain blood-borne substances. In several mammalian species (e.g., rat, dog, cat, and rabbit), the area postrema is thought to be a chemoreceptive zone (Borison, 1974; Roth and Yamamoto, 1968). The area postrema is neurally coupled to the vomiting center in the lateral reticular formation, and as such may be an important component of the circuitry subserving the UCS.

Additional interest in the area postrema arises because the region is one of the so-called circumventricular organs which can be distinguished from other regions of the brain by the more rapid rate of exchange of some substances between the cerebral blood vessels and the interstitial fluid (Oldendorf, 1975). The reciprocal neural connections with the nucleus of the solitary tract (Morest, 1960), and the fact that the area postrema is outside the blood–brain barrier and therefore capable of being influenced by a wide range of blood-borne substances, some of which do not easily gain access to other regions of the brain, suggests that the area postrema may be a receptive region for the UCS in taste aversion learning.

The rat does not vomit (for discussion of this issue, see Hatcher and Weiss, 1923). However, it has been assumed that the area postrema serves the same type of chemoreceptive function in the rat as it does in species that can vomit. Berger et al. (1973) have shown that cauterization of the area postrema prevents the acquisition of a taste aversion when methylscopolamine is used as a UCS. Methylated compounds do not easily pass the blood-brain barrier (Iversen and Iversen, 1975), and thus Berger et al. (1973) concluded that aversions conditioned with methylscopolamine act through the chemoreceptive area postrema. In contrast, they found that elimination of the area postrema did not prevent the acquisition of an aversion when $d$-amphetamine was used as a UCS. Amphetamine, which does pass the blood–brain barrier, may therefore act directly at peripheral as well as central nervous system loci. Berger et al. (1973) conclude that different drugs produce aversions by different mechanisms. Attenuation of taste aversion acquisition following lesions to the area postrema appears to hold for intraperitoneally injected LiCl, apomorphine, and $CuSO_4$ (Hartley, 1977; J. Rauschenberger, unpublished observations) as well. Recalling the reports of Wang and Borison (1952) that the locus of action of $CuSO_4$ depends upon the route of administration, i.e., oral administration of $CuSO_4$ exerts its effect through the visceral afferent nerves in contrast to intravenous administration which is dependent upon an intact area postrema, it would be expected that the aversion-inducing effect of $CuSO_4$ delivered via stomach tube should not be prevented by area postrema lesions, while aversions induced by intraperitoneally injected $CuSO_4$ should be prevented by these lesions. Precisely these results were found in recent studies by J. Rauschenberger (unpublished) in our laboratory. In these studies, Rauschenberger lesioned the area postrema of rats and after a 2-month recovery period tested them, using our standard experimental procedures (Nachmen, 1970a) for their ability to learn a taste aversion using $CuSO_4$ administered intraperitoneally versus administration by stomach tube. $CuSO_4$ given intraperitoneally is far more effective in producing a learned taste aversion than is $CuSO_4$ given by stomach tube. In terms of effectiveness, with normal rats a dose of 5 mg/kg given intraperitoneally produces about the same degree of aversion as a 50 mg/kg dose given by stomach tube. Rauschenberger found that rats with lesions of the area postrema did not learn an aversion when an intraperitoneal dose of 5 mg/kg was used, but did learn the aversion when a 10 or 50 mg/kg dose was given by stomach tube. Thus, it appears that $CuSO_4$ given intraperitoneally, which becomes blood-borne, acts via the area postrema to produce aversions, whereas $CuSO_4$ given by stomach tube does not act via the area postrema. This latter interpretation is consistent with the work of Coil *et al.* (1978b), discussed earlier, which showed that vagotomy attenuated aversions learned with stomach tubed $CuSO_4$ but not aversions learned with $CuSO_4$ given intraperitoneally.

When considering the neuronal substrate of taste aversion learning, the nucleus of the solitary tract has usually been implicated solely because of the convergence of the gustatory and visceral pathways. However, the nucleus of the solitary tract appears to have a pivotal function in a general arousal system (Koella, 1974) as well, and these functions may also be important for acquisition of a taste aversion. Efferents of the area postrema project to the nucleus of the solitary track (Morest, 1960), and both of these regions have been implicated in the induction of electrocortical synchronization and sleep (Key and Mehta, 1977; Koella, 1974). Furthermore, fibers from the nucleus of the solitary tract establish synaptic contact with the dorsal raphe nucleus (Aghajanian and Wang, 1977) which exerts inhibitory control over the amygdala and possibly other telencephalic structures via serotonin-containing axons (Wang and Aghajanian, 1977). Thus, it is interesting to note that afferents of gustatory and visceral pathways, in addition to their sensory role, project directly to and are presumably involved in the activity of regions known to have a role in the regulation of physiological and behavior states of arousal.

In a recent investigation of the role of the serotonergic network in taste aversion learning, Lorden and Margules (1977) found that either electrolytic lesions of the raphe nuclei or depletion of raphe serotonin with 5,7–dihydroxytryptamine actually facilitated the magnitude of taste aversion learning. Conversely, in lesioned rats systemic administration of the serotonin precursor 5–hydroxytryptophan blocked the facilitation of taste aversion, but also tended to suppress CS intake to a level below that of intact controls (Lorden and Oltmans, 1978). When administered to intact animals, 5–hydroxytryptophan also resulted in an attenuated aversion. These findings suggest a role for the raphe nuclei and serotonin in modulating taste aversion learning. As discussed by Lorden and Margules lesions to the medial septal nucleus, which receives a strong serotonergic projection from the raphe nuclei (Conrad *et al.*, 1974), also result in an enhanced taste aversion learning (McGowan *et al.*, 1969). Much work is yet to be done, but these findings suggest that extensive investigation of the function of this serotonergic network in the acquisition of learned taste aversions may be particularly fruitful.

Other studies have focused on the action of different drugs at specific loci in the brain to produce learned taste aversions. A recent report suggests that the central mechanisms involved in the acquisition of a taste aversion may vary depending upon the nature of the UCS (Amit *et al.*, 1977). These investigators report that aversions to saccharin can be established with morphine, ethanol, or $\triangle^9$-tetrahydrocannabinol ($\triangle^9$-THC) when the UCS was given by intraperitoneal injection. However, when infused into the dorsal hippocampus only $\triangle^9$-THC was functional as a UCS. Furthermore, the effectiveness of infused $\triangle^9$-THC was specific to the hippocampus; infusion of $\triangle^9$-THC or morphine into the caudate nucleus was ineffective in establishing saccharin aversion while morphine infusions into the cerebral ventricles were said to be effective.

Acquisition of a learned taste aversion may also proceed via UCS pathways that apparently do not involve chemical unconditioned stimuli. In an attempt to overcome the difficulties encountered in specifying the anatomical pathway of the UCS when chemicals are used, Hartley (1977) sought to utilize vestibular stimulation as a UCS. Following ingestion of a novel solution, rats were placed in an apparatus designed to emulate the coriolis forces and pattern of vestibular stimulation thought to accompany motion sickness. Presumably such stimulation would also initiate the constellation of physiological responses found in motion sickness. Hartley reports that motion-induced learned taste aversions are easily produced and depend upon an intact labyrinth but not an intact area postrema. The latter finding suggests that the UCS effect is primarily mediated by neural activity and that vestibular stimulation does not release substances into the circulation that secondarily function as unconditioned stimuli via the area postrema. Additionally, Hartley found that lesions of the area postrema attenuate learned taste aversions induced by LiCl. Thus while area postrema lesions did not affect aversions learned with motion sickness the lesions did have an effect on aversions learned with LiCl suggesting that the primary action of LiCl as a UCS may be via the area postrema. Such a hypothesis would be consistent with the fact that salts, such as LiCl, in their dissociated form do not readily traverse the blood–brain barrier (Iversen and Iversen, 1975).

## IV. Central Modulation of Taste Aversion Learning

The ease of formation of a learned taste aversion has led to the suggestion that the organism is more "prepared" to acquire habits that are biologically relevant than those that have only limited biological value in the natural environment (Seligman, 1970). When an animal undergoes an experience, learning is only one of a wider complex of physiological responses that may occur. Arousal, attention, stress, and motor responses are all just as likely to be initiated, and it is also likely that these responses are coupled to associative mechanisms (Gold and McGaugh, 1975). One of the major by-products of learned taste aversion research has been the reemphasis on the importance of understanding the total animal in elucidating the principles of associative formation. In neurobiological terms, "preparedness" may be interpreted as a measure of the degree of coordination of learning mechanisms with ongoing physiological processes. The appropriate presentation of any CS or UCS will initiate a wide variety of physiologic responses of varying time course, including those necessary for learning. The distinctive features of taste aversion learning such as one-trial learning and the long CS–UCS interval suggest that the nature of the stimuli used set these events in motion and that they aid in creating the appropriate conditions for learning the association. Stimuli that initiate internal consequences that are smoothly coupled to the on-going physiology of the animal should result in the most robust learning and thus the animal will appear to be especially "prepared" for the acquisition of this learning. Also the rapid learning and the nature of gustatory and visceral stimuli hint at a strong autonomic component of taste aversion learning, and autonomic responses have typically been shown to condition faster than somatic responses when longer CS–UCS intervals are used (Dykman, 1967).

Hence, a strategy characterized by examination of interrelationships between physiological responses could perhaps lead to new insight into the process of taste aversion acquisition. For example, in view of the important relationship between neophobia and taste aversion learning (Krane et al., 1976; Nachman and Ashe, 1974) the neural correlates of neophobia and an understanding of their relationship to the distinctive features of taste aversion may lead to a broader and potentially more productive conceptual basis for understanding learned taste aversions. Neophobia, among other things, is likely to be indicative of a change in the motivational state of the organism and as such may be reflected in alterations of neural activity, e.g., the rate of tonic neuronal discharge in various brain regions (Bambridge and Gijsbers, 1977). Knowledge of the physiological basis and duration of neophobic reactions may provide important clues to the nature of taste aversions. Likewise, one would also like to know how modification of on-going autonomic processes by gustatory stimuli affects the central processing of subsequent information conveyed centrally via autonomic afferents or hormonal pathways. However, much of this work is yet to be done.

A variety of studies have been undertaken in an effort to identify central nervous system loci that may be involved in learned taste aversion.

The large majority of these studies have used ablation and electrical stimulation techniques. In these studies, usually the ablation of a particular area is followed by taste aversion training and the consequent deficits in performance are described. However, in some instances lesions are made between the learning and testing of the aversion. To date, the literature consists of an abundance of reports, some of which are conflicting, of the effects of lesions of the neocortex (Braun *et al.*, 1972; Hankins *et al.*, 1974; Lorden, 1976), olfactory bulbs (Hankins *et al.*, 1973; Hobbs *et al.*, 1976), amygdala (Kemble and Nagel, 1973; McGowan *et al.*, 1972; Nachman and Ashe, 1974; Rolls and Rolls, 1973), septal nuclei (Hobbs *et al.*, 1974; McGowan *et al.*, 1972), hippocampus (Best and Orr, 1973; Krane *et al.*, 1976; McGowan *et al.*, 1972; Miller *et al.*, 1975; Miller *et al.*, 1971; Murphy and Brown, 1974; Nachman and Ashe, 1974), hypothalamus (Gold and Proulx, 1972; Peters and Reich, 1973; Roth *et al.*, 1973; Schwartz and Teitelbaum, 1974; Weisman, *et al.*, 1972), and area postrema (Berger *et al.*, 1973; Hartley, 1977). The bulk of these studies have recently been reviewed and categorized (Gaston, 1978).

Of the various cortical and subcortical regions investigated in relation to learned taste aversions, the most systematic study and consistent findings have been for the amygdalar complex. The amygdalar complex is one of the principal nuclear regions of convergence of gustatory and visceral afferents (Dell and Olson, 1951; Eleftheriou, 1972; Norgren, 1976), and is also a region known to be involved in autonomic and endocrine functions (Eleftheriou, 1972). Thus, it is of particular interest that studies of the effects of damage to the amygdala have been consistent in reporting deficits in taste aversion learning (Kemble and Nagel, 1973; McGowan *et al.*, 1972; Nachman and Ashe, 1974; Rolls and Rolls, 1973), although it is also the case that lesions of the amygdala result in deficits in other types of learning as well, e.g., active and passive avoidance (Eleftheriou, 1972). The nature of the taste aversion deficit produced by lesions of the amygdala does not appear to be an inability to learn per se but more of a perceptual deficit. Nachman and Ashe (1974) found that rats with lesions of the basolateral amygdala were impaired on their ability to learn a specific aversion to sucrose, but showed a greater generalized aversion to water when compared to intact animals. These results plus the findings that (*a*) rats with amygdala lesions showed a diminished neophobic response when presented with a novel solution, and (*b*) rats with amygdala lesions learned an aversion to a novel solution which was comparable to the aversion acquired by intact rats to a familiar solution, were interpreted as indicating that rats with amygdala lesions are deficient in recognizing the significance of gustatory stimuli. Parenthetically, it is noteworthy that the amygdalar complex is also intricately involved in the orienting responses of most mammals (Kaada, 1972). Lesions of the amygdala eliminate the autonomic components of the orienting reflex (Kaada, 1972), and it is also likely that amygdala ablation disrupts the motivational components of the orienting reflex (as seen by diminution of neophobia, Nachman and Ashe, 1974) including those aspects directly related to the situational relevance of stimuli (Velden, 1978).

Another example of the important role of the amygdala in taste aversion learning is the recent finding that unilateral electrical stimulation of the basolateral nuclei can provide an effective CS when paired with intraperitoneally administered LiCl injection (Phillips and LePiane, 1978). When mild electrical stimulation of the amygdala concurrent with water ingestion was followed by LiCl injection, rats, in a later test, avoided drinking water while electric current was being passed to the amygdala. LiCl injection following water ingestion alone or physiological saline injection following amygdala stimulation alone were ineffective for conditioning. These findings demonstrate that electrical stimulation of the basolateral amygdalar nuclei can be an effective cue for aversion learning. The significance of this study lies partially in the finding that amygdala stimulation combined with water ingestion can produce sufficient information for aversion learning. This is in contrast to the findings that stimulation with light and sound combined with water ingestion, as in the Garcia and Koelling (1966) "bright-noisy water" experiment, is not sufficient for learning a taste aversion. However, the exact nature of the cue produced by amygdala stimulation as in the Phillips and LePiane study remains undetermined; conceivably the electrical stimulus could have imparted a distinctive "taste" to the water. Of equal importance, the same study demonstrated that similar stimulation of the caudate nucleus was ineffective as a CS, indicating at least some specificity of the amygdalar effect.

Electrical stimulation of the amygdala is also effective for the modulation of taste aversion learning when interposed within the CS–UCS interval. However, the exact nature of the effect is far from clear. Kesner et al. (1975) report that subseizure threshold stimulation of the amygdala within the CS–UCS interval is ineffective in disrupting taste aversion learning, but if stimulation is administered 1 minute to 3 hours after the UCS, taste aversion learning is blocked or attenuated. On the other hand, Arthur (1975) using stimulation strengths above the seizure threshold reported converse results, namely, that amygdala stimulation given within the CS–UCS interval disrupted taste aversion acquisition, but stimulation given 15 minutes after the UCS did not disrupt the learning. Thus, it appears that electrical stimulation of the amygdala can be disruptive to taste aversion learning; however, it is difficult to reach firm conclusions regarding the type of deficit involved, and parametric investigations are certainly warranted.

It can be seen that the behavioral effects of altering the functional integrity of the amygdala provides an excellent example of the potential role of processes such as arousal and perceptual discrimination in taste aversion learning. The effect of modulation of the amygdala may reflect the disruption of correlated physiological functions, rather than associative mechanisms per se, and as such is indicative of the need to understand the mode of integration of various physiological processes.

## V. Summary

Recent advances in behavioral research have established taste aversion learning as an important phenomenon suggestive of specialized learning mechanisms. In parallel with these influential behavioral studies, others have focused on the neural basis of taste aversion learning. However, the nature of the underlying neural mechanisms still remains a matter of considerable conjecture. Nevertheless, these studies have served the purpose of highlighting some of the important and basic questions concerning taste aversion learning.

The cardinal question is whether the gustatory and visceral systems are unique in their interaction with each other, and if unique interactions do exist, whether they form the basis of taste aversion learning. In relation to this issue, an attempt has been made to examine the implications of the fact that the gustatory and visceral sensory systems converge at the same initial CNS nucleus. However, the functional relevance of this anatomical convergence remains unknown. As an alternative to the idea of a specialized direct interaction of gustatory and visceral stimuli, it may be that these two afferent systems do not interact directly, any more than do any other two sensory systems, but may for other reasons be especially effective in modulating the on-going physiology of the animal in a manner necessary for subsequent learning.

Another question that has been addressed concerns the neural basis for the long CS–UCS interval. At this juncture only a few neuronal models are available that can account for the long CS–UCS interval seen in taste aversion learning. Whether such enduring neuronal mechanisms may have a role in long-delay taste aversion learning remains for future investigation. Nonetheless, it appears likely that the time-spanning processes reflected in the extended CS–UCS interval are initiated by the gustatory stimulus. Evidently, the memory of gustatory input is stored in a manner that is readily accessible, and in an associable form, for the later association with a visceral UCS.

Research concerned with the neuroanatomical substrate of taste aversion learning has consisted primarily of the ablation of discrete nuclei of the CNS. For the most part, these studies have not been particularly enlightening, but it is encouraging that various lines of evidence have converged to strongly implicate a region of the limbic system, the amygdalar complex, in taste aversion learning. In addition to being an important region of gustatory–visceral convergence, the amygdala has been implicated partly because of its contribution to alerting reactions (neophobia) and to general arousal. It will undoubtedly prove profitable to our knowledge of the neural basis of taste aversion learning, to extend out understanding of the neural correlates of neophobia and the relationship that they may bear to the acquisition of this learning. Likewise, future research will surely inquire more fully into the nature of gustatory–visceral afferents at the primary sensory level, i.e., the nucleus of the solitary tract.

We are also encouraged by the apparent first signs of movement toward examination of the functional role in taste aversion learning of specific neuroanatomical systems as defined by their common neurotransmitters. We envision that this trend will broaden to encompass the study of the modulating effect that one neurotransmitter may have upon the subsequent postsynaptic action of another neurotransmitter as such interactions may have unusual significance for the initiation of enduring neuronal changes.

## References

Aghajanian, G. K., and Wang, R. Y. (1977). Habenular and other midbrain raphe afferents demonstrated by a modified retrograde tracing technique. *Brain Research* **122**, 229–242.

Alger, B. E., and Teyler, T. J. (1976). Long-term and short-term plasticity in the CA1, CA3, and dentate regions of the rat hippocampal slice. *Brain Research* **110**, 463–480.

Amit, Z., and Baum, M. (1970). Comment on the increased resistance-to-extinction of an avoidance response induced by certain drugs. *Phychological Reports,* **27**, 310.

Amit, Z., Levitan, D. E., Brown, Z. W., and Rogan, F. (1977). Possible involvement of central factors in the mediation of conditioned taste aversion. *Neuropharmacology* **16**, 121–124.

Arthur, J. B. (1975). Taste aversion learning is impaired by interpolated amygdaloid stimulation but not by posttraining amygdaloid stimulation. *Behavioral Biology* **13**, 369–376.

Baker, L. J., Baker, T. B., and Kesner, R. P., (1977). Taste aversion learning in young and adult rats. *Journal of Comparative and Physiological Psychology* **91**, 1168–1178.

Bambridge, R., and Gijsbers, K. (1977). The role of tonic neural activity in motivational processes. *Experimental Neurology* 56, 370–385.

Barker, L. M. (1976). CS duration, amount, and concentration effects in conditioning taste aversions. *Learning and Motivation* 7, 265–273.

Barker, L. M., Best, M. R., and Domjan, M. (Eds.) (1977). "Learning Mechanisms in Food Selection." Baylor University Press, Waco, Texas.

Barnett, S. A. (1975). "The Rat: A Study in Behavior" (rev. ed.). University of Chicago Press, Chicago.

Berger, B. D. (1972). Conditioning of food aversions by injections of phychoactive drugs. *Journal of Comparative and Physiological Psychology* 81, 21–26.

Berger, B. D., Wise, C. D., and Stein, L. (1973). Area postrema damage and bait shyness. *Journal of Comparative and Physiological Psychology* 82, 475–479.

Best, P. J., and Orr, J. (1973). Effects of hippocampal lesions on passive avoidance and taste aversion conditioning. *Physiology and Behavior* 10, 193–196.

Bliss, T. V. P., and Gardner-Medwin, A. R. (1973). Long-lasting potentiation of synaptic transmission in the dentate area of the unanaesthetized rabbit following stimulation of the perforant path. *Journal of Physiology* 232, 357–374.

Bliss, T. V. P., and Lómo, T. (1973). Long-lasting potentiation of synaptic transmission in the dentate area of the anaesthetized rabbit following stimulation of the perforant path. *Journal of Physiology* 232, 331–356.

Blomquist, A. J., and Antem, A. (1965). Localization of the terminals of the tongue afferents in the nucleus of the solitary tract. *Journal of Comparative Neurology* 124, 127–130.

Borison, H. L. (1974). Area postrema: Chemoreceptor trigger zone for vomiting—is that all? *Life Sciences* 14, 1807–1817.

Borison, H. L., and Wang, S. C. (1949). Functional localization of central coordinating mechanism for emesis in cat. *Journal of Neurophysiology* 12, 305–313.

Braun, J. J., and McIntosh, H. (1973). Learned taste aversions induced by rotational stimulation. *Physiological Psychology* 1, 301–304.

Braun, J. J., and Rosenthal, B. (1976). Relative salience of saccharin and quinine in long-delay taste aversion learning. *Behavioral Biology* 16, 341–352.

Braun, J. J., Slick, T. B., and Lorden, J. F., (1972). Involvement of gustatory neocortex in the learning of taste aversions. *Physiology and Behavior* 9, 637–641.

Brauth, S. E., and Olds, J. (1977). Midbrain unit activity during classical conditioning. *Brain Research* 134, 73–82.

Braveman, N. S. (1977). What studies on preexposure to pharmacological agents tell us about the nature of the aversion-inducing agent. *In* "Learning Mechanisms in Food Selection" (L. M. Barker, M. R. Best, and M. Domjan, eds.), pp. 511–530. Baylor University Press, Waco, Texas.

Brodal, A. (1969). "Neurological Anatomy" (2nd ed.). Oxford University Press, New York.

Brown, D. L., and Glusman, M. (1971). Conditioned gustatory aversion produced with anesthetic and convulsive agents. *Psychonomic Science* 25, 49.

Bures, J., Buresová, O., and Fifková, E. (1961). The effect of cortical and hippocampal spreading depression on activity of bulbopontine reticular units in the rat. *Archives Italiennes de Biologie* 99, 23–32.

Buresová, O., and Bures, J. (1973). Cortical and subcortical components of the conditioned saccharin aversion. *Physiology and Behavior* 11, 435–439.

Buresová, O., and Bures, J. (1974). Functional decortication in the CS-US interval decrease efficiency of taste learning. *Behavioral Biology* 12, 357–364.

Buresová, O., and Bures, J. (1977). The effect of anesthesia on acquisition and extinction of conditioned taste aversion. *Behavioral Biology* 20, 41–50.

Cappell, H., and LeBlanc, A. E. (1971). Conditioned aversion to saccharin by single administrations of mescaline and $d$-amphetamine. *Psychopharmacologia* 22, 352–356.

Cappell, H. D., LeBlanc, A. E., and Endrenyi, L. (1973). Aversive conditioning by psychoactive drugs: Effects of morphine, alcohol, and chlordiazepoxide. *Psychopharmacologia* **29**, 239–246.

Carey, R. J., and Goodall, E. B. (1974). A conditioned taste aversion induced by $\alpha$-methyl-$p$-tyrosine. *Neuropharmacology* **13**, 595–600.

Coil, J. D., Hankins, W. G., Jenden, D. J., and Garcia, J. (1978a). The attenuation of a specific cue-to-consequence association by antiemetic agents. *Psychopharmacology* **56**, 21–25.

Coil, J. D., Rogers, R. C., Garcia, J., and Novin, D. (1978b). Conditioned taste aversions: Vagal and circulatory mediation of the toxic unconditioned stimulus. *Behavioral Biology* **24**, 509–519.

Conrad, L. C. A., Leonard, C. M., and Pfaff, D. W. (1974). Connections of the median and dorsal raphe nuclei in the rat: An autoradiographic and degeneration study. *Journal of Comparative Neurology* **156**, 179–206.

Deadwyler, S. A., Gribkoff, V., Cotman, C. W., and Lynch, G. (1976). Long-lasting changes in the spontaneous activity of hippocampal neurons following stimulation of the entorhinal cortex. *Brain Research Bulletin* **1**, 1–7.

Dell, P., and Olson, R. (1951). Projections "secondaires" mésencéphaliques, diencéphaliques et amygdaliennes des afférences viscérales vagales. *Societé de Biologie Comptes Rendus* **145**, 1088–1091.

de Wied, D. (1974). Pituitary-adrenal system hormones and behavior. *In* "The Neurosciences: Third Study Program" (F. O. Schmitt and F. G. Worden, eds.), pp. 653–666. MIT Press, Cambridge.

Douglas, R. M., and Goddard, G. V. (1975). Long-term potentiation of the perforant path-granule cell synapse in the rat hippocampus. *Brain Research* **86**, 205–215.

Dykman, R. A. (1967). On the nature of classical conditioning. *In* "Methods in Psychophysiology" (C. C. Brown, ed.), pp. 234–290. Wilkins & Wilkins, Baltimore.

Eccles, J. C. (1964). "The Physiology of Synapses." Academic Press, New York.

Eleftheriou, B. E. (ed.) (1972). "The neurobiology of the Amygdala." Plenum, New York.

Etscorn, F., and Stephens, R. (1973). Establishment of conditioned taste aversion with a 24-hour CS-US interval. *Physiological Psychology* **1**, 251–253.

Freedman, R., Hoffer, B. J., Woodward, D. J., and Puro, D. (1977). Interaction of norepinephrine with cerebellar activity evoked by mossy and climbing fibers. *Experimental Neurology* **55**, 269–288.

Gamzu, E. (1977). The multifaceted nature of taste-aversion-inducing agents: Is there a single common factor? *In* "Learning Mechanisms in Food Selection" (L. M. Barker, M. R. Best, and M. Domjan, eds.), pp. 477–509. Baylor University Press, Waco, Texas.

Garcia, J., and Ervin, F. R. (1968). Gustatory-visceral and telereceptor-cutaneous conditioning: Adaptation in internal and external milieus. *Communications in Behavioral Biology* **1** 389–415.

Garcia, J., Koelling, R. A. (1966). Relation of cue to consequence in avoidance learning. *Psychonomic Science* **4**, 123–124.

Garcia, J., and Kimeldorf, D. J., and Koelling, R. A. (1955). Conditioned aversion to saccharin resulting from exposure to gamma radiation. *Science* **122**, 157–158.

Garcia, J., Ervin, F. R., and Koelling, R. A. (1966). Learning with prolonged delay of reinforcement. *Psychonomic Science* **5**, 121–122.

Gaston, K. E. (1978). Brain mechanisms of conditioned taste aversion learning: A review of the literature. *Physiological Psychology* **6**, 340–353.

Gold, P. E., and McGaugh, J. L. (1975). A single-trace, two process view of memory storage processes. *In* "Short-Term Memory" (D. Deutsch and J. A. Deutsch, eds.), pp. 335–378. Academic Press, New York.

Gold, R. M., and Proulx, D. M. (1972). Bait-shyness acquisition is impaired by VMH lesions that produce obesity. *Journal of Comparative and Physiological Psychology* **79**, 201–209.

Greenberg, D., Dowdy, E. E., and Peacock, L. J. (1977). Disruption of lithiumchloride-induced taste aversion by subdiaphragmatic vagotomy. *Bulletin of the Psychonomic Society* **18**, 254.

Hankins, W. G., Garcia, J., and Rusiniak, K. W. (1973). Dissociation of odor and taste in bait shyness. *Behavioral Biology* **8**, 407–419.

Hankins, W. G., Garcia, J., and Rusiniak, K. W. (1974). Cortical lesions: Flavor illness and noise-shock conditioning. *Behavioral Biology* **10**, 173–181.

Hartley, P. L. (1977). Motion-induced learned taste aversions in rats and the role of the area postrema. Unpublished dissertation. University of California, Riverside.

Hatcher, R. A., and Weiss, S. (1923). Studies on vomiting. *Journal of Pharmacology and Experimental Therapeutics* **22**, 139–193.

Herrick, C. J. (1948). "The Brain of the Tiger Salamander: *Ambystoma tigrinum.*" University of Chicago Press, (1976). Chicago.

Hobbs, S. H., Elkins, R. L., and Peacock, L. J. (1974). Taste-aversion conditioning in rats with septal lesions. *Behavioral Biology* **11**, 239–245.

Hobbs, S. H., Clingerman, H. K., and Elkins, R. L. (1976). Illness-induced taste aversions in normal and bulbectomized hamsters. *Physiology and Behavior* **17**, 235–238.

Ionescu, E., and Buresová, O. (1977). Failure to elicit conditioned taste aversion by severe poisoning. *Pharmacology Biochemistry and Behavior* **6**, 251–254.

Iversen, S. D., and Iversen, L. L. (1975). "Behavioral Pharmacology." Oxford University Press, New York.

Kaada, B. R. (1972). Stimulation and regional ablation of the amygdaloid complex with reference to functional representations. *In* "The Neurobiology of the Amygdala" (B. E. Eleftheriou, ed.), pp. 205–281. Plenum, New York.

Kemble, E. D., and Nagel, J. A. (1973). Failure to form a learned taste aversion in rats with amygdaloid lesions. *Bulletin of the Psychonomic Society* **2**, 155–156.

Kesner, R. P., Berman, R. F., Burton, B., and Hankins, W. G. (1975). Effects of electrical stimulation of amygdala upon neophobia and taste aversion. *Behavioral Biology* **13**, 349–358.

Key, B. J., and Mehta, V. H. (1977). Changes in electrocortical activity induced by the perfusion of 5-hydroxytryptamine into the nucleus of the solitary tract. *Neuropharmacology* **16**, 99–106.

Koella, W. P. (1974). Serotonin—a hypnogenic transmitter and an antiwaking agent. *Advances in Biochemical Psychopharmacology* **11**, 181–186.

Kral, P. A. (1971). Electroconvulsive shock during taste-illness interval: Evidence for induced disassociation. *Physiology and Behavior* **7**, 667–670.

Krane, R. V., and Wagner, A. R. (1975). Taste aversion learning with a delayed shock US: Implications for the "generality of the laws of learning." *Journal of Comparative and Physiological Psychology* **88**, 882–889.

Krane, R. V., Sinnamon, H. M., and Thomas, G. J. (1976). Conditioned taste aversions and neophobia in rats with hippocampal lesions. *Journal of Comparative and Physiological Psychology* **90**, 680–693.

Levy, C. J., Carroll, M. E., and Smith, J. C. (1974). Antihistamines block radiation-induced taste aversions. *Science* **186**, 1044–1046.

Libet, B. (1970). Generation of slow inhibitory and excitatory postsynaptic potentials. *Federation Proceedings* **29**, 1945–1956.

Libet, B. (1979). Dopaminergic synaptic processes in the superior cervical ganglion: Models for synaptic actions. In "The Neurobiology of Dopamine " (A. Horn, J. Korf, and B.H.C. Westerink, eds.), pp. 453–474. Academic Press, New York.

Libet, B., and Owman, C. (1974). Concomitant changes in formaldehyde-induced fluorescence of dopamine interneurones and in slow inhibitory postsynaptic potentials of the rabbit superior cervical ganglion, induced by stimulation of the preganglionic nerve or by a muscarinic agent. *Journal of Physiology* 237, 635–662.

Libet, B., and Tosaka, T. (1970). Dopamine as a synaptic transmitter and modulator in sympathetic ganglia: A different mode of synaptic action. *Proceedings of the National Academy of Sciences* 67, 667–673.

Libet, B., Kobayashi, H., and Tanaka, T. (1975). Synaptic coupling into the production and storage of a neuronal memory trace. *Nature (London)* 258, 155–157.

Lorden, J. F. (1976). Effects of lesions of the gustatory neocortex on taste aversion learning in the rat. *Journal of Comparative and Physiological Psychology* 90, 665–679.

Lorden, J. F., and Margules, D. L. (1977). Enhancement of conditioned taste aversions by lesions of the midbrain raphe nuclei that deplete serotonin. *Physiological Psychology* 5, 273–279.

Lorden, J. F., and Oltmans, G. A. (1978). Alteration of the characteristics of learned taste aversion by manipulation of serotonin levels in the rat. *Pharmacology Biochemistry and Behavior* 8, 13–18.

McGaugh, J. L., and Gold, P. E. (1974). The effects of drugs and electrical stimulation of the brain on memory storage processes. In "Neurohumoral Coding of Brain Function" (R. D. Myers and R. R. Drucker-Colin, eds.), pp. 189–206. Plenum, New York.

McGowan, B. K., Garcia, J., Ervin, F. R., and Schwartz, J. (1969). Effects of septal lesions on bait shyness in the rat. *Physiology and Behavior* 4, 907–909.

McGowan, B. K., Hankins, W. G., and Garcia, J. (1972). Limbic lesions and control of the internal and external environment. *Behavioral Biology* 7, 841–852.

Makous, W., Nord, S., Oakley, B., and Pfaffman, C. (1963). The gustatory relay in the medulla. In "Olfaction and Taste" (Y. Zotterman, ed.), pp. 381–393. Pergamon, New York.

Martin, J. R., Cheng, F. Y., and Novin, D. (1978). Acquisition of learned taste aversion following bilateral subdiaphragmatic vagotomy in rats. *Physiology and Behavior* 21, 13–17.

Miller, C. R., Elkins, R. L., and Peacock, L. J. (1971). Disruption of a radiation induced preference shift by hippocampal lesions. *Physiology and Behavior* 6, 283–285.

Miller, C. R., Elkins, R. L., Fraser, J., Peacock, L. J., and Hobbs, S. H. (1975). Taste aversion and passive avoidance in rats with hippocampal lesions. *Physiological Psychology* 3, 123–126.

Morest, D. K. (1960). A study of the structure of the area postrema with golgi methods. *American Journal of Anatomy* 107, 291–303.

Morest, D. K. (1967). Experimental study of the projections of the nucleus of the tractus solitarius and the area postrema in the cat. *Journal of Comparative Neurology* 130, 277–300.

Murphy, L. R., and Brown, T. S. (1974). Hippocampal lesions and learned taste aversion. *Physiological Psychology* 2, 60–64.

Nachman, M. (1963). Learned aversion to the taste of lithium chloride and generalization to other salts. *Journal of Comparative and Physiological Psychology* 56, 343–349.

Nachman, M. (1970a). Learned taste and temperature aversions due to lithium chloride sickness after temporal delays. *Journal of Comparative and Physiological Psychology* 73, 22–30.

Nachman, M. (1970b). Limited effects of electroconvulsive shock on memory of taste stimulation. *Journal of Comparative and Physiological Psychology* **73**, 31-37.

Nachman, M., and Ashe, J. H. (1973). Learned taste aversions in rats as a function of dosage, concentration, and route of administration of LiCl. *Physiology and Behavior* **10**, 73-78.

Nachman, M., and Ashe, J. H. (1974). Effects of basolateral amygdala lesions on neophobia, learned taste aversions, and sodium appetite in rats. *Journal of Comparative and Physiological Psychology* **87**, 622-643.

Nachman, M., and Hartley, P. L. (1975). Role of illness in producing learned taste aversions in rats: A comparison of several rodenticides. *Journal of Comparative and Physiological Psychology* **89**, 1010-1018.

Nachman, M., Rauschenberger, J., and Ashe, J. H. (1977a). Stimulus characteristics in food aversion learning. In "Food Aversion Learning" (N. W. Milgram, L. Krames, and T. M. Alloway, eds.), pp. 105-131. Plenum, New York.

Nachman, M., Rauschenberger, J., and Ashe, J. H. (1977b). Studies of learned aversions using non-gustatory stimuli. In "Learning Mechanisms in Food Selection" (L. M. Barker, M. R. Best, and M. Domjan, eds.), pp. 395-417. Baylor University Press, Waco, Texas.

Newman, P. P. (1974). "Visceral Afferent Functions of the Nervous System." Edward Arnold, London.

Norgren, R. (1976). Taste pathways to hypothalamus and amygdala. *Journal of Comparative Neurology* **166**, 17-30.

Norgren, R., and Leonard, C. M. (1973). Ascending central gustatory pathways. *Journal of Comparative Neurology* **150**, 217-238.

Norgren, R., and Wolf, G. (1975). Projections of thalamic gustatory and lingual areas in the rat. *Brain Research* **92**, 123-129.

O'Brien, J. H., and Fox, S. S. (1969). Single-cell activity in cat motor cortex. II. Functional characteristics of the cell related to conditioning changes. *Journal of Neurophysiology* **32**, 285-296.

Oldendorf, W. H. (1975). Permeability of the blood-brain barrier. In "The Nervous System. Vol. I: The Basic Neurosciences" (D. B. Tower, ed.) pp. 279-289. Raven Press, New York.

Oleson, T. D., Ashe, J. H., and Weinberger, N. M. (1975). Modification of auditory and somatosensory system activity during pupillary conditioning in the paralyzed cat. *Journal of Neurophysiology* **38**, 1114-1139.

Perrotto, R. S., and Scott, T. R. (1976). Gustatory neural coding in the pons. *Brain Research* **110**, 283-300.

Peters, R. H., and Reich, M. J. (1973). Effects of ventromedial hypothalamic lesions on conditioned sucrose aversions in rats. *Journal of Comparative and Physiological Psychology* **84**, 502-506.

Phillips, A. G., and LePiane, F. G. (1978). Electrical stimulation of the amygdala as a conditioned stimulus in a bait-shyness paradigm. *Science* **201**, 536-538.

Prosser, C L., Painter, E. E., Lisco, H., Brues, A. M., Jacobson, L. O., and Swift, M. N. (1947). The clinical sequence of physiological effects of ionizing radiation in animals. *Radiology* **49**, 299-313.

Reader, T. A., Ferron, A., and Descarries, L. (1977). Modulation of the unitary activity of cortical neurons by the biogenic amines: A microiontophoretic study. *Society for Neuroscience Abstracts* **3**, 257.

Revusky, S. H., (1968). Aversion to sucrose produced by contingent x-irradiation: Temporal and dosage parameters. *Journal of Comparative and Physiological Psychology* **65**, 17-22.

Revusky, S. H., and Garcia, J. (1970). Learned associations over long delays. *In* "Psychology of Learning and Motivation: Advances in Research and Theory" (G.H. Bower and J. T. Spence, eds.), Vol. IV, pp. 1-84. Academic Press, New York.

Rigter, H., and Popping, A. (1976). Hormonal influences on the extinction of conditioned taste aversion. *Psychopharmacologia* 46, 255-261.

Riley, A. L., and Baril, L. L. (1976). Conditioned taste aversions: A bibliography. *Animal Learning and Behavior* 4, 1S-13S.

Rolls, B. J., and Rolls, E. T. (1973). Effects of lesions in the basolateral amygdala on fluid intake in the rat. *Journal of Comparative and Physiological Psychology* 83, 240-247.

Roth, G. I., and Yamamoto, W. S. (1968). The microcirculation of the area postrema in the rat. *Journal of Comparative Neurology* 133, 329-340.

Roth, S. R., Schwartz, M., and Teitelbaum, P. (1973). Failure of recovered lateral hypothalamic rats to learn specific food aversions. *Journal of Comparative and Physiological Psychology* 83, 184-197.

Rozin, P. (1969). Central or peripheral mediation of learning with long CS-US intervals in the feeding system. *Journal of Comparative and Physiological Psychology* 67, 421-429.

Rozin, P., and Ree, P. (1972). Long extension of effective CS-US interval by anesthesia between CS and US. *Journal of Comparative and Physiological Psychology* 80, 43-48.

Schuster, C. R., and Thompson, T. (1969). Self administration of and behavioral dependence on drugs. *Annual Review of Pharmacology* 9, 483-502.

Schwartz, M., and Teitelbaum, P. (1974). Dissociation between learning and remembering in rats with lesions in the lateral hypothalamus. *Journal of Comparative and Physiological Psychology* 87, 384-398.

Seligman, M. E. P. (1970). On the generality of the laws of learning. *Psychological Review* 77, 406-418.

Smith, J. C. (1971). Radiation: Its detection and its effects on taste preferences. *In* "Progress in Physiological Psychology" (E. Stellar and J. M. Sprague, eds.), Vol. IV pp. 53-118. Academic Press, New York.

Smith, J. C., and Roll, D. L. (1967). Trace conditioning with X-rays as an aversive stimulus. *Psychonomic Science* 9, 11-12.

Smotherman, W. P., and Levine, S. (1978). ACTH and $ACTH_{4-10}$ modification of neophobia and taste aversion responses in the rat. *Journal of Comparative and Physiological Psychology* 92, 22-33.

Smotherman, W. P., Hennessy, J. W., and Levine, S. (1976). Plasma corticosterone levels as an index of the strength of illness induced taste aversions. *Physiology and Behavior* 17, 903-908.

Testa, T. J. (1974). Causal relationships and the acquisition of avoidance responses. *Psychological Review* 81, 491-505.

Thompson, R. F. (1976). The search for the engram. *American Psychologist* 31, 209-227.

Torvik, A. (1956). Afferent connections of the sensory trigeminal nuclei, the nucleus of the solitary tract and adjacent structures. An experimental study in the rat. *Journal of Comparative Neurology* 106, 51-141.

Velden, M. (1978). Some necessary revisions of the neuronal model concept of the orienting response. *Psychophysiology* 15, 181-185.

Wang, R. Y., and Aghajanian, G. K. (1977). Inhibition of neurons in the amygdala by dorsal raphe stimulation: Mediation through a direct serotonergic pathway. *Brain Research* 120, 85-102.

Wang, S. C., and Borison, H. L. (1952). A new concept of organization of the central emetic mechanism: Recent studies on the sites of action of apomorphine, copper sulfate and cardiac glycosides. *Gastroenterology* **22**, 1-12.

Weisman, R. N., Hamilton, L. W., and Carlton, P. L. (1972). Increased conditioned gustatory aversion following VMH lesions in rats. *Physiology and Behavior* **9**, 801-804.

Winn, F. J., Kent, M. A., and Libkuman, T. M. (1975). Learned taste aversion induced by cortical spreading depression. *Physiology and Behavior* **15**, 21-24.

Yoshii, N., and Ogura, N. (1960). Studies on the unit discharge of brainstem reticular formation in the cat. *Medical Journal of Osaka University* **11**, 1-17.

Young, R. A., Cegavske, C. F., and Thompson, R. F. (1976). Tone-induced changes in excitability of abducens motoneurons and of the reflex path of nictitating membrane response in rabbit (*Oryctolagus cuniculus*). *Journal of Comparative and Physiological Psychology* **90**, 424-434.

PROGRESS IN PSYCHOBIOLOGY AND PHYSIOLOGICAL PSYCHOLOGY, VOL. 9

# Thirst: The Initiation, Maintenance, and Termination of Drinking

Barbara J. Rolls, Roger J. Wood, and Edmund T. Rolls

*The Department of Experimental Psychology*
*University of Oxford, Oxford, Great Britain*

## I. Introduction

Body water is contained within two compartments, the cellular (approximately 40%of body weight) and extracellular (approximately 20% of body weight, divided between the blood plasma and the interstitial fluid). These compartments can be selectively depleted and a reduction in the fluid content of either the cellular or extracellular fluid compartment stimulates thirst as well as fluid conservation by the kidneys. Studies of the physiological significance of these cellular and extracellular stimuli in relation to drinking form an important part of this article. The particular concern here is to what extent these depletions are present and actually produce normal drinking by animals, either after water deprivation or during spontaneous drinking when the animal has continual free access to water. If fluid deficits are insufficient to account

263

Copyright © 1980 by Academic Press, Inc.
All rights of reproduction in any form reserved.
ISBN 0-12-542109-5

for normal drinking, other possibilities to be considered are that by habit drinking normally occurs in anticipation of the development of deficits in the cellular and extracellular fluid compartments (Mogenson and Phillips, 1976; Toates, 1979), peripheral factors such as a dry mouth normally provide the stimulus to drink, and fluid is taken at meal times to facilitate the ingestion of food.

Once drinking is initiated, the question arises as to which factors maintain the drinking. Do animals drink because removal of physiological deficits is sensed and is rewarding or do animals drink because of oropharyngeal sensations such as taste, or because gastric or intestinal stimulation is rewarding? These questions can be answered by using gastric, duodenal, and intravenous cannulae to isolate these factors experimentally. Investigations in which this has been done are described.

Drinking that is in progress can be terminated by removal of fluid deficits in the two main compartments following absorption or by "feedforward" mechanisms such as oral metering, or activation of receptors in the gut or hepatic portal circulation. We have measured how rapidly the cellular and extracellular stimuli of drinking diminish during drinking to determine whether they decrease sufficiently rapidly to account for the termination of drinking in cannulated preparations.

Many of these investigations require repeated withdrawal of blood to estimate changes in the cellular and extracellular fluid compartments. For this reason, and also because the different patterns of drinking in different species can highlight the ways in which various factors contribute to drinking, the questions raised have been investigated in the dog and in the monkey in addition to the more commonly used laboratory rat. Investigations in the monkey are of particular interest, in that, despite clinical problems of thirst in man, relatively little of the physiology of drinking has been investigated in any primate. Some recent studies on the controls of drinking in man himself are also described. We first consider the initiation of drinking.

## II. The Initiation of Drinking

A. Cellular Stimuli

*1. Cellular Dehydration as a Thirst Stimulus*

The drinking which occurs when the body fluids become concentrated appears to be initiated by cellular dehydration. For example, administration (intravenously or intraperitoneally) of hypertonic sodium chloride leads to withdrawal of water from the cells by osmosis, and produces drinking. The effective change appears to be cellular dehydration and not absolute osmotic pressure (i.e., osmolality, as measured by freezing point depression), in that administration of substances such as sodium chloride and sucrose which remain outside the cells and therefore cause cellular dehydration do cause drinking, whereas administration of substances such as glucose, urea, and methyl glucose, which cross the cell membrane and do not therefore lead to cellular dehydration, stimulate little or no drinking (Gilman, 1937; Fitzsimons, 1961). The degree of cellular dehydration is monitored accurately in that there is a precise relation between the amount of sodium chloride administered and the amount drunk in nephrectomized rats in which the stimulus cannot be modified by urine production (Fitzsimons, 1961).

Recently, the cellular dehydration theory has been challenged by Andersson and his colleagues (Andersson and Olsson, 1973; Andersson, 1978). They suggest that the critical event may be a change in the sodium concentration of the cerebrospinal fluid. They agree that the receptors for cellular thirst are located in the central nervous sytem, but propose that they respond to changes in the sodium concentration of the cerebrospinal fluid (CSF) rather than to cellular dehydration. A critical test of this theory is to apply an osmotically active substance other than sodium to the receptors in the brain and to determine whether drinking follows. Blass and Epstein (1971) and Peck and Novin (1971) found that the direct application of sucrose to central osmoreceptors stimulates drinking in the rat and rabbit. In a different type of test the sodium content of the cerebrospinal fluid was measured and manipulated. It was found that drinking correlates poorly with the measured concentration of sodium in the cerebrospinal fluid (Epstein, 1978). Instead drinking was related to withdrawal of water from the cells during ventricular infusions of sodium or sucrose (Thrasher et al., 1978). So we have come full circle back to Gilman's sugestion that dehydration of cells is a crucial stimulus of thirst, and is sensed rather than sodium concentration or absolute osmotic pressure.

Before proceeding to the question of where the receptors for cellular thirst are located it is essential to clarify one point. We have just reviewed the evidence which indicates that cellular dehydration and not general increases in osmolality or sodium concentration constitutes the crucial thirst stimulus. In practice, however, plasma sodium concentration and plasma osmolality are highly correlated (Wood et al., 1977) and both give a good indication of the degree of cellular dehydration. This is because sodium and its attendant anions account for 95% of plasma osmolality so that changes in sodium concentration acting through cellular dehydration will be the most important factor in cellular thirst.

In the past the cells which respond to cellular dehydration have been referred to as "osmoreceptors" and we will continue this convention.

## 2. Localization of the Osmoreceptors

It is thought that there are specific osmoreceptors for thirst similar to those described by Verney (1947) for the release of antidiuretic hormone. A wide variety of possible locations for such thirst receptors have been suggested, including the stomach, gut, hepatic portal circulation, and mast cells in the peritoneal cavity (see Section II,A,4). Since 1953, when Andersson found that injections of hypertonic sodium chloride directly into the hypothalamus caused drinking in the goat, it has been presumed that there are osmoreceptors for thirst in the central nervous system. Andersson's doses of saline were, however, large and outside the physiological range so that the thirst could have been due to nonspecific stimulation.

One way of establishing clearly whether there are receptors in the brain which respond to dehydration is to increase the tonicity of the blood perfusing the brain. This technique provides a more physiological stimulus than does direct application of substances to the brain, and has been utilized by Wood et al. (1977). The main blood supply to the forebrain is provided by the carotid arteries, and, in a large animal such as the dog, carotid loops can be prepared. This is a simple surgical procedure in which the arteries are exteriorized and then the loose skin of the neck is sewn around them.

The arteries are thus readily accessible for injections or infusions. An advantage of this technique is that the osmolality of the blood perfusing the brain can be altered with little change in the osmolality of the rest of the body. Dogs which had been prepared with bilateral carotid loops were infused for 10 minutes with hypertonic sodium chloride in doses designed to elevate central osmolality within the physiological range. A graded increase in drinking was obtained with increasing concentration of the saline (see Fig. 1). It was shown by plasma samples taken from the jugular vein that the infusions which elicited drinking did elevate central osmolality within the range which can occur normally after, for example, water deprivation, and it was also shown that these small carotid infusions had no significant effect on peripheral systemic osmolality. Control intravenous (as opposed to intracarotid) infusions of 0.3 $M$ NaCl at the same rate did not cause drinking. Thus these results show clearly that there are receptors for thirst in the brain and that they are located within the area supplied with blood from the carotid arteries (Wood et al., 1977).

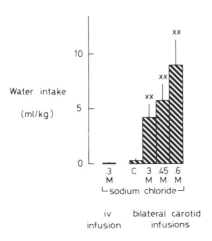

FIG. 1. Water intake during infusions of hypertonic solutions in eight fluid-replete dogs. Means and SEM are shown. All carotid infusions were bilateral at a total rate of 0.6 ml kg$^{-1}$ min$^{-1}$ for 10 minutes and water intake was measured for the last 5 minutes. Control infusion (C) was 0.15 $M$ NaCl. xx, Significant at $p < 0.01$ when compared to control. Modified from Wood *et al.* (1977).

## 3. Osmoreceptors in the Central Nervous System

Further evidence that there are central osmoreceptors for drinking comes from studies in which osmotically active solutions have been injected intracranially. Relatively small volumes (0.5–2.0 μl) of mildly hypertonic (0.18–0.30 $M$ or more) saline injected bilaterally into the lateral preoptic area produced drinking in the rat (Blass and Epstein, 1971) and rabbit (Peck and Novin, 1971). The effect of the injections is specific in that eating was not elicited by the injections. The effect is ascribed to cellular dehydration and not to activation of a sodium receptor in that similar injections of hypertonic sucrose also elicited drinking. Further, equimolar injections of urea, which do not cause cellular dehydration because the urea crosses the cell membrane, did not elicit drinking. The effective injection sites were dispersed relatively widely, from the anterior commissure anteriorly to the zona incerta posteriorly (Blass, 1974; Peck and Blass, 1975), so that the osmoreceptors themselves could be widely distributed in the lateral preoptic and lateral hypothalamic areas. Intraventricular injections have been found to be less effective (in terms of the minimal effective concentration) in eliciting drinking, so that the effective injections in the lateral preoptic and hypothalamic areas probably do not act by spread of fluid through the ventricles to a different osmoreceptor region (Blass, 1974). Because the thirst-inducing action of these injections does not always correspond with their effect on antidiuretic hormone (ADH) release, it is possible that osmoreceptors for ADH release and for thirst are separate, but contiguous (Peck and Blass, 1975). Thus this evidence suggests that there are osmoreceptors in the brain with a rather widespread distribution in the lateral preoptic and lateral hypothalamic areas whose activation can lead to drinking.

Apparently consistent with the view that there are osmoreceptors for drinking in the lateral preoptic area is the report that bilateral lesions of the lateral preoptic area abolish drinking to systemic loads of sodium chloride in the rat (Blass and Epstein, 1971) and rabbit (Peck and Novin, 1971). However, the effect of the lesions is complex in that in some animals there is a specific deficit to cellular dehydration alone whereas in others both cellular and extracellular thirst are impaired (Blass and Epstein, 1971; B. J. Rolls, 1975). Recently, interpretation of the preoptic area lesion studies has been complicated by the finding that if instead of allowing rats just 4 hours to drink to an osmotic load of sodium chloride delivered intraperitoneally, a longer period of time is allowed, rats with such lesions drink almost exactly what they need for osmoregulation (Coburn and Stricker, 1978), as if they can respond to osmotic stimuli. A similar conclusion was reached independently by B. J. Rolls who observed that ip injections of $2\ M$ NaCl reduced the activity of the lesioned rats, as if they were particularly sensitive to the stress of this procedure, and therefore measured drinking to ip injections of a smaller osmotic load ($1\ M$ NaCl) over a longer period (6 hours). She found that the lesioned rats did drink to the osmotic load, but that the drinking was slow. Thus rats with lateral preoptic lesions can drink to osmotic loads, although with intraperitoneal injections a long observation period and the use of a saline solution which is not too hypertonic may be necessary to show this. It should be noted, however, that in these extended tests it is possible that in excreting the solute load, the rats became hypovolemic, and thus drank in response to this stimulus. It would be informative to repeat these studies in nephrectomized rats. However, further evidence that large intraperitoneal salt loads may inhibit behavior through stress is that if hypertonic salt was administered either in the food or intravenously, the lesioned rats drank amounts similar to those taken by control animals (Coburn and Stricker, 1978).

Thus the lesion evidence does not provide useful support for the hypothesis that osmoreceptors for drinking are in the lateral preoptic area. Lesions more medial, in the periventricular tissue at preoptic and hypothalamic levels, particularly in the anteroventral part of the third ventricle (AV3V), can reduce drinking to osmotic as well as some other thirst challenges (Buggy and Johnson, 1977), but the deficits are not fully understood as yet. The function of this region of the brain in drinking is considered in Section II,B,2.

The hypothesis that cells in the preoptic region have a function in response to osmotic changes receives some support from electrophysiological investigations. It has been shown in a number of studies that infusions (in most studies intracarotid) of hypertonic saline influence the activity of some neurons in the preoptic area and hypothalamus, as well as in the supraoptic nucleus, of the rat (Cross and Green, 1959; Blank and Wayner, 1975; Malmo and Mundl, 1975; Weiss and Almli, 1975), the monkey (Hayward and Vincent, 1970; Vincent *et al.*, 1972; see also Hayward, 1977), and the cat (Emmers, 1973). Of the responsive neurons, some in the supraoptic nucleus itself were antidromically activated from the posterior pituitary and are neurosecretory cells for antidiuretic hormone, and others close to the supraoptic nucleus which did not respond to other nonosmotic stimuli could be osmoreceptors in synaptic contact with neuroendocrine cells (Hayward and Vincent 1970; Vincent *et al.*, 1972; Arnauld *et al.*, 1975). Other neurons scattered through the lateral preoptic region and the hypothalamus which responded to the hypertonic infusions could be involved in drinking, but there is no proof of this. Whether these cells responded directly to the hypertonic saline (i.e., were osmoreceptors) or were instead influenced by other osmoreceptor cells is not known, but Oomura *et al.* (1969) did suggest that some neurons in the lateral hypothalamus which responded to the iontophoretic ejection of $Na^+$ were osmoreceptors. Thus there is electrophysiological evidence that neurons in the preoptic area and hypothalamus could be involved in responses to osmotic changes, but whether their activation is involved in drinking is not yet clear.

### 4. Peripheral Osmoreceptors

As shown by intracranial injections and intracarotid infusions of solutions, the osmoreceptors in the central nervous system respond directly to changes in the tonicity of cerebral blood. It is possible that peripheral thirst receptors also feed information about the hydrational state of the rest of the body into the brain. Receptors which respond to changes in osmolality are widely distributed in the stomach, gut (Hunt, 1956), and hepatic-portal system. It has even been suggested that mast cells which are abundant around small blood vessels might act as receptors for cellular dehydration-induced drinking (Goldstein and Halperin, 1977). Of the possible peripheral osmoreceptors those in the hepatic-portal system have received the most attention. Such receptors were originally studied in relation to the secretion of antidiuretic hormone (Haberich, 1968), but there are now studies on both the dog and the rat which suggest that hepatic-portal osmoreceptors may be involved in the control of drinking. In the dog infusions of water into the hepatic-portal vein elevate the threshold for drinking to cellular dehydration produced by systemic hypertonic sodium chloride infusions (Kozlowski and Drzewiecki, 1973). Information about peripheral hydration appears to travel to the central nervous system via the vagus nerve since vagotomy abolishes the effect of these hepatic infusions on drinking in the dog (Kozlowski and Drzewiecki, 1973), and disrupts drinking to a hypertonic challenge in the rat (Kraly *et al.*, 1975). It has also been shown electrophysiologically that perfusion of the portal vein with solutions which alter the osmolality of the blood reaching the liver caused changes in the discharge of the hepatic vagus nerve (Adachi, 1977) and of certain lateral hypothalamic neurons (Schmitt, 1973).

To investigate the role of peripheral osmoreceptors in drinking, we determined whether increased peripheral tonicity can arouse drinking when the blood perfusing central osmoreceptors remains isotonic. In dogs with bilateral carotid loops water intake was measured while an intravenous infusion of hypertonic saline which elevated both systemic and central osmolality (to a degree similar to that which occurs after water deprivation) was combined with intracarotid infusion of water, which kept the blood perfusing the brain isotonic. With such selective peripheral activation the dogs did not drink. Thus peripheral hyperosmolality alone at levels which occur after water deprivation is not sufficient for drinking (Wood *et al.*, 1977). It has also been concluded that the peripheral hyperosmolality produced by water deprivation is not sufficient alone to induce drinking, on the basis of similar experiments in the water-deprived dog in which central hyperosmolality has been attenuated by carotid water infusions (see Section II,C,2,b). These findings, taken with the findings previously described on the drinking induced by central elevation of osmotic pressure alone, indicate that information from peripheral osmoreceptors is not necessary for, and is not sufficient when acting alone for the initiation of drinking in response to physiological levels of cellular dehydration. If peripheral osmoreceptors are involved in the initiation of drinking, their effects must be dependent on the state of central osmoreceptors.

## B. Extracellular Thirst Stimuli

Thus far we have considered only the effect of loss of fluid from inside cells on thirst. Although the amount of fluid in the extracellular fluid compartment is less than that in the cells, it is vital that the extracellular fluid be vigorously defended to avoid debilitating changes in vascular fluid volume and pressure. In addition to the complex physiological and hormonal (e.g., baroreceptor reflexes, antidiuretic hormone, and aldosterone) mechanisms which contribute to the maintenance of extracellular fluid volume, behavioral responses ensure that plasma volume does not fall to dangerously low levels. It is thought that the same type of baro-(i.e., pressure) receptor in the circulatory system which controls the release of antidiuretic hormone is also involved in the control of fluid intake. It is clearly established that hypovolemia (reduction of plasma volume) initiates drinking (see Fitzsimons, 1972; or Stricker, 1973, for review), and there is some evidence from vagosympathectomy studies (Kozlowski and Szczepanska-Sadowska, 1975), and atrial crushing experiments (Zimmerman *et al.*, 1979) that vascular receptors near the heart are involved.

### 1. Angiotensin as a Thirst Stimulus

There is abundant evidence that renal receptors are important in extracellular thirst. Reduced perfusion of the kidney releases renin from that organ. Renin acts on plasma substrate to form angiotensin I, which is then converted to angiotensin II, the vasoactive octapeptide. The stimulation of the central nervous sytem by elevated levels of angiotensin results in increased fluid intake. The suggestion that the kidney may have a role in extracellular thirst was first clearly stated by Fitzsimons (1964) after he found that reduction of levels of circulating angiotensin by bilateral removal of the kidneys reduced drinking to some extracellular thirst challenges. That the effect was hormonal was suggested by the fact that renal extracts stimulated drinking (Fitzsimons, 1969). Fitzsimons and B. Rolls showed that the active dipsogen was probably angiotensin II since intravenous infusions of that substance caused copious drinking (Fitzsimons and Simons, 1969). This then raised the question of how angiotensin elicits drinking. The hypothesis tested by Epstein *et al.* (1970) was that it acts directly on receptors in the central nervous system. They found that the direct application of angiotensin to the brain caused rats in water balance to drink large quantities of water.

The effect of angiotensin is very specific. Drinking is the only behavioral response which follows its administration. For example, after intracranial angiotensin, a sleeping rat woke and went immediately to water. Also, a rat which had been deprived of food, but not of water, stopped feeding to drink (Epstein *et al.,* 1970; McFarland and Rolls, 1972; Rolls and McFarland, 1973). The drinking following angiotensin is highly motivated. After intracranial angiotensin, rats pressed a lever as many as 64 times for a single reward of 0.1 ml of water (Rolls *et al.,* 1972). All species tested with angiotensin (e.g., the rat, gerbil, rabbit, guinea pig, cat, dog, monkey, goat, sheep, Barbary dove, pigeon, sparrow, chicken, marsupial possum, and iguana) have shown a copious drinking response (see Schwob and Johnson, 1977).

## 2. Localization of the Angiotensin Receptors

Since the initial discovery that intracranial angiotensin stimulates drinking, much work has been aimed at precisely localizing the receptive site. In their original work Epstein *et al.* (1970) found the preoptic area to be the most sensitive site, but since angiotensin does not normally penetrate the blood–brain barrier it was difficult to see how the substance would reach its receptors unless the barrier in this region was permeable to angiotensin. A possible answer to this problem is provided by the circumventricular organs. These organs on the surface of the ventricles are part of the brain but lie outside the blood–brain barrier. The importance of the ventricles for the dipsogenic response was indicated by the work of Johnson and Epstein (1975) which showed that intracranial angiotensin stimulated drinking only if the cannulae for its injection passed through a ventricle. Several circumventricular organs have been suggested as receptive sites for angiotensin. Local application of angiotensin to the subfornical organ stimulated drinking and the threshold dose was very low—between 0.1 and 1.0 pg. Furthermore, lesions there or local application of a competitive angiotensin inhibitor abolished drinking to intravenous angiotensin (Simpson and Routtenberg, 1973; Simpson *et al.,* 1977) without affecting drinking to cellular thirst stimuli. Electrophysiological studies have identified angiotensin-sensitive units in the subfornical organ (Felix and Akert, 1974; Phillips and Felix, 1976).

A controversial issue which has been raised by the work on the subfornical organ is whether this site is unique in containing cells sensitive to angiotensin acting as a dipsogen. Lesions of the subfornical organ completely blocked drinking to intravenous angiotensin, but it has been reported that ablation of another circumventricular organ, the organum vasculosum of the lamina terminalis (OVLT) in the anteroventral region of the third ventricle (AV3V) also blocked drinking to angiotensin as well as to other thirst stimuli (Buggy and Johnson, 1977). Furthermore, low doses of angiotensin (down to 50 fg) elicit drinking when applied to the OVLT (Phillips, 1978). Phillips proposes that both ventricular organs contain angiotensin receptors, with the subfornical organ responding to angiotensin in the blood and not the cerebrospinal fluid (CSF) and with the OVLT responding to angiotensin in both the blood and CSF.

In addition to the controversy over whether the subfornical organ or the OVLT might be the sole receptive site or the more important site for angiotensin dipsogenesis, Swanson *et al.* (1978) have continued to pursue the possibility that the preoptic area might contain angiotensin receptors. They found that injections into the preoptic area of small volumes of angiotensin (0.01 $\mu$l containing approximately 6.8 ng), through cannulae which were angled not to pass through the ventricles, stimulated drinking. Radioactive substances injected through the same cannula did not enter the ventricles. They propose that the preoptic area and the circumventricular organs contain duplicate receptors for angiotensin dipsogenesis which respond in different ways since lesions in the lateral hypothalamus decrease drinking to injections in the preoptic area but have little effect on ventricular injections.

Most of the work on the localization of angiotensin receptors has been done in the rat. However, by using a larger animal such as the dog a specific site can be stimulated more precisely and the spread of the injected solution to other areas becomes less of a problem. Recently, using the dog, Fitzsimons and Kucharczyk (1978) have found that both the preoptic area and subfornical organ are very sensitive dipsogenic sites for angiotensin and that the behavior following preoptic area stimulation is not simply due to spread of the injectate to the ventricular organs. They also concluded that there are duplicate receptors for angiotensin dipsogenesis in the preoptic area.

A problem with the preoptic area as a receptive site is still that of the blood–brain barrier. To overcome this problem it has been suggested that the preoptic area might be responsive to the angiotensin generated within the brain (Kucharczyk *et al.*, 1976). However, the current status of the proposal for a brain renin system is controversial (Hirose *et al.*, 1978; Ramsay, 1979). The renin-like activity found in brain extracts does not occur at physiological pH (Day and Reid, 1976) and intracerebroventricular administration of naturally occurring renin substrate is relatively ineffective in stimulating drinking (Fitzsimons and Kucharczyk, 1978; Simpson *et al.*, 1978).

Part of the problem in interpreting the evidence for various receptor sites for angiotensin is that the interconnections of the several proposed receptive areas are not understood. It may be that when the functional anatomy is clearer the main controversies will resolve themselves. Such anatomical studies are now beginning (Mogenson and Kucharczyk, 1978). Swanson *et al.* (1978) have shown that an efferent pathway from the angiotensin-sensitive sites in the preoptic area follows the medial forebrain bundle to the midbrain. Miselis *et al.* (1977) found that the subfornical organ sends efferent connections to both the OVLT and the preoptic area. It may be that the three areas act as an integrated system which must be intact for angiotensin dipsogenesis to occur. It is also possible that understanding the anatomy will lead to the discovery of more receptive sites.

Another important issue concerning angiotensin is what role it plays in normal drinking. Is the drinking observed after angiotensin due to pharmacological manipulation of normal behavior or does it indicate an important role for angiotensin in thirst? This issue will be discussed in relation to drinking following water deprivation (see Section II,C,5). First, the body fluid changes which influence drinking following deprivation will be described.

## C. The Initiation of Drinking
### Following Water Deprivation

We have studied water deprivation in detail because it is a relatively natural way to produce thirst, and could reveal the physiological changes which might act to initiate drinking in animals in normal nonlaboratory situations. In the standard experiment water, but not food, was withdrawn for 21 to 24 hours. The work described indicates that such thirst is initiated by depletion of both the cellular and extracellular fluid compartments. It thus provids evidence for a double-depletion mechanism of thirst, consistent with the hypothesis proposed by Epstein (1973).

### 1. The Effect of Water Deprivation on the Cellular and Extracellular Fluid

The effect of the 21–24 hour water deprivation on body fluid balance is shown for the four different species we have investigated (Table I) (data from Ramsay *et al.*, 1977a, b; R. J. Wood, B. J. Rolls, and E. T. Rolls, in preparation; B. J. Rolls, R. J. Wood, E. T. Rolls, H. Lind, R. W. Lind, and J. Ledingham, in preparation). In the rat, dog, monkey,

TABLE I

CHANGES IN BODY FLUID VARIABLES PRODUCED BY WATER DEPRIVATION IN FOUR SPECIES[a]

| | Rat ($N$ = 15) | Dog ($N$ = 8) | Monkey ($N$ = 5) | Man ($N$ = 5) |
|---|---|---|---|---|
| Osmolality (mOsm/kg $H_2O$) | | | | |
| Nondeprived | 299.6 ± 0.5 | 298.5 ± 0.7 | 297.8 ± 2.4 | 282.4 ± 2.2 |
| Deprived | 306.1 ± 0.6*** | 310.3 ± 0.9*** | 311.0 ± 4.5*** | 290.8 ± 1.8*** |
| Sodium (mEq/liter) | | | | |
| Nondeprived | 138.9 ± 0.5 | 147.3 ± 0.7 | 143.0 ± 1.7 | 140.4 ± 0.7 |
| Deprived | 139.9 ± 0.5 | 153.7 ± 0.7*** | 149.2 ± 2.0*** | 143.3 ± 0.6*** |
| Hematocrit (%) | | | | |
| Nondeprived | 42.2 ± 0.7 | 42.4 ± 2.0 | 36.6 ± 1.9 | 47.2 ± 1.8 |
| Deprived | 46.2 ± 0.6*** | 47.3 ± 2.1*** | 35.8 ± 1.1 | 48.2 ± 2.3 |
| Plasma protein (g%) | | | | |
| Nondeprived | 7.5 ± 0.2 | 5.5 ± 0.1 | 7.1 ± 0.2 | 7.3 ± 0.2 |
| Deprived | 7.8 ± 0.1*** | 6.1 ± 0.1*** | 7.4 ± 0.2 | 7.7 ± 0.2*** |

[a] The means (± SEM) are shown for plasma osmolality, sodium concentration, protein concentration, and hematocrit, measured before and after deprivation. The periods of water deprivation (with food available) were 21 hours for the rat and 24 hours for the dog, monkey, and man. Significant differences between predeprivation and postdeprivation values are indicated: ** $p < 0.01$; *** $p < 0.001$.

and man there was depletion of both the cellular fluid compartment (indicated by the elevation of plasma osmolality or sodium concentration) and the extracellular fluid compartment (assessed by the elevated hematocrit or raised plasma protein levels).

Given that the cellular and extracellular fluid compartments are depleted by water deprivation, the next question is to what extent these depletions contribute to the drinking following water deprivation. This has been investigated in laboratory animals by selective replacement of the deficits produced by water deprivation, using infusions of water to replace the cellular deficit and infusions of isotonic solution to reexpand the extracellular fluid volume. After confirming that the selective replacement had been successful, the residual drinking was measured. These investigations are described in the next section.

## 2. Effects of Selective Replacement of the Cellular or Extracellular Deficits on the Drinking following Deprivation

The purpose of our experiments was to examine the relative contribution of cellular and extracellular depletions to deprivation-induced thirst by selectively rehydrating the two fluid compartments and measuring the residual fluid intake. Three different species have been studied, the rat, the dog, and the monkey. This type of study has not yet been extended to man.

*a. Preloads in the Deprived Rat.* In the rat selective replacement was achieved by administering preloads of water or a balanced isotonic salt solution via different routes (Ramsay *et al.*, 1977b). Intragastric loads were employed because they are simple, do not require surgery, and are relatively untraumatic. Intravenous loads were also used to ensure that any reduction of drinking was due to plasma changes and not to oropharyngeal or gastric cues. Rats were also given "oral preloads" in which they were offered a given volume of fluid to drink and the effect of this consumption on later intake was determined. This oral preload controlled for the possibility that stress from the other types of preloads affected drinking. The results indicated that the route of administration of the load had little effect on intake and it was found that a preload of 10 ml of water which brought plasma osmolality down to predeprivation levels but had little effect on plasma volume reduced the total intake of water in one hour by 64–69% (Table II). If the plasma volume was restored with an isotonic balanced salt solution which had little effect on osmolality, drinking was reduced by 20–26% after 1 hour (Table II). This reduction of drinking was a graded effect, correlating with the volume of the preload of balanced salt (Fig. 2).

TABLE II

THE EFFECT ON DRINKING OF REMOVING
THE CELLULAR AND EXTRACELLULAR DEFICITS
THAT FOLLOW WATER DEPRIVATION IN THREE SPECIES[a]

|  | Percentage reduction in water intake | | |
| --- | --- | --- | --- |
|  | Rat | Dog | Monkey |
| Removal of cellular thirst stimulus | 64–69 | 72[b] | 85 |
| Removal of extracellular thirst stimulus | 20–26 | 27 | 5 |

[a]Water intake is expressed as a percentage of the intake in control conditions where the deficits are not restored. Since the precise effect depends on the route of administration of preloads in the rat, the range is given ($N$ = 15). The mean reduction is given for the dog ($N$ = 8) and monkey ($N$ = 3).
[b]Only the central osmoreceptors were rehydrated.

In rats with intact kidneys there was always the possibility that by the production of a hypertonic urine some osmotic dilution of plasma would occur after the saline infusions and that this could be the reason for reduced fluid intake. To control for this possibility intragastric preloads were given to rats that had urine production blocked by either nephrectomy or ureteric ligation. The effects of the preloads of water and balanced salt were the same as in rats with intact kidneys. Thus the reduction of drinking following isotonic balanced salt must be due to extracellular fluid volume expansion.

These results show that after water deprivation in the rat, changes in both the cellular and extracellular fluid compartments contribute to drinking. The changes in the cellular compartment make the largest contribution to thirst, but the changes in the extracellular compartment do significantly affect drinking (Ramsay et al., 1977b).

b. Preloads in the Deprived Dog. Our technique for studying deprivation-induced drinking in the dog was somewhat different from that in the rat in that the larger size of the animal allowed the preparation of carotid loops (Ramsay et al., 1977a). Since the carotid arteries provide the main blood supply to the brain, we were able to manipulate the osmolality of the blood perfusing the brain with little change in the concentration of the blood in the rest of the body. The tonicity of the blood perfusing the brain was monitored via a catheter in the jugular vein, the main exit route of blood from the brain. Peripheral plasma changes were monitored via a catheter in a leg vein. It was found that carotid infusions had to be made bilaterally to stimulate both halves of the brain equally. With unilateral infusions there were marked differences between the concentration of plasma in the jugular veins ipsi-

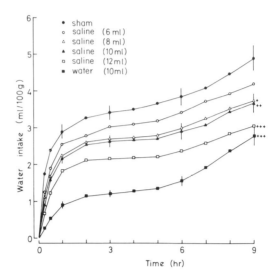

FIG. 2. The mean cumulative water intake of 19 water-deprived rats, used as their own controls, after intragastric preloads of 6, 8, 10, or 12 ml balanced salt, 10 ml deionized water, or a sham load. Standard errors of the means are indicated by vertical bars. The levels of significance are calculated from a comparison between the preload and sham conditions ($+$, $p < 0.05$; $+ +$, $p < 0.01$; $+ + +$, $p < 0.001$). From Ramsay et al. (1977b).

and contralateral to the infusion. This probably reflected inadequate distribution of the infusate in the Circle of Willis. On the other hand we found that the dog with bilateral carotid loops was an excellent subject for the selective rehydration of the postulated central osmoreceptors. Since the dog took less than 5 minutes to rehydrate after deprivation the effects of the infusions could be determined immediately.

After overnight deprivation of water, we found that bilateral intracarotid infusions of water at a rate which brought jugular plasma osmolality down to predeprivation levels reduced water intake by 72% (Table II) compared to control infusions of isotonic saline (Ramsay et al., 1977a). The effect of higher and lower rates of infusion showed the reduction in drinking to be dose-related (see Fig. 3). Since control infusions of isotonic saline at different rates did not affect intake, and the dogs would eat normally if offered food during water infusions, there was no indication that the reduction of water intake was due to discomfort. Analysis of peripheral venous samples showed that the carotid infusions did not significantly change systemic plasma osmolality. Also, infusing water at the same rate intravenously did not reduce intake, so it is concluded that the reduction of drinking was due to removal of the central stimulus. The 72% reduction in intake is particularly impressive when it is remembered that because systemic cellular dehydration and hypovolemia persisted, the dogs were still out of fluid balance when they terminated their drinking. Thus central cellular dehydration appears to be the factor which accounts for the greater part of drinking after water deprivation in the dog.

The reduction in extracellular fluid volume (Table I) which followed water deprivation in the dog might also initiate drinking. We tested this

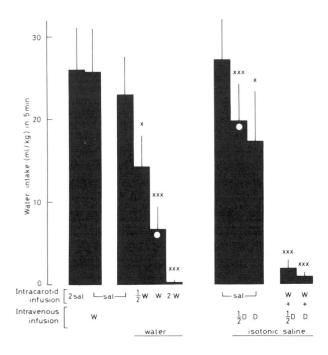

FIG. 3. Mean (± SEM) water intake in eight 24-hour water-deprived dogs during stimulus removal experiments. Left to right; control treatments, intracarotid water infusions, intravenous saline infusions, and combined water and saline infusions. Intracarotid water infusions attenuate the central cellular thirst stimulus and intravenous saline infusions attenuate the extracellular thirst stimulus. White circles indicate treatments that restore central plasma tonicity and systemic plasma volume to predeprivation values. *Intracarotid infusions* (bilateral, 10 minutes): water infusions at a total rate of 0.6 ml kg$^{-1}$ min$^{-1}$ (W) or at half ($\frac{1}{2}$W) or twice (2W) this rate. Intracarotid isotonic (0.15 $M$ NaCl) saline infusions (sal) were a control procedure to replicate any discomfort of the water infusions, and they accompanied all intravenous infusions. *Intravenous infusions* (40 minutes): isotonic (0.15 $M$ NaCl) saline given in volumes equivalent to half ($\frac{1}{2}$D) or all (D) of the total fluid loss, by weight, during deprivation. Water (W) given intravenously at 0.6 ml kg$^{-1}$ min$^{-1}$ was to control for peripheral effects of equivalent intracarotid water infusions. Significant differences: x, $p < 0.05$; xxx, $p < 0.001$, compared to control. Modified from Ramsay *et al.* (1977a).

by expanding the extracellular fluid volume with an intravenous infusion of isotonic saline prior to drinking following water deprivation (Ramsay *et al.*, 1977a). Infusion of 0.15 *M* (isotonic) sodium chloride in an amount sufficient to restore the extracellular fluid volume to predeprivation levels, as shown by the restoration of the plasma protein concentration to normal, reduced drinking by water-deprived dogs by 27% (Table II). Note that this isotonic infusion did not alter plasma osmolality. This effect, although significant, was not as marked as that observed when the central osmotic stimulus was removed. Doubling the volume of the saline infused reduced the plasma protein level to below normal but did not further reduce drinking. Thus restoration of the volume of the extracellular compartment to normal reduced intake but there was no indication that hypervolemia can satiate the remaining thirst. It did not inhibit a persisting cellular stimulus (see Fig. 3).

If both the central hypertonicity and the hypovolemia were removed simultaneously by giving both carotid water infusions and intravenous saline, there was no significant drinking. Half the dogs showed no interest in the water; the other half drank small amounts. It appears that in the dog the mechanisms which control drinking after 24 hours of water deprivation can be accounted for in terms of the raised central plasma osmolality and the reduced extracellular fluid volume, with the raised plasma osmolality making the largest contribution (Ramsay *et al.*, 1977a).

*c. Preloads in the Deprived Monkey.* In both the rat and dog the relative contribution of the cellular and extracellular deficits to thirst following water deprivation was similar (Table II). In the monkey, both cellular and extracellular deficits resulted from water deprivation as in the other species studied (Table I). The contribution of these changes to thirst has been studied in monkeys which had been prepared with a chronic jugular catheter (R. J. Wood, B. J. Rolls, and E. T. Rolls, in preparation). The monkeys were deprived of fluid for 24 hours and then infused with different volumes of water in order to rehydrate the cellular fluid compartment to different extents before the animals were allowed to drink. The effect of the infusions on drinking was dose-related in a linear fashion (Fig. 4). Infusion of a volume of water which returned plasma sodium and osmolality to predeprivation levels reduced drinking by a mean value of 85% (Table II) in the three monkeys so far tested. Larger infusions reduced plasma concentration to below normal and virtually abolished drinking. Infusions of isotonic saline were also given to selectively attenuate the extracellular fluid deficit before allowing the animals to drink. A volume of saline which restored plasma volume to predeprivation levels reduced the mean water intake by only 5% (Table

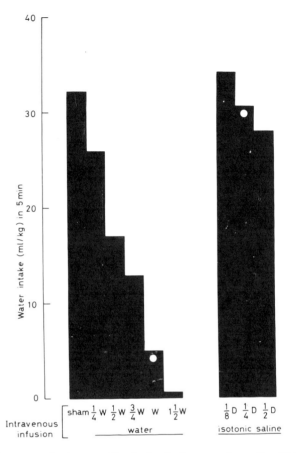

FIG. 4. Mean water intake over 15 minutes in three monkeys after 24-hour water deprivation during stimulus removal experiments. *Intravenous infusions* (infusion for 40 minutes); W, water infusion at 0.7 ml kg$^{-1}$ min$^{-1}$; $\frac{1}{4}$W, $\frac{1}{2}$W, $\frac{3}{4}$W, $1\frac{1}{2}$W, water infusions at rates proportional to W. D is total body fluid deficit calculated from weight loss during deprivation; $\frac{1}{8}$D, $\frac{1}{4}$D, $\frac{1}{2}$D, infusions of isotonic 0.15 $M$ NaCl equal in volume to a proportion of the deficit. White circles indicate treatments that restore measures of cellular hydration (water infusion) or extracellular hydration (isotonic saline infusion) to predeprivation values.

II) in the monkeys. A smaller volume had no effect, and larger volumes which expanded plasma volume above normal without debilitating the animals produced a similarly small further reduction in intake. Thus, in the monkey the cellular stimulus to thirst is even more important in relation to the extracellular stimulus than in the rat or dog.

In man the role of the observed cellular and extracellular fluid deficits in initiating drinking after water deprivation has not been definitively established by stimulus removal experiments such as those we have performed in the rat, dog, and monkey. Nevertheless, the fact that the drinking threshold to a cellular fluid deficit produced by intravenous infusions of hypertonic sodium chloride solutions in man 1-2%, Wolf, 1950) is less than the magnitude of the change we found in plasma sodium (2.1%) produced by water deprivation (see Table I) makes it likely that the cellular fluid deficit is an important stimulus for drinking.

## 3. The Importance of Other Factors in Regulating Body Fluid Homeostasis

The stimulus removal experiments just described for the rat, dog, and monkey indicate that approximately 64-85% of the drinking following deprivation is due to cellular dehydration, whereas hypovolemia accounts for 5-27% of the drinking (Table II). Thus we can conclude that although cellular dehydration makes a major contribution to thirst, it is not the only stimulus following deprivation. That factors other than the degree of cellular dehydration are important in regulating water intake is demonstrated in Fig. 5. Water intake is plotted against plasma sodium concentration for two conditions: after water deprivation, and after hypertonic sodium chloride infusions given to fluid-replete animals. In both the dog and the monkey, equivalent increases in plasma sodium, and thus in cellular dehydration, initiated significantly different volumes of water intake in the two conditions. Water deprivation is clearly a much more effective stimulus than is indicated by a given sodium change, demonstrating that multiple factors must be involved in drinking after water deprivation as suggested previously by Adolph et al. (1954). Hypovolemia is one such factor, as we have shown, but even after the selective removal of this stimulus there is still a marked difference in the drinking response under the two conditions. Thus there could be factors other than the level of cellular dehydration and hypovolemia which contribute to deprivation-induced drinking. It is possible that the overall bodily distribution of cellular dehydration and its duration might influence drinking.

## 4. The Relation between Water Intake and Excretion in Body Fluid Homeostasis

The kidney may also contribute to rehydration following drinking either by removing excess salts and thereby reducing the cellular deficit or by removing water if intake is in excess of needs. The importance of

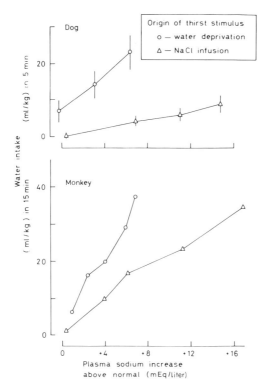

Fig. 5. Mean water intake in the dog ($N = 8$) and the monkey ($N = 2$) during two different treatments which elevate plasma sodium concentration above normal. o, Drinking by water-deprived animals when the elevation of plasma sodium concentration due to deprivation is varied by means of water infusions (intracarotid in the dog, intravenous in the monkey). △, Drinking by fluid-replete animals when plasma sodium concentration is elevated by means of hypertonic NaCl infusions (intracarotid in the dog, intravenous in the monkey).

renal mechanisms in the rehydration process, and an indication of how precise the regulation of drinking is, can be derived by measuring changes in excretion which occur during water deprivation and subsequent drinking.

In the rat, drinking following water deprivation typically leads to a rapid and significant plasma dilution. The hypo-osmolality with respect to predeprivation levels may be involved in the termination of drinking despite a persistent hypovolemia (Blass and Hall, 1976; Hatton and Bennett, 1970). The eventual restoration of body fluid balance to normal in the rat will depend on renal mechanisms to excrete the excess water. Behavioral regulation is therefore not sufficient to ensure homeostasis in this species.

The effects of drinking on excretion in the water-deprived dog are not as marked as in the rat. There is some variance in the excretory response following drinking. Some animals produced a hypotonic urine and the maximum volume of urine excreted in excess of normal in any dog was equivalent to 17% of initial intake (Rolls and Wood, 1977b; R. J. Wood and B. J. Rolls, in preparation). Some errors in water intake regulation do then occur in the dog, but in most individuals these are remarkably small when it is considered that the dog must rely heavily on preabsorptive mechanisms to control the rapid initial intake of water. Renal mechanisms do not contribute to the removal of the cellular fluid deficit following drinking in the dog since the rates of excretion of sodium and potassium do not increase during the rehydration period. The role of the kidney in the process of rehydration is therefore of a secondary nature in this species, serving merely to make relatively small adjustments to fluid balance, when small errors in water intake occur.

During our studies of water deprivation in man, we also measured the effects of drinking on excretion. As in the dog, there was some significant individual variation in the renal response to water ingestion after water deprivation. In two of the five subjects used in this experiment, urine flow and composition returned to predeprivation values following drinking without any excess urine being excreted. The other three subjects exhibited a marked water diuresis during the second hour after the start of drinking, such that the total volume of urine excreted above normal was equivalent to up to 30% of the initial water intake. As in the dog, the excretion of salts following drinking did not increase significantly above normal so that the removal of the cellular fluid deficit was not a result of renal processes. These results show that fluid excretion following deprivation is variable, so that while some humans are liable to overhydrate to a significant degree after water deprivation, others rehydrate with some precision.

It should be noted that all of our studies on excretion were carried out with no food available. Normally the ingestion of dietary salts would serve to moderate the diluting effects of water absorption on the body fluids. For example, the osmotic dilution and persisting hypovolemia experienced by the rat after drinking is obviated by allowing access to food (Rowland, 1977).

## 5. Role of Angiotensin in Deprivation-Induced Drinking

We have shown in our experiments on rats and dogs that the decrease in extracellular fluid volume is an important component of deprivation-induced drinking. As stated earlier, hypovolemia might stimulate drinking in two ways. First, a low venous return will lead to a reduction in the stimulation of both cardiac distension receptors and arterial baroreceptors. Second, a reduction in blood volume may release renin and lead to the formation of angiotensin. Since the first possibility is still largely hypothetical, we will concentrate on the role of angiotensin in thirst.

We have already seen that injections of angiotensin produce highly motivated drinking in a wide variety of species. As yet, however, no physiological role for angiotensin in normal thirst has been proven (Rolls and Wood, 1977a; Stricker, 1978). One of the most common techniques to show that a system is involved in the control of a particular behavior is to remove an essential component of the system and observe the behavioral changes. Thus if we use water deprivation as our model for normal thrist, knowing already that reduced extracellular volume contributes to the rehydration, we might expect that removal or blockade of the angiotensin system would reduce drinking by an appropriate amount. We know from our rehydration experiments that the extracellular component of deprivation-induced drinking accounts for 20 to 26% of the drinking of the rat. If extracellular thirst under these conditions does involve the angiotensin system, the contribution of this factor in terms of the percentage of fluid intake during rehydration would be relatively small—20 to 26% at most.

Since the level of circulating angiotensin is supposed to be an important influence on drinking, we removed the kidneys, the source of circulating angiotensin. To control for the possibility that either the anuria or the surgery influenced intake, another group of rats had their ureters ligated. This was a particularly useful control because ureteric ligation is reported to elevate angiotensin levels. It can be seen in Fig. 6 that bilateral nephrectomy or ureteric ligation after overnight water deprivation did not differ in their effect on rehydration in spite of differences in circulating angiotensin. Further, the rehydration achieved after 3 hours by these animals was similar to that of unoperated control rats. Thus water deprivation-induced thirst was not affected by the removal of the renal renin-angiotensin system (Rolls and Wood, 1977a).

It has been suggested that nephrectomy may be an inappropriate procedure for investigating the role of angiotensin in thirst since it could undermine an animal's general capacity to behave (Stricker *et al.*, 1976). However, nephrectomy did not have this effect on our deprived rats in that they drank normally following the water deprivation. Furthermore, experiments using the competitive blocker of angiotensin, saralasin acetate (P-113), led to the same conclusion. Injections or infusions of P-113 into the third ventricle of the dog (Ramsay and Reid, 1975), sheep (Abraham *et al.*, 1976), or rat (Lee *et al.*, 1978) did not affect deprivation-induced drinking.

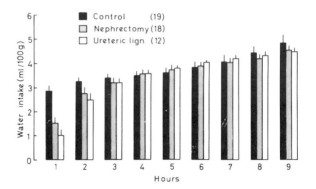

FIG. 6. The mean cumulative hourly water intake (ml/100 g initial body weight) after 21-hour water-deprivation by control rats that had not undergone surgery, by rats that were bilaterally nephrectomized, and by rats with both ureters ligated. The vertical bars show the SE of the mean. The number of rats in each group is given in parenthesis. From Rolls and Wood (1977a).

There has been one report claiming a physiological role for angiotensin in deprivation-induced drinking (Malvin *et al.,* 1977), based on the finding that intraventricular infusion of P-113 reduced deprivation-induced drinking; however, the infusions appear to have nonspecifically depressed the rats, perhaps through stress. This is evident in the data, in that when drinking was affected it was totally suppressed for varying lengths of time. As indicated above, removal of the angiotensin system should not reduce deprivation-induced drinking by more than 20–26% since most drinking following deprivation is due to cellular dehydration.

Thus the bulk of the evidence indicates that angiotensin is not an essential mediator of deprivation-induced water intake in the species so far studied in this context. That angiotensin is not essential does not necessarily imply that angiotensin does not normally play a role in deprivation-induced drinking. It may be that in drinking, as in other physiological systems, there is redundancy of mechanisms so that when one is removed, others take over. We have already seen that after deprivation the fluid changes are complex and various receptors may be involved. It may be that normally these receptors work together but that if one type is removed the remaining receptors can take over the lost function. As it is essential to maintain fluid balance, redundancy would be an advantage. A recent experiment (Hoffman *et al.,* 1978) supports the redundancy hypothesis. It was found that blocking either angiotensin receptors or cholinergic receptors (which it is suggested may mediate cellular dehydration-induced drinking) had no effect on deprivation-induced drinking. However, combined blockade of both receptors reduced deprivation-induced drinking by 70%. They suggest that the two receptors are independently capable of maintaining thirst.

If the removal experiments do not provide conclusive evidence that angiotensin is involved in deprivation-induced thirst, a remaining approach is to correlate changes in angiotensin levels with behavior. Angiotensin has been infused both centrally and peripherally in rats and dogs which were in fluid balance and has been found to cause significant drinking at levels which could occur physiologically (Trippodo *et al.*, 1976; Hsiao *et al.*, 1977; Fitzsimons, *et al.*, 1978). Thus there is no doubt that angiotensin is an extremely potent dipsogen. Also, the elevations in circulating renin and angiotensin levels after water deprivation are similar to those which probably result from dipsogenic doses of exogenous angiotensin (Abdelaal *et al.*, 1976). We have recently found that renin activity is also elevated by water deprivation in man (B. J. Rolls, R. J. Wood, E. T. Rolls, H. Lind, R. W. Lind, and J. Ledingham, in preparation). This increase in plasma renin activity ($1.7 \pm 0.6$ to $3.2 \pm 0.8$ ng ml$^{-1}$ hr$^{-1}$) is probably physiologically significant because the basal values we observed are within the normal range for humans (Laragh and Leaf, 1973), and the higher values are similar to those found when increased renin activity is associated with significant changes in fluid balance and sodium excretion following salt restriction (Leenen *et al.*, 1978).

## 6. Role of Angiotensin in Clinical Syndromes

Whether angiotensin in involved in normal drinking or not, it seems clear that the renin-angiotensin system could provide an emergency mechanism for protecting plasma volume in some pathological conditions. The uncontrollable thirst observed in patients with chronic renal failure occurs in spite of reduced plasma sodium, and appears to be correlated with elevated renin. Bilateral nephrectomy reduces both renin levels and thirst in these patients. Thirst and elevated renin are also found in hyperaldosteronism, and secondary hyperaldosteronism accompanying pregnancy, hemorrhage, and sodium depletion (Brown *et al.*, 1969).

We have also shown that two pathological conditions in the dog are associated with both elevated angiotensin and excessive water intake. Constriction of the thoracic inferior vena cava to produce experimental heart failure elevated water intake which led to excessive edema (Fig. 7). Water intake was also significantly increased in dogs with hypertension due to the constriction of one renal artery with a Goldblatt clamp (Rolls and Ramsay, 1975).

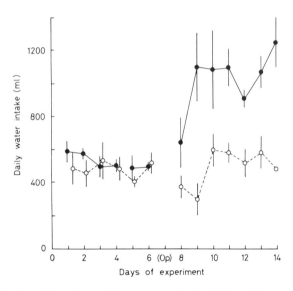

Fig. 7. The effect of caval constriction on water intake in dogs. Points represent values of mean daily water intake, for the experimental group ( ● ) with thoracic caval constriction ($N$ = 5), and the control group (o) with abdominal caval constriction ($N$ = 5). Vertical bars indicate the standard error of the mean. OP indicates the day of operation. The excessive drinking by the experimental group let to the development of edema, which could be prevented by restriction of fluid intake. From Ramsay *et al.* (1973).

As we have already mentioned, changes in the vascular fluid compartment could initiate drinking in two ways, either by increasing the level of circulating angiotensin or by reducing the rate of stimulation of cardiac distention receptors and arterial baroreceptors. During the development of low-output experimental cardiac failure, such as that seen in our dogs, either of these mechanisms could have stimulated drinking since there was an increase in the angiotensin level and a decrease in the rate of stimulation of cardiac distension receptors and arterial baroreceptors (Fig. 8). We have shown, however, that the elevated intake is more likely to have been due to increased levels of circulating angiotensin since the competitive angiotensin inhibitor, P-113 or saralasin acetate, reduced the water intake of the dogs in experimental heart failure. Thus the elevated angiotensin in experimental cardiac failure leads to primary hyperdipsia, and it is of interest that the edema which is produced is alleviated by restriction of fluid intake (Ramsay *et al.,* 1975). In the development of renal hypertension the situation is somewhat different. There was a marked increase in angiotensin levels, but, in addition, volume and pressure receptor input was also increased in our dogs (Fig. 8), and this would normally inhibit drinking. The fact that drinking still occurred in-

|  | Experimental cardiac failure | Benign renal hypertension |
|---|---|---|
| Angiotensin level | ↑ | ↑ |
| Volume and pressure receptor input | ↓ | ↑ |

FIG. 8. Changes in the vascular fluid compartment could stimulate drinking in two ways, either by increasing the level of circulating angiotensin or by reducing the rate of stimulation of cardiac distension receptors and arterial baroreceptors. During the development of experimental cardiac failure either of these signals could possibly stimulate drinking, but the increase in angiotensin is more likely to be responsible since a competitive angiotensin inhibitor reduced the excessive intake. In renal hypertension only the change in angiotensin is in the right direction to stimulate drinking.

dicates that angiotensin is an important dipsogen in renal hypertension as well as in experimental cardiac failure. Furthermore, angiotensin may be involved in the etiology of hypertension in that lesions in the region of the anteroventral third ventricle, which is thought to be a site for angiotensin-induced drinking and pressor responses, prevented the development of renal hypertension in rats (Buggy *et al.*, 1977).

## III. The Maintenance of Drinking

So far we have considered physiological factors which can initiate drinking. We now consider how drinking is maintained. Do animals drink in order to remove thirst stimuli, for example, in order to dilute their plasma or expand their extracellular fluid volume? Or do they drink in order to obtain oropharyngeal sensations such as the taste of water?

### A. THE ROLE OF OROPHARYNGEAL, GASTRIC, AND INTESTINAL FACTORS, AND POSTABSORPTIVE FACTORS IN THE MAINTENANCE OF DRINKING

One way in which these factors can be separated is in the sham-drinking preparation, in which, for example, the animal may drink water and receive oropharyngeal sensations, but other factors do not operate because the ingested water drains through an esophageal or gastric fistula. It was found that such sham-drinking was maintained, that is, there was at least as much water ingested when the fistula was open as when it was closed. In fact, the drinking was maintained very convincingly, in that animals usually sham-drank very large quantities of water. This has been shown in the horse (Bernard, 1856), in the dog (Bellows, 1939; Towbin, 1949; Adolph, 1950), and more recently in the rat (Mook, 1963; Blass and Hall, 1976). An example of sham-drinking in the 18-hour water-deprived rat with a gastric fistula open is shown in Fig. 9 (from unpublished experiments of B. J. Rolls, E. A. Rowe, J. G. Gibbs, E. T. Rolls, and S. Maddison, 1977). It is clear that oropharyngeal factors such as the taste of water and perhaps swallowing are sufficient to maintain drinking, that is, to provide the incentive for drinking, in the rat. It is not necessary for water to reach the intestine, or for it to be absorbed.

In order to throw light on the relative importance of these factors in

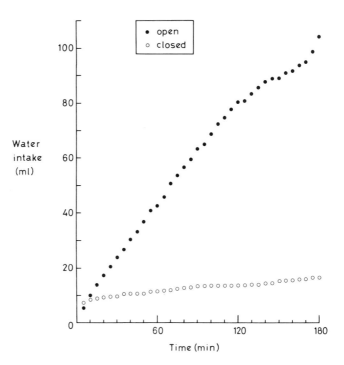

FIG. 9. Drinking by a rat after 18-hour water-deprivation with the gastric fistula either open or closed. In the open condition drainage from the fistula exceeded intake throughout the test and visual inspection showed the fistula to be draining freely.

maintaining drinking in primates, sham-drinking has been investigated in the rhesus monkey (Maddison *et al.*, 1977, 1980). The monkeys were equipped with a gastric cannula and a duodenal cannula relatively close to the pylorus (see Fig. 10), both of which were normally closed. When both the cannulae were closed, the 22.5-hour water-deprived monkeys drank approximately 135 ml in the 1-hour test session (Fig. 11). When the gastric or the duodenal cannula was open so that water did not reach the intestine and was not absorbed, drinking still occurred (Fig. 11). (In fact there was much more drinking than with the cannulae closed—see Section IV,B,3.) Thus the monkeys did drink when oropharyngeal factors such as taste were provided by the water, but no water was absorbed, or entered the intestine. This shows that in the primate, as well as in the dog, horse, and rat, the animal works to obtain oropharyngeal and other sensations provided by drinking the water, and that the gradual dilution of plasma or expansion of extracellular fluid volume produced by the ingestion of water is not necessary for the maintenance of drinking. It thus appears that animals normally drink to obtain oropharyngeal and other sensations provided by water, and not primarily because body fluid deficits are being removed. This view is strengthened by the evidence that animals have difficulty in learning to self-administer water intragastrically (Epstein, 1960), or intravenously (Nicolaïdis and Rowland, 1974), in that relatively large volumes (e.g., normally 1 ml, but in the range 0.25–2 ml) of water must be delivered for

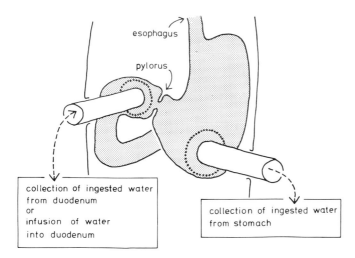

Fig. 10. Diagram showing the cannulated preparation used in monkeys for the investigation of peripheral factors in drinking.

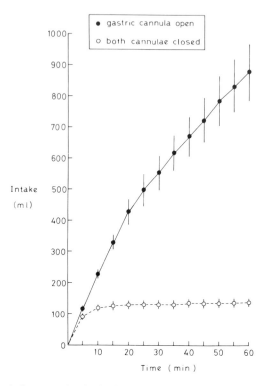

F<small>IG</small>. 11. Cumulative water intake in five monkeys after 22.5-hour water-deprivation, with the gastric and duodenal cannulae both closed (o), and with the gastric cannula open ( ● ). Means ( ± S EM ) are shown. From Maddison *et al.* (1980).

every bar-press if the animal is to learn to self-administer water that does not pass through the oropharynx. In contrast, if an animal can taste the water, then it readily learns to perform a response to obtain a much smaller volume of water. It is in this sense that oropharyngeal factors guide and maintain (or provide the reward or incentive for) intake normally, and this view is in line with the fact that oropharyngeal, e.g., taste, receptors are specialized for the rapid and sensitive detection of small quantities of substances which may be rewarding, such as water for the thirsty animal. In the course of evolution, or perhaps as a result of learning, animals must have adapted to work for sensations such as the taste of water when they are thirsty, that is, for sensations which precede the removal of fluid deficits by the ingested water. This clearly provides a more sensitive and more rapid mechanism to guide behavior than that which could be provided by changes in systemic fluid balance.

## B. HOW OROPHARYNGEAL FACTORS MAY
MAINTAIN DRINKING

The experiments just described show that, normally, oropharyngeal sensations guide intake (so that water-deprived animals drink water rather than hypertonic saline, for example), and maintain intake, and thus provide the incentive, or in this sense the reward, for drinking in the thirsty animal. The subjective sensations underlying this reward value which water has for the thirsty animal have been investigated in experiments in which human subjects gave a rating of how pleasant water tasted after overnight water deprivation, and during and following drinking. It was found that the subjects in the water-deprived state gave a high rating to the pleasantness of the taste of water immediately before drinking (see Fig. 12). At the termination of drinking to satiety, which the subjects reached after drinking for 2–7 minutes, the pleasantness was considerably less (by a ratio of 0.76—see Fig. 12, from experiments by E. T. Rolls, B. J. Rolls, and J. Seton). The pleasantness of the taste of water continued to diminish for 20 minutes following the drinking. It is suggested that an action of thirst stimuli is to make the oropharyngeal sensations produced by water pleasant, and that this underlies the incentive or reward which water has for the thirsty animal. Conversely, satiety mechanisms produce a decrease in the pleasantness of the taste of water, and this underlies the reduction in the incentive or reward which water has as the animal becomes satiated. It is of interest that some alliesthesia (literally "changing sensation," cf. Cabanac, 1971) was found when the humans simply rinsed their mouths with water, and were not allowed to drink to satiety (see Fig. 12 ). Thus some minor alleviation of thirst by oropharyngeal stimulation alone can occur. Thirst apears to modulate the subjective sensations and the reward produced by oropharyngeal stimulation with water. This analysis suggests that the subjective phenomenon just described, namely, alliesthesia, is an important mechanism in the control of drinking.

This finding of modulation in the pleasantness of the taste of water by thirst receives support from a second experiment in humans, in which estimates of the hydration of the cellular and extracellular fluid compartments were made. It was found that the rating (again on a visual analog scale) of "how pleasant would it be to drink some water now" was elevated very significantly (compared to the nondeprived state) toward pleasantness, following 24-hour water deprivation (Fig. 21). Also the pleasantness returned rapidly toward the baseline nondeprived value in the 5- to 10-minute period in which most of the drinking occurred (Fig. 21) (B. J. Rolls, R. J. Wood, E. T. Rolls, H. Lind, R. W. Lind,

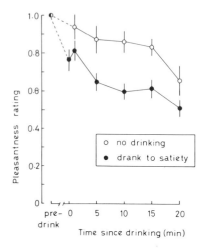

FIG. 12. Alliesthesia and drinking. Human subjects deprived of water overnight (until testing at 11 am) rated the pleasantness of the taste of water on a visual analog scale (the subjects marked the subjective pleasantness of the taste on a 100-mm line labeled at one end "very pleasant" and at the other "very unpleasant"). This rating is shown as the "predrink" rating of 1 on the graph. Then one group ( ● ) of subjects ($N = 20$) was allowed to drink water to satiety. Their ratings of the pleasantness of the taste of small samples of water at different times since the drinking are shown and it is clear that the taste of water became less pleasant following drinking to satiety ($p < 0.001$). The ratings at each time are expressed as a ratio of the predrink rating, and the means ( ± SEM) are shown. In a second group (o) of subjects ($N = 12$), no drinking of the water to satiety was allowed, but ratings of the pleasantness of the taste of small samples of water at different times after the start of testing were made for comparison with the control group. In this group, being allowed to taste the water without ingestion did make water taste a little less pleasant, but the effect was smaller than in the group allowed to drink the water ($p < 0.025$ for the difference between the two groups).

and J. Ledingham, in preparation). The increase in the pleasantness rating was associated with the depletions of the cellular and extracellular compartments shown in Fig. 17. Evidence on how this modulation of reward value contributes to the regulation of feeding is described elsewhere (E. T. Rolls, 1975, 1976; Rolls and Rolls, 1977), but only a little of its neurophysiological basis with respect to drinking has yet been investigated (Rolls *et al.,* 1979; E. T. Rolls, 1980). In this context, it is of interest that in the lateral and dorsal hypothalamus of the monkey, neurons have been found which decreased their firing rates when thirsty monkeys were drinking water, and which in contrast increased their firing rates as a result of water deprivation or the intracarotid infusion of hypertonic saline (Vincent *et al.,* 1972; Arnauld *et al.,* 1975). Neurons which respond to oropharyngeal stimulation by water, yet whose activity is also dependent on internal osmotic stimulation, have also been described in the rat (Nicolaïdis, 1969).

## C. PALATABILITY AND BODY FLUID HOMEOSTASIS

The experiments previously described show that thirsty animals normally work in order to obtain oropharyngeal sensations such as the taste of water. The importance of oropharyngeal sensations in maintaining or providing the incentive for fluid intake is seen very dramatically in experiments in which the palatability of the fluid is enhanced. For example, making the fluid taste sweet by the addition of saccharine makes it so rewarding that even nondeprived rats drink large quantities of it (Ernits and Corbit, 1973; Rolls et al., 1978). This effect is seen to be very powerful in a clinically relevant paradigm (Rolls et al., 1978), in which the ability of the rats to produce a dilute urine was impaired by the administration of antidiuretic hormone. When the rats, which were in fluid balance at the start of the experiment, were offered saccharine solution, they drank so much of it that they went markedly into positive fluid balance (Fig. 13), and their plasma was diluted by an average of 22 mOsm/kg $H_2O$ (which resulted in hemolysis in some animals). Thus inhibitory signals from plasma dilution must be relatively ineffective

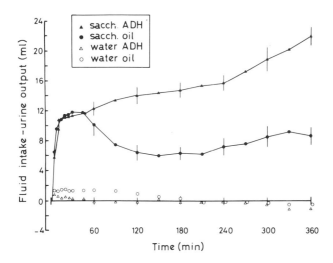

FIG. 13. Mean fluid balance (fluid intake minus urine output) of 12 rats drinking either saccharine solution or water after an injection of either antidiuretic hormone (ADH) or oil vehicle. The rats which were in fluid balance at the start of the experiment were each tested in all four conditions. Means (± SEM) are shown. From Rolls et al. (1978).

against the consumption of a palatable saccharine solution. The clinical relevance of this is that if excretion is impaired, for example, because of high levels of antidiuretic hormone, polydipsia may cause plasma dilution and hyponatremic convulsions (Hobson and English, 1963; Pickering and Hogan, 1971; Peterson and Marshall, 1975). Palatability appears to be one factor which leads to overdrinking and can exacerbate clinical problems of inappropriate fluid intake. For example, we (J. G. G. Ledingham, B. J. Rolls, and J. G. Gibbs) have observed a patient with hyponatremic convulsions who drinks little water but consumes up to 100 cups of tea a day (over 15 liters). Because the mammalian kidney excretes excess fluid rapidly in a dilute urine, large volumes can normally be consumed without seriously affecting fluid balance. When excretion of water is impaired, the effect of palatability may lead, despite plasma dilution, to pathological fluid intake.

D. Effects of Variety on Fluid Intake

We have just seen that giving liquids a pleasant taste significantly increases fluid consumption. Another factor unrelated to physiological need which may affect intake is the variety of fluids available. It has been shown that offering foods with a variety of flavors significantly increases feeding (Le Magnen, 1956; B. J. Rolls, 1979). To determine whether this effect is found for drinking, we offered rats that were in fluid balance either water for an hour, water with one of four artificial essences added (orange, raspberry, malt, and peach supplied by Barnett & Foster) for an hour, or water with a different essence every 15 minutes over the hour (i.e., they had orange, raspberry, malt, and peach in succession over an hour). It can be seen in Fig. 14 that offering rats a variety of fluids to consume significantly increased intake (B. J. Rolls and R. J. Wood, unpublished).

Similar results have been obtained in humans (B. J. Rolls, E. T. Rolls, and A. Pringle, unpublished). Nondeprived subjects, under the pretext of a tasting experiment, consumed three drinks successively, with a 10-minute period allowed for each drink, under three different conditions: three different flavors (low calorie orange, lemon, and lime drinks), one flavor only, or water alone with no flavor. More was consumed in the three-flavor than in the one-flavor condition, and more in the one-than in the no-flavor condition (see Fig. 15). Thus the experiments in both rats and man show that offering a variety of fluids over a short period stimulates significantly more intake than is needed for homeostatic control. These experiments provide another demonstration of how oropharyngeal sensations are important in providing the reinforcement for fluid intake.

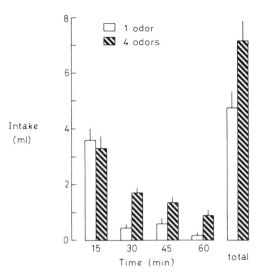

FIG. 14. Over 1 hour, 15 nondeprived rats were offered either water with one artificial essence added (orange, raspberry, peach, or malt), or all four essences in succession for 15 minutes each. These rats had consumed 2.5 ± 0.4 ml plain water in the same situation. Adding just one essence to water increased intake by 88% ($p < 0.001$) compared with plain water and changing the smell every 15 minutes over an hour increased intake by 182% ($p < 0.001$) compared with plain water and by 50% ($p < 0.001$) compared with just one essence. Means (± SEM) are shown.

## IV. The Termination of Drinking

We have described measurable physiological events which may account for the initiation of drinking. Satiation or the termination of drinking is more difficult to define behaviorally than is the onset of drinking, and thus the physiological events involved in the termination of drinking have been more difficult to analyze. Also, drinking is easily disrupted by experimental manipulation, so if an animal does not drink it is difficult to know if it is no longer thirsty or is in some way upset by an experimental regime. Our observation of a satiety sequence for drinking in the monkey, in which drinking is followed by a period of sleepiness (similar to that observed after feeding; Antin *et al.*, 1975), and our measurement of subjective reports as satiety is reached in man, are helpful in determining true satiety as compared with interference with drinking.

Various mechanisms may be involved in the termination of drinking. One possible mechanism is that animals may meter the amount consumed using signals from the mouth, the esophagus, the stomach, or

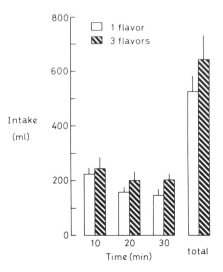

FIG. 15. Over 30 minutes, 18 nondeprived people were offered either one low-calorie fruit drink (orange, lemon, or lime) or all three in succession for 10 minutes each. Twelve of these subjects consumed 265 ± 68 ml of plain water when tested in the same situation. Adding just one flavor to water increased intake by 99% ($p < 0.001$) compared with water, and giving three different flavors increased intake by 143% ($p < 0.001$) compared with plain water and by 22% ($p < 0.001$) compared with just one flavor. Means (± SEM) are shown.

the duodenum. A second possibility is that osmoreceptors in these areas or in the vasculature, e.g., in the hepatic-portal system, may signal to the brain that sufficient dilution has occurred or is occurring. A third possibility is that drinking may continue until the body fluid deficits that initiated the behavior are repleted, that is, until central osmoreceptors are rehydrated or levels of circulating angiotensin are reduced through restoration of plasma volume.

## A. THE PATTERN OF DRINKING

In attempting to define the crucial events for stopping drinking it is particularly informative to compare species that drink at different rates, and to examine the pattern of drinking in a particular species for clues about the possible mechanisms which terminate drinking in that species (Adolph, 1950). The pattern of water intake in the four species with which we have worked is shown in Fig. 16. The intake was measured after a standard 21- to 24-hour overnight water-deprivation period. The

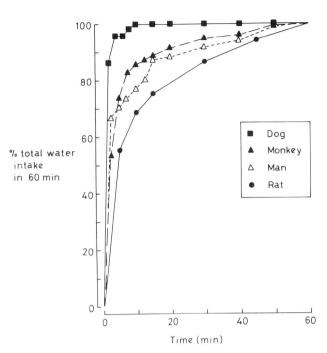

Fɪɢ. 16. Water intake plotted as a percentage of the total intake in 1 hour after over-night water but not food deprivation. The dog is a rapid drinker, completing its drinking within 10 minutes, whereas the rat drinks comparatively slowly. The monkey and man fall between those extremes.

dog is a very rapid drinker, typically consuming almost all of its re-quirements in 2–3 minutes of the onset of drinking (Adolph, 1939). Some form of peripheral metering thus seems a probable mechanism for the termination of drinking in the dog. In contrast, the rat is a relatively slow drinker, and after the initial drinking bout continues to drink inter-mittently during the full 1-hour period following the start of drinking (see Fig. 16). Given this slow time course, it is possible that the removal of thirst signals as water is absorbed accounts for the eventual slowing of the drinking rate and the termination of drinking in the rat. The monkey and man are relatively rapid drinkers, consuming most of their intake within 10 minutes, but continuing to have small drinking bouts in the remainder of the 1-hour test period (Fig. 16). To determine how the different mechanisms contribute to the termination of drinking in the different species, we have performed experiments in which changes in fluid balance have been assessed repeatedly during rehydration by the dog, the monkey, and man, as described in the next section.

B. SYSTEMIC AND PERIPHERAL FACTORS IN
RELATION TO THE TERMINATION OF DRINKING

*1. The Termination of Drinking in the Rat*

In the rat it is difficult to study possible systemic factors involved in drinking termination because the small size of the animal makes continuous assessment of plasma composition impractical (Rolls and Wood, 1979). Nevertheless, Hatton and Bennett (1970) found from single plasma samples taken at the end of drinking that the termination of drinking coincided with a significant reduction in plasma osmolality, whereas plasma protein was still elevated. Thus it appears that in the rat drinking proceeds at a rate which is slow enough for significant absorption to take place before drinking terminates. The removal of the cellular fluid deficit may be the most important factor in the termination of drinking in this species.

*2. The Termination of Drinking in the Dog*

In the dog, which completes drinking within 2 to 3 minutes, it is unlikely that rehydration could have taken place before drinking stops. We examined this by allowing overnight water-deprived dogs to drink normally and by determining the rate at which plasma volume and composition returned to normal. Almost all of the drinking was completed within 2–3 minutes of the start of drinking (see Fig. 16), but there was no significant change in plasma sodium (which assessed cellular dehydration), or plasma protein (which assessed plasma volume), until 10 minutes after the start of drinking (Fig. 17). After that time there was a steady fall in these variables, the rehydration of both fluid compartments being completed at about 50 min after the onset of drinking (Fig. 17) (Ramsay *et al.,* 1977a). The accuracy of the dog's rehydration is emphasized by the data on excretion (see Section II,C,4).

In the dog the termination of drinking occurred before the restoration by absorption of the cellular or extracellular fluid deficits. As originally proposed by Bellows (1939) the dogs were able to meter water intake so that enough water was ingested to replenish the body fluids successfully. Dogs with an esophageal fistula will terminate drinking, but under these sham-drinking conditions, water intake greatly exceeds normal (Bellows, 1939; Towbin, 1949). Thus oropharyngeal stimulation is probably involved in the termination of drinking, but this factor is not sufficient to account for the normal termination of water intake.

It is possible that some metering of fluid intake could occur at the

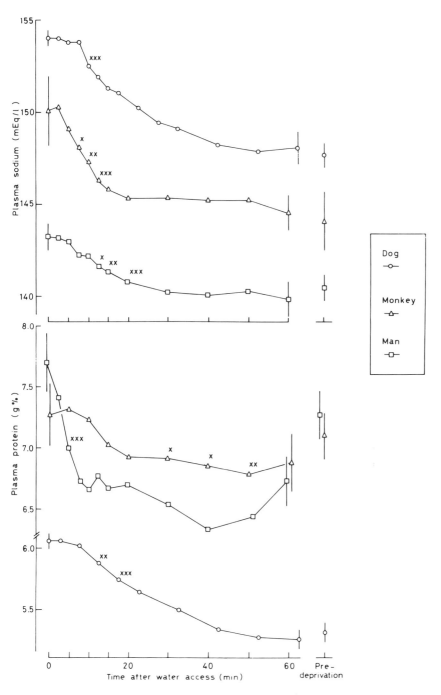

FIG. 17. Changes in plasma sodium concentration and plasma protein concentration during and following drinking in 24-hour water-deprived dogs (o), $N = 8$, monkeys, ($\triangle$), $N = 5$, and humans ($\square$), $N = 5$. The subjects were allowed access to water at the start of the hour. Means ($\pm$ SEM) are shown. Significant differences from initial values: x, $p < 0.05$; xx, $p < 0.01$; xxx, $p < 0.001$.

level of the stomach; however, Adolph (1950) noted that distension of the stomach by balloon inflation had a relatively small effect on drinking in the dog compared with other species. Sobocinska (1978) has also found that intragastric balloon inflation has little effect on drinking following a hypertonic saline load. Another possibility for metering is that peripheral receptors in either the duodenum or hepatic-portal system, such as those we describe below in the monkey, are involved in the rapid termination of drinking in the dog. Studies using radioactively labeled water given via the mouth indicate that water enters the hepatic-portal circulation within 2 to 3 minutes (Kozlowski and Drzewiecki, 1973), so that a duodenal or hepatic-portal signal would be sufficiently rapid to have a role in the termination of drinking. (In the rat, it has been shown that hepatic-portal infusions of osmotically active fluids do influence the activity of hypothalamic neurons—Schmitt, 1973). In the dog, oral metering and duodenal or hepatic-portal metering probably combine to account for the termination of drinking.

### 3. The Termination of Drinking in the Monkey

In the water-deprived monkey, the initial bout of relatively rapid drinking typically lasted for about 7.5 minutes. After that time, further intake was smaller and more sporadic (Fig. 16). Following the start of drinking, plasma sodium concentration fell rapidly, the change becoming significant by 7.5 minutes (Fig. 17). Plasma protein concentration fell appreciably during the first 20 minutes, but this change did not become statistically significant until 30 minutes. Thus in the monkey the absorption of water is relatively rapid and cellular dehydration (as assessed by plasma sodium) as a thirst stimulus is starting to change at the time when drinking is being attenuated. However, it takes 20 minutes or more for the major change in both the cellular and extracellular fluid compartments to be completed so that some factor other than this may contribute to the termination of drinking in the primate. Some signal such as preabsorptive metering may be required to restrain drinking for the period 7.5–30 minutes after the onset of drinking. The possibility of such metering in the primate has been investigated using the sham-drinking preparation.

We found first that oropharyngeal factors alone are not sufficient to produce normal termination of drinking in the monkey (see Section III,A). This is clear from the massive overdrinking which occurred in the monkey when a gastric or duodenal cannula was opened to permit drainage of water, allowing normal oropharyngeal stimulation by the ingested water but preventing its absorption by the gut (Maddison et al.,

1977, 1980; see, e.g., Fig. 11). This massive overdrinking in the primate, as in the dog and in the rat when gastric drainage prevents absorption of the ingested water, shows that drinking is not terminated simply by oral metering or by oropharyngeal factors in general.

To assess the importance of intestinal factors as well as absorption in the termination of drinking in the primate, duodenal infusions of water were given in the next series of experiments. Using gastric sham-drinking (i.e., drinking with a gastric cannula open) to provide a steady baseline of drinking, it was shown that slow intraduodenal infusions of water did reduce drinking. The effects of the infusion are illustrated in Figs. 18 and 19. Even relatively small volumes of water (25–30 ml, compared to 130 ml normally consumed with both cannulae closed) were able to slow and usually even to stop drinking for a short period (Maddison *et al.*, 1980). The inhibition of drinking did not appear to be due to nonspecific stress, in that intraduodenal infusions of larger volumes of isotonic saline (e.g., 100 ml) did not stop drinking, and in that during the infusions of water, the monkeys would still eat. The periods for which the different infusions stop drinking in individual drinking tests are shown in Fig. 20. The volumes infused were not as large as those normally ingested by the monkey and drinking did resume later. This experiment raises the possibility that stimuli at the level of the intestine (intestinal or hepatic-portal receptors) as well as the central effects of the infused water could contribute to the termination of drinking. This possibility is being investigated by giving slow intravenous infusions of water at a rate to match the absorption of water from the duodenum, in order to determine whether central rehydration alone terminates the drinking, or whether duodenal or hepatic-portal mechanisms also play a role (R. J. Wood, S. Maddison, E. T. Rolls, and B. J. Rolls, in preparation). So far, it appears that intravenous infusions which produce changes in plasma composition that are equivalent to those produced by duodenal infusions, may not be as effective as the duodenal infusions in terminating drinking. An additional important factor in the initial rapid termination of drinking in the monkey may be gastric distension, for if monkeys are allowed to drink until they stop, and then a gastric cannula is opened allowing drainage of gastric contents, drinking resumes almost immediately (S. Maddison, B. J. Rolls, E. T. Rolls, and R. Wood, 1980). Thus, gastric and duodenal or hepatic-portal signals probably combine with partial plasma fluid repletion to terminate drinking. In addition, although oropharyngeal factors alone are not sufficient for the termination of drinking, they may make a contribution to the early termination of drinking. Within 30 minutes of the start of drinking in the monkey, the major body fluid deficits have been

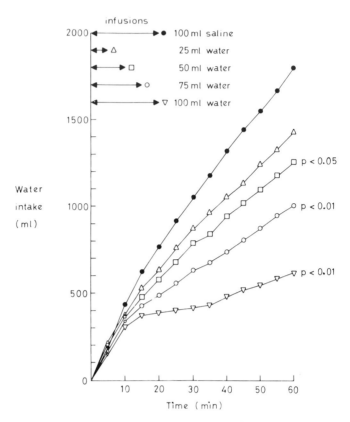

FIG. 18. Cumulative water intake in five monkeys after 22.5-hour water-deprivation, with the gastric cannula open. The curves represent drinking when different volumes of water were infused through the duodenal cannula at a rate of 5 ml min$^{-1}$. As a control, a volume of isotonic saline equal to the largest water infusion was administered. Significant differences from the control intake are indicated on the figure by $p$ values. From Maddison et al. (1980).

replenished, and preabsorptive or hepatic-portal signals are no longer necessary to stop drinking.

## 4. The Termination of Drinking in Man

Man is a relatively rapid drinker, drinking much of his total intake in the first 2.5 minutes following 24-hour water deprivation, but continuing to ingest small volumes of water during the remainder of a 1-hour test (Fig. 16). Plasma dilution (shown by osmolality and sodium concentration changes) associated with this drinking has a slower time course, with some dilution apparent 7.5 minutes after access to water, but con-

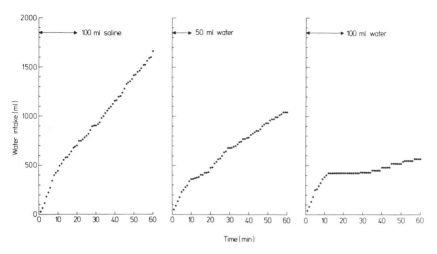

FIG. 19. Typical records of cumulative water intake for the monkey after 22.5-hour water-deprivation, with the gastric cannula open. The curves represent drinking when isotonic saline, and two different volumes of water, were infused through the duodenal cannula at a rate of 0.5 ml kg⁻¹ min⁻¹. From Maddison *et al.* (1980).

sistent and significant changes are not apparent until about 12.5 minutes after access to water (Fig. 17). Thus replenishment of the cellular fluid deficit cannot account for the termination of drinking in man, although by 12.5–20 minutes it is probably an important factor in limiting further drinking. The change in plasma protein concentration following drinking was remarkably rapid in this experiment (B. J. Rolls, R. J. Wood, E. T. Rolls, H. Lind, R. W. Lind, and J. Ledingham, in preparation) (Fig. 17), indicating that the extracellular fluid (plasma volume) deficit was repaired within 5 minutes of the start of drinking, and that by 7.5 minutes hypervolemia occurred, which then persisted for the remainder of the hour. This rapid repletion of plasma volume following drinking may have resulted from food being present in the gut so that drinking water produced an isotonic fluid which was rapidly absorbed, or from a shift of extracellular fluid into the vasculature, as well as from absorption of some water. Whether this rapid hypervolemia contributes to the termination of drinking in man is uncertain, but it is unlikely to be a major factor in view of our observation that elevation of plasma volume to normal in the monkey following water deprivation reduced drinking by only 5%, and that only a similarly small further reduction in drinking was produced by a marked plasma hypervolemia (see Section II,C,2,c). Thus in man cellular rehydration does not appear to be sufficiently rapid to account for the early decrease in the rate of drinking, but may con-

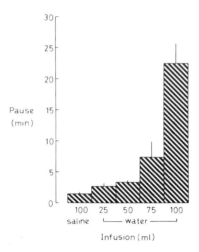

FIG. 20. Effect of intraduodenal infusions of water on drinking in five monkeys after 22.5-hour water-deprivation with the gastric cannula open. The durations of the pauses in drinking provided by the different volumes of water infused, as compared to a control infusion of isotonic saline, are shown. Means (± SEM) are shown.

tribute to satiety after 12.5 minutes. Expansion of plasma volume, although rapid, may not be a powerful factor in terminating drinking. Therefore, a contribution of other factors to the early termination of drinking must be suspected.

Some information about the role of peripheral factors in terminating drinking in man comes from subjective reports and ratings made by our human subjects during rehydration. The subjects consistently rated stomach fullness (which perhaps reflected general distension of the gut) as high within 2.5 minutes of the start of the drinking, and this continued for 20–30 minutes, so that this sensation may be a factor in the early termination of drinking (see Fig. 21). It is interesting to recall that in the monkey, drinking restarts if gastric distension is relieved by opening a gastric cannula. Another consistent observation was that humans rated their mouths as being dry following the water deprivation, with rapid relief following access to water (see Fig. 21), but reported feelings of mouth dryness and an unpleasant taste later in the 1-hour drinking test and promptly drank a few milliliters of water to relieve this. This subjective sensation may arise because rehydration of the body fluids, particularly of peripheral tissues, is not yet complete. In a different experiment, on alliesthesia (see Section III,B), it was also found that repeated rinsing of the mouth with water every few minutes produced some decrease in the pleasantness of the taste of water (see Fig. 12). This

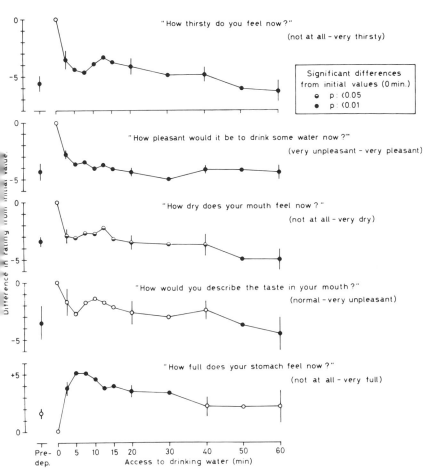

FIG. 21. Changes in subjective ratings during 24-hour water-deprivation and rehydration in man. The curves represent ratings on a 10 cm visual analog scale. The mean data shown are the differences in ratings from initial ratings at the start of the rehydration period. Open symbols indicate nonsignificant differences, and the closed and partially closed symbols, the different levels of significance.

is consistent with the view that oropharyngeal factors contribute to the termination of drinking in man, and suggest that diminished subjective pleasantness of the taste of water produced by a sensory satiety mechanism is part of a mechanism for the operation of these factors.

We conclude that, in the dog, oropharyngeal mechanisms combined with intestinal or hepatic-portal mechanisms are the major factors in the early termination of drinking. In the monkey, which drinks more slowly, there is time for absorption of fluid to bring about some plasma dilution before drinking slows or stops in the period 7.5–20 minutes after the onset of drinking, but it is likely that preabsorptive or hepatic-portal factors contribute to the termination of drinking. In these species the peripheral factors probably include duodenal or hepatic-portal signals, as well as oropharyngeal metering, as the latter is not sufficient to terminate drinking.

In man, also, systemic factors do not seem to be sufficient to account for the early termination of drinking. Thus it is likely that a combination of oropharyngeal factors, gut distension, perhaps osmotic effects of water in the gut and hepatic-portal system, and dilution and expansion produced by absorbed water, normally terminate drinking, and it may be that temporal contiguity between these factors is important for their full effectiveness (see Blass and Hall, 1976). Factors such as oropharyngeal stimulation by water and gut distension may be relatively important early in satiety, and effects of absorbed water may be relatively more important later in maintaining satiety. In the rat, drinking is even slower, so that absorption of fluid and replacement of fluid deficits may be more important for the termination of drinking than in the dog, monkey, and man.

## V. Physiological Mechanisms and *ad Libitum* Drinking

### A. Spontaneous Drinking in Relation to Body Fluid Balance in the Dog

We have considered water deprivation as a model for thirst because it is a common thirst challenge and because it can be used to investigate drinking that is similar to that which can occur in the natural environment. We found that animals drinking to fluid deprivation respond to specific deficits in both the cellular and extracellular compartments and drink amounts appropriate to reverse them. When animals have free access to water, they may not drink only when significant fluid deficits occur. Drinking in the rat is strongly coupled to feeding behavior and the ingestion of water anticipates needs under these circumstances (Fitzsimons and Le Magnen, 1969). Rats may also drink more than is necessary for body fluid homeostasis (Dicker and Nun, 1957; Mogenson and Phillips, 1976) because of this reliance on secondary controls of fluid intake. Man also may prevent significant fluid deficits from occurring under normal circumstances by consuming palatable fluids in quantities which are in excess of immediate requirements. It is not established to what extent fluid intake determined by secondary factors and exemplified by periprandial drinking, drinking due to habit or circadian rhythms of activity, or fluid intake because of palatability, is a typical pattern of ingestion in mammals. To investigate the importance of secondary factors, as against physiological deficits for initiating spontaneous drinking, it is necessary to examine the pattern of physiological changes in body fluid balance in the freely behaving animal with its normal access to water.

One useful index of fluid balance is the nature of the urine excreted. By measuring the effects of spontaneous drinking on the flow of urine and the excretion of water, the extent to which intake exceeds that necessary to maintain normal fluid balance can be assessed. This has been determined in dogs following water deprivation-induced drinking (see Section II,C,4), and following *ad libitum* drinking (Rolls and Wood, 1977b; R. J. Wood and B. J. Rolls, in preparation). In the animals studied with free water access, the pattern of excretion associated with drinking was seen to vary during the day such that at times close to feeding the excretion of electrolytes was particularly high and the urine was relatively concentrated even after drinking. At other times, the effect of drinking on excretion was generally to decrease urine concentration, and on some occasions to produce a transient hypotonic urine. In about 25% of the observed instances when significant volumes of water were drunk, a dilute urine resulted. Thus drinking sometimes resulted in overhydration, but the volumes of urine excreted in excess of normal were relatively small, with no dog excreting an excess of more than 15% of initial water intake. These levels of excess probably represent errors in, rather than a lack of, physiological regulation. If drinking had typically occurred because of secondary factors without reference to needs, the incidence of a dilute urine being excreted and the magnitude of the diuresis following drinking would be much higher than that observed. The fact that in the majority of dogs we have studied the pattern of daily water intake under *ad libitum* access conditions was characterized by relatively infrequent but substantial bouts of drinking is consistent with an interpretation of drinking behavior as the result of a depletion–repletion cycle of body fluid balance with deficits arising because of metabolic activity, in particular because of the processes associated with the digestion and absorption of food.

Typical patterns of daily water intake for two dogs are shown in Fig. 22. One feature of the drinking pattern of the dogs was that little water was drunk before and during feeding, but significant drinking usually started some time between 20 and 60 minutes after the meal. It should be noted that these dogs were not eating dry food. So that they did not ex-

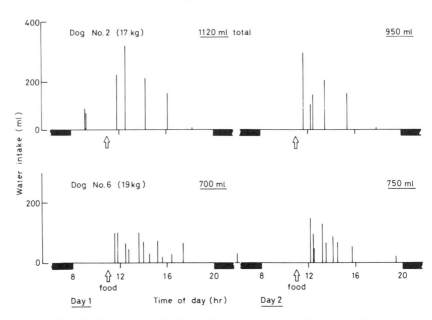

Fig. 22. Individual records of drinking by two dogs over a 48-hour period when water was freely available in the home kennel. Food was given at 11.00 hours and artificial lighting was on from 8.00 to 20.00 hours each day.

perience any difficulty in swallowing the dry synthetic diet, their daily meal consisted of dry food and water mixed in a 4:1 ratio by weight.

## B. PLASMA CHANGES DURING SPONTANEOUS DRINKING IN THE DOG

Studies of excretion do not indicate the nature of the initiating stimuli for thirst under *ad libitum* conditions. For this it is necessary to monitor the patterns of change in body fluid balance continuously while the animal is free to drink (R. J. Wood, and B. J. Rolls, in preparation). Dogs were prepared with indwelling venous catheters and blood was drawn every half hour, and immediately after every drinking bout, throughout the dog's normal period of activity. Plasma sodium levels during drinking and nondrinking periods are shown in Table III. the nondrinking plasma values were selected from samples taken during periods dissociated from drinking (at least 40 minutes before the next drinking bout, and 90 minutes since the previous drinking bout to ensure that any plasma overdilution due to the drinking had been eliminated by excretion). It is shown in Table III that plasma sodium was higher at the

## TABLE III

### The Relationship between *ad libitum* Water Intake and Plasma Sodium Changes in the Dog[a]

|  | Feeding time | First drink after feeding | All drinking bouts | All nondrinking periods | Drinking to threshold dose of intravenous NaCl |
|---|---|---|---|---|---|
| Water intake (ml/kg) |  | 8.0 ± 1.1 | 7.6 ± 0.8 |  | 2.5 ± 0.1 |
| Plasma Na (mEq/liter) | 144.3 ± 1.4 | 149.3 ± 1.1 | 148.4 ± 1.1 | 144.2 ± 1.3 | 149.5 ± 0.7 |
| Plasma Na change (mEq/liter) | 4.9 ± 0.6 |  | 4.2 ± 0.4 |  | 3.6 ± 0.4 |

[a]Means (± SEM) are shown for water intake, plasma sodium concentration, and plasma sodium changes between conditions, for 11 dogs over 24-hour periods with free access to water in the home kennel. The minimum change in plasma sodium concentration necessary to evoke drinking in the same animals (*N* = 10) during intravenous NaCl infusions is also shown. Individual data making up the mean figures in the table were derived from at least three complete daily records of drinking with associated plasma measured for each animal. The water intake data refer only to drinking bouts considered to be of a significant volume, excluding any less than 2 ml/kg body weight. In the dog, very little of the total water intake is due to drinking of less than this magnitude.

time of drinking (148.4 mEq/liter) than in nondrinking periods (144.2 mEq/liters). To determine whether this increase in cellular dehydration (equivalent to 4.2 mEq/liter of plasma sodium) is of sufficient magnitude to initiate drinking, the plasma sodium change (produced by intravenous infusion of hypertonic sodium chloride) that was just necessary to initiate drinking in fluid replete animals was also measured. This was 3.6 mEq/liter, so it can be concluded that the cellular dehydration present when the dog drinks under *ad libitum* conditions is of sufficient magnitude to induce drinking. These experiments provide evidence that in the dog *ad libitum* drinking may not be simply anticipatory, and that fluid deficits do occur under these conditions, can be sensed physiologically, and are large enough to produce drinking.

It is also shown in Table III that the effect of feeding the dogs was to elevate plasma sodium. At the time when substantial drinking first occurred, the increase in plasma sodium concentration (+4.9 mEq/liter) was greater than the threshold change sufficient to evoke drinking. This indicates that the osmotic consequences of feeding in producing cellular dehydration may provide a physiological stimulus for drinking of importance in the natural environment. To test this further, the dogs were fed a low-sodium meal, to minimize the osmotic effects of feeding. It was found that the latency to drink from the time of feeding was increased in the dogs on the low sodium diet (from 48 ± 5 to 244 ± 44 minutes, $N = 10$), and that the total daily volume of water ingested was decreased (from 42 ± 5 to 21 ± 5 ml/kg).

It is interesting to note that changes in plasma volume may also be associated with drinking. In the sheep, feeding leads to a rapid reduction in plasma volume and elevated plasma renin (Blair-West and Brook, 1969). The clearest plasma volume change in the dogs used in this study was at the time when drinking first occurred after feeding. Thus, plasma protein concentration increased from a mean value of 5.2 ± 0.1 to 5.5 ± 0.1 g% during the interval between feeding and drinking, equivalent to a change of about 6% in plasma volume. It has not been established whether this order of change in plasma volume is an effective thirst stimulus in the dog, but these observations further emphasize that the physiological changes which arise because of the ingestion of food are among the reasons for drinking under natural conditions.

The pattern of water intake which we have described for the dog may represent behavior driven by significant physiological needs incurred as a result of the ingestion of food. This may be compared to the rat which drinks just before and just after meals, thereby moderating the postingestional effects of feeding on fluid balance (Fitzsimons and Le Magnen, 1969). The extent to which drinking in different species may be due to physiologically significant deficits in body fluid balance, or may be secondary or anticipatory, is of particular interest when considering physiological mechanisms and normal behavior. Species differences in drinking apparent in the laboratory may reflect adaptation to environmental constraints during evolution, in particular the nature of the diet and water resources. Future research, embracing studies of the natural drinking behavior and ecology of animals, would be useful to further our understanding of the relation of physiological thirst mechanisms to normal behavior. Surprisingly, studies of man in this regard are even less common than in other species.

## VI. Conclusions

Drinking can be initiated by depletion of the cellular or extracellular fluid compartments. The work reviewed here shows that both cellular and extracellular thirst stimuli are produced by water deprivation in a variety of mammalian species, including man. The experiments in which either the cellular or the extracellular stimuli produced by water deprivation are selectively replaced indicate that 64–85% of the drinking following water deprivation is due to cellular dehydration, whereas hypovolemia accounts for 5–27% of the drinking. These figures include the findings for the rat, dog, and monkey; within these species hypovolemia is relatively less significant in the monkey than in the rat and dog. It is also found that fluid deficits are frequently present in the dog at the time when drinking is initiated under *ad libitum* conditions, and that the deficits are of a magnitude which may be sufficient to stimulate drinking. These fluid deficits arise not only from ongoing fluid losses, but are also seen particularly clearly when osmotic (or cellular) stimuli arise as a consequence of feeding. In addition to being within the physiologically detectable range, it has been shown that the cellular fluid deficits which arise as a consequence of feeding are important in the control of spontaneous drinking, in that reducing the osmotic effects of food by removing sodium from the diet results in a longer latency to drink, and a reduced daily water intake in the dog. These findings thus show that in the dog depletion of body fluid is important in the initiation of spontaneous drinking, occurring, for example, under *ad libitum* conditions or following water deprivation. The possible dependence of *ad libitum* drinking on physiological deficits is a new finding. It is not yet known to what extent normal drinking in other species may similarly be due to physiologically detected fluid deficits, or may be in anticipation of, or in addition to, such needs.

The investigations of sham-drinking make it clear in the dog and rat, and for the first time in the primate, the rhesus monkey, that drinking is normally maintained or rewarded by oropharyngeal factors, and not directly by replacement of physiological fluid deficits. The way in which the incentive for drinking is normally provided by factors such as taste is illustrated by the excessive drinking which occurs when the fluid is made especially palatable, for example, by the addition of saccharine. Because of taste, animals (probably including man) in which excretion is impaired will drink themselves markedly and dangerously into positive fluid balance. It was also shown that simply increasing the variety of the available fluids can lead to enhanced fluid intake in rats and men. The incentive or reward value which water has for the thirsty animal may have as a basis the subjective sensations of pleasantness produced by the taste of water, for it is shown in the human drinking studies that the ratings of the pleasantness of the taste of water are increased by water deprivation, and decreased as the subjects drink to satiety. It may be through such a mechanism that thirst signals modulate the reward or incentive value of oropharyngeal sensations, and lead to acceptance of water when thirsty and rejection when satiated.

The main factor which terminates drinking cannot be oropharyngeal metering, since the dog, rat, and monkey all overdrink with an open esophageal or gastric fistula. In the rat, a relatively slow drinker, the absorption of fluid and the repletion of the cellular fluid deficit is probably sufficiently rapid to make a major contribution to the termination of drinking. In the monkey, the absorption of fluid and replacement of fluid deficits is also rapid, but drinking slows or terminates at a time when significant cellular and extracellular fluid deficits remain. Absorption alone may not be sufficient to account for the satiety. It appears that there is a feed-forward contribution from peripheral receptors to satiety in this early period. The signals for short-term satiety may originate in the duodenum or hepatic-portal system, as well as from oropharyngeal mechanisms. In the dog, which drinks to satiety very rapidly in a few minutes, oropharyngeal mechanisms and intestinal or hepatic-portal receptors are required to explain the early termination of drinking. It should be emphasized that the mechanisms which terminate fluid intake are not powerful. For example, rats offered saccharine overdrink massively, and dangerously, if excretion is impaired. Similarly, in man the wide variety of palatable fluids available to drink may result in considerably more drinking than necessary for the requirements of fluid homeostasis alone. One reason why powerful satiety mechanisms for thirst may not have developed is that overdrinking is not normally a problem, as excessive water intake can normally be excreted as hypotonic urine.

These different signals which initiate, maintain, and terminate drinking must be integrated by the brain. There is evidence that cells in and
near the preoptic area sense cellular dehydration, and evidence that
some circumventricular organs such as the subfornical organ sense an
elevation in angiotensin, and thus that these regions are important in initiating drinking. There is evidence that there are cells in the lateral
hypothalamus and preoptic area which respond to the oropharyngeal
sensory stimulation produced by water, and some evidence that the
responsiveness of these cells may depend on the presence of thirst
stimuli, so that it is possible that these neurons are involved in maintaining drinking. Relatively rapid signals important in the early termination
of drinking may reach the hypothalamus and preoptic area, and effects
of gut distension and hepatic portal infusions on hypothalamic neurons
have been described. Over a longer term, satiety could be prolonged by
the postabsorptive effects of the ingested water, which by this time are
producing major repletion of the body fluid compartments and removing the original thirst stimuli.

### Acknowledgments

We would like to thank all of our colleagues who have collaborated on the experiments
described. Our research was supported by the Medical Research Council of Great Britain.

### References

Abdelaal, A. E., Mercer, P. F., and Mogenson, G. J. (1976). Plasma angiotensin II
    levels and water intake following b-adrenergic stimulation, hypovolemia, cellular
    dehydration and water deprivation. *Pharmacology, Biochemistry and Behavior* **4**,
    317-321.
Abraham, S. F., Denton, D. A., and Weisinger, B. S. (1976). Effect of an angiotensin
    antagonist, Sar¹-Ala⁸-Angiotensin II on physiological thirst. *Pharmacology,
    Biochemistry and Behavior* **4**, 243-247.
Adachi, A. (1977). On hepatic osmoreceptors in the rat. Proceedings of the Sixth
    International Conference on the Physiology of Food and Fluid Intake, Paris, France.
Adolph, E. F. (1939). Measurements of water drinking in dogs. *American Journal
    of Physiology* **125**, 75-86.
Adolph, E. F. (1943). "Physiological Regulations." Jacques Cattell Press, Lancaster, Pa.
Adolph, E. F. (1950). Thirst and its inhibition in the stomach. *American Journal of
    Physiology* **161**, 374-386.
Adolph, E. F., Barker, J. P., and Hoy, P. A. (1954). Multiple factors in thirst.
    *American Journal of Physiology* **178**, 538-562.
Andersson, B. (1953). The effect of injections of hypertonic NaCl solutions into
    different parts of the hypothalamus of goats. *Acta Physiologica Scandinavica* **18**,
    188-201.

Andersson, B. (1978). Regulation of water intake. *Physiological Reviews* **58**, 582–603.
Andersson, B., and Olsson, K. (1973). On central control of body fluid homeostasis. *Conditional Reflex* **8**, 147–159.
Antin, J., Gibbs, J., Holt, J., Young, R. C., and Smith, G. P. (1975). Cholecystokinin elicits the complete behavioral sequence of satiety in rats. *Journal of Comparative and Physiological Psychology* **89**, 784–790.
Arnauld, E., Dufy, B., and Vincent, J. D. (1975). Hypothalamic supraoptic neurones: Rates and patterns of action potential firing during water deprivation in the unanaesthetized monkey. *Brain Research* **100**, 315–325.
Bellows, R. T. (1939). Time factors in water drinking in dogs. *American Journal of Physiology* **125**, 87–97.
Bernard, C. (1856). "Lecons de physiologie expérimentale appliquée à la médecine," Vol. II, p. 51. Baillière, Paris.
Blair-West, J. R., and Brook, A. H. (1969). Circulatory changes and renin secretion in sheep in response to feeding. *Journal of Physiology (London)* **204**, 15–30.
Blank, D. L., and Wayner, M. J. (1975). Lateral preoptic single unit activity: Effects of various solutions. *Physiology and Behavior* **15**, 723–730.
Blass, E. M. (1974). Evidence for basal forebrain thirst osmoreceptors in rat. *Brain Research* **82**, 69–76.
Blass, E. M., and Epstein, A. N. (1971). A lateral preoptic osmosensitive zone for thirst in the rat. *Journal of Comparative and Physiological Psychology* **76**, 378–394.
Blass, E. M., and Hall, W. G. (1976). Drinking termination: Interactions among hydrational, orogastric, and behavioral controls in rats. *Psychological Review* **83**, 356–374.
Brown, J. J., Curtis, J. R., Lever, A. F., Robertson, J. I. S., DeWardener, H. E., and Wing, A. J. (1969). Plasma renin concentration and the control of blood pressure in patients on maintenance hemodialysis. *Nephron* **6**, 329–349.
Buggy, J., and Johnson, A. K. (1977). Anteroventral third ventricle periventricular ablation: Temporary adipsia and persisting thirst deficits *Neuroscience Letters* **5**, 177–182.
Buggy, J., Fink, G. D., Johnson, A. K., and Brody, M. J. (1977). Prevention of the development of renal hypertension by anteroventral third ventricular tissue lesions. *Circulation Research,* Supplement 1 **40**, 1–110–1–117.
Cabanac, M. (1971). Physiological role of pleasure. *Science* **173**, 1103–1107.
Coburn, P. C., and Stricker, E. M. (1978). Osmoregulatory thirst in rats after lateral preoptic lesions. *Journal of Comparative and Physiological Psychology* **92**, 350–361.
Cross, B. A., and Green, J. D. (1959). Activity of single neurones in the hypothalamus: Effects of osmotic and other stimuli. *Journal of Physiology (London)* **148**, 554–569.
Day, R. P., and Reid, I. A. (1976). Renin activity in dog brain: Enzymological similarity to Cathepsin D. *Endocrinology* **99**, 93–100.
Dicker, S. E., and Nunn, J. (1957). The role of antidiuretic hormone during water deprivation in rats. *Journal of Physiology (London)* **136**, 235–248.
Emmers, R. (1973). Interaction of neural systems which control body water. *Brain Research* **49**, 323–347.
Epstein, A. N. (1960). Water intake without the act of drinking. *Science* **131**, 497–498.
Epstein, A. N. (1973). Epilogue: Retrospect and prognosis. *In* "The Neuropsychology of Thirst: New Findings and Advances in Concepts" (A. N. Epstein, H. R. Kissileff, and E. Stellar, eds.), pp. 315–332. Wiley, New York.
Epstein, A. N. (1978). Consensus, controversies, and curiosities. *Federation Proceedings* **37**, 2711–2716.

Epstein, A. N., Fitzsimons, J. T., and Rolls, B. J. (1970). Drinking induced by injection of angiotensin into the brain of the rat. *Journal of Physiology (London)* 210, 457–474.

Ernits, T., and Corbit, J. D. (1973). Taste as a dipsogenic stimulus. *Journal of Comparative and Physiological Psychology* 83, 27–31.

Felix, D., and Akert, K. (1974). The effect of angiotensin II on neurones of the cat subfornical organ. *Brain Research* 76, 350–353.

Fitzsimons, J. T. (1961). Drinking by nephrectomized rats injected with various substances. *Journal of Physiology (London)* 155, 563–579.

Fitzsimons, J. T. (1964). Drinking caused by constriction of the inferior vena cava in the rat. *Nature (London)* 204, 479–480.

Fitzsimons, J. T. (1969). The role of renal thirst factor in drinking induced by extracellular stimuli. *Journal of Physiology (London)* 201, 349–368.

Fitzsimons, J. T. (1972). Thirst. *Physiological Review* 52, 468–561.

Fitzsimons, J. T., and Kucharczyk, J. (1978). Drinking and haemodynamic changes induced in the dog by intracranial injection of components of the renin-angiotensin system. *Journal of Physiology (London)* 276, 419–434.

Fitzsimons, J. T., and Le Magnen, J. (1969). Eating as a regulatory control of drinking. *Journal of Comparative and Physiological Psychology* 67, 273–283.

Fitzsimons, J. T., and Simons, B. J. (1969). The effects on drinking in the rat of intravenous infusion of angiotensin, given alone or in combination with other stimuli of thirst. *Journal of Physiology (London)* 203, 45–57.

Fitzsimons, J. T., Kucharczyk, J., and Richards, G. (1978). Systemic angiotensin-induced drinking in the dog: A physiological phenomenon. *Journal of Physiology (London)* 276, 435–448.

Gilman, A. (1937). The relation between blood osmotic pressure, fluid distribution and voluntary water intake. *American Journal of Physiology* 120, 323–328.

Goldstein, D. J., and Halperin, J. A. (1977). Mast cell histamine and cell dehydration thirst. *Nature (London)* 267, 250–252.

Haberich, F. J. (1968). Osmoreception in the portal system. *Federation Proceedings* 27, 1137–1141.

Hatton, G. I., and Bennett, C. T. (1970). Satiation of thirst and termination of drinking: Roles of plasma osmolality and absorption. *Physiology and Behavior* 5, 579–587.

Hayward, J. N. (1977). Functional and morphological aspects of hypothalamic neurons. *Physiological Review* 57, 574–658.

Hayward, J. N., and Vincent, J. D. (1970). Osmosensitive single neurones in the hypothalamus of unanaesthetized monkeys. *Journal of Physiology (London)* 210, 947–971.

Hirose, S., Yokosawa, H., and Inagami, T. (1978). Immunochemical identification of renin in rat brain and distinction from acid proteases. *Nature (London)* 274, 392–393.

Hobson, J. A., and English, J. T. (1963). Self-induced water intoxication. Case study of a chronically schizophrenic patient with physiological evidence of water retention due to inappropriate release of antidiuretic hormone. *Annals of Internal Medicine* 58, 324–332.

Hoffman, W. E., Ganten, U., Phillips, M. I., Schmid, P. G., Schelling, P., and Ganten, D. (1978). Inhibition of drinking in water-deprived rats by combined central angiotensin II and cholinergic receptor blockade. *American Journal of Physiology* 234, F41–F47.

Hsiao, S., Epstein, A. N., and Camardo, J. S. (1977). The dipsogenic potency of peripheral angiotensin II. *Hormones and Behavior* 8, 129–140.

Hunt, J. N. (1956). Some properties of an alimentary osmoreceptor mechanism. *Journal of Physiology (London)* **132**, 267–288.

Johnson, A. K., and Epstein, A. N. (1975). The cerebral ventricles as the avenue for the dipsogenic action of intracranial angiotensin. *Brain Research* **86**, 399–418.

Kozlowski, S., and Drzewiecki, K. (1973). The role of osmoreception in portal circulation in control of water intake in dogs. *Acta Physiologica Polonica* **24**, 325–330.

Kozlowski, S., and Szczepanska-Sadowska, E. (1975). Mechanisms of hypovolaemic thirst and interactions between hypovolaemia, hyperosmolality and the antidiuretic system. *In* "Control Mechanisms of Drinking" (G. Peters, J. T. Fitzsimons, and L. Peters-Haefeli, eds.), pp. 25–35. Springer-Verlag, Berlin.

Kraly, F. S., Gibbs, J., and Smith, G. P. (1975). Disordered drinking after abdominal vagotomy in rats. *Nature (London)* **258**, 226–228.

Kucharczyk, J., Assaf, S. Y., and Mogenson, G. J. (1976). Differential effects of brain lesions on thirst induced by the administration of angiotensin II to the preoptic region, subfornical organ and anterior third ventricle. *Brain Research* **108**, 327–337.

Laragh, J. H., and Leaf, A. (1973). The renin-angiotensin-aldosterone hormonal system and the regulation of sodium, potassium and blood pressure homeostasis. *In* "Handbook of Physiology, Section 8, Renal Physiology" (J. Orloff and R. W. Berliner, eds.), pp. 831–908. Waverly Press, Washington, D.C.

Lee, M. C., Thrasher, T. N., and Ramsay, D. J. (1978). The effect of intracerebroventricular infusion of saralason on drinking following caval ligation, hypertonic saline and water deprivation in rats. *Abstracts of the Society for Neuroscience.*

Leenan, F. H. H., Boer, P., and Geyskes, G. G. (1978). Sodium intake and the effects of isoproterenol and exercise on plasma renin activity in man. *Journal of Applied Physiology* **45**, 870–874.

Le Magnen, J. (1956). Hyperphagie provoquée chez le rat blanc par altération du mécanism de satiété périphérique. *Comptes rendus de la Société de Biologie* **150**, 32–35.

McFarland, D. J., and Rolls, B. J. (1972). Suppression of feeding by intracranial injections of angiotensin. *Nature (London)* **236**, 172–173.

Maddison, S., Rolls, B. J., Rolls, E. T., and Wood, R. J. (1977). Analysis of drinking in the chronically cannulated monkey. *Journal of Physiology (London)* **272**, 4–5P.

Maddison, S., Wood, R. J., Rolls, E. T., Rolls, B. J., and Gibbs, J. (1980). Drinking in the rhesus monkey: Peripheral factors. *Journal of Comparative and Physiological Psychology, in press.*

Maddison, S., Rolls, B. J., Rolls, E. T., and Wood, R. J. (1980). The role of gastric factors in drinking termination in the monkey. *Journal of Physiology (London)*, in press.

Malmo, R. B., and Mundl, W. J. (1975). Osmosensitive neurons in the rat's preoptic area: Medial-lateral comparison. *Journal of Comparative and Physiological Psychology* **88**, 161–175.

Malvin, R. L., Mouw, D., and Vander, A. J. (1977). Angiotensin: Physiological role in water-deprivation-induced thirst in rats. *Science* **197**, 171–173.

Miselis, R. R., Hand, P. J., and Berger, R. (1977). An autoradiographic study of the efferent connectivity of the subfornical organ. Proceedings of the Sixth International Conference on the Physiology of Food and Fluid Intake, Paris, France.

Mogenson, G. J., and Kucharczyk, J. (1978). Central neural pathways for angiotensin-induced thirst. *Federation Proceedings* **37**, 2683–2688.

Mogenson, G. J., and Phillips, A. G. (1976). Motivation: A psychological construct in search of a physiological substrate. *Progress in Psychobiology and Physiological Psychology* **6**, 189–243.

Mook, D. G. (1963). Oral and postingestional determinants of the intake of various solutions in rats with esophageal fistulas. *Journal of Comparative and Physiological Psychology* **56**, 645–659.

Nicolaïdis, S. (1969). Early systemic responses to orgastric stimulation and the regulation of food and water balance: Functional and electrophysiological data. *Annals of the New York Academy of Sciences* **151**, 1176–1203.

Nicolaïdis, S., and Rowland, N. (1974). Long-term intravenous "drinking" in the rat. *Journal of Comparative and Physiological Psychology* **87**, 1–15.

Oomura, Y., Ono, T., Ooyama, H., and Wayner, M. J. (1969). Glucose and osmosensitive neurones of the rat hypothalamus. *Nature (London)* **222**, 282–284.

Peck, J. W., and Blass, E. M. (1975). Localization of thirst and antidiuretic osmoreceptors by intracranial injections in rats. *American Journal of Physiology* **228**, 1501–1509.

Peck, J. W., and Novin, D. (1971). Evidence that osmoreceptors mediating drinking in rabbits are in the lateral preoptic area. *Journal of Comparative and Physiological Psychology* **74**, 134–147.

Peterson, D. T., and Marshall, W. H. (1975). Polydipsia and inappropriate secretion of antidiuretic hormone associated with hydrocephalus. *Annals of Internal Medicine* **83**, 675–676.

Phillips, M. I. (1978). Angiotensin in the brain. *Neuroendocrinology* **25**, 354–377.

Phillips, M. I., and Felix, D. (1976). Specific angiotensin II receptive neurones in the cat subfornical organ. *Brain Research* **109**, 531–540.

Pickering, L., and Hogan, G. (1971). Voluntary water intoxication in a normal child. *Journal of Pediatrics* **78**, 316–318.

Ramsay, D. J. (1979). The brain renin angiotensin system: A reevaluation. *Neuroscience* **4**, 313–321.

Ramsay, D. J., and Reid, I. A. (1975). Some central mechanisms of thirst in the dog. *Journal of Physiology (London)* **253**, 517–525.

Ramsay, D. J., Rolls, B. J., and Wood, R. J. (1973). Increased drinking in dogs during congestive heart failure. *Journal of Physiology (London)* **234**, 48–50 P.

Ramsay, D. J., Rolls, B. J., and Wood, R. J. (1975). The relationship between elevated water intake and oedema associated with congestive cardiac failure in the dog. *Journal of Physiology (London)* **244**, 303–312.

Ramsay, D. J., Rolls, B. J., and Wood, R. J. (1977a). Thirst following water deprivation in dogs. *American Journal of Physiology* **232**, R93–R100.

Ramsay, D. J., Rolls, B. J., and Wood, R. J. (1977b). Body fluid changes which influence drinking in the water-deprived rat. *Journal of Physiology (London)* **266**, 453–469.

Rolls, B. J. (1975). Interaction of hunger and thirst in rats with lesions of the preoptic area. *Physiology and Behavior* **14**, 537–543.

Rolls, B. J. (1979). How variety and palatability can stimulate appetite. *Nutrition Bulletin* **5**, 78–86.

Rolls, B. J., and McFarland, D. J. (1973). Hydration releases inhibition of feeding produced by intracranial angiotensin. *Physiology and Behavior* **11**, 881–884.

Rolls, B. J., and Ramsay, D. J. (1975). The elevation of endogenous angiotensin and thirst in the dog. *In* "Control Mechanisms of Drinking" (G. Peters, J. T. Fitzsimons, and L. Peters-Haefeli, eds.), pp. 74–78. Springer-Verlag, Heidelberg.

Rolls, B. J., and Wood, R. J. (1977a). The role of angiotensin in thirst. *Pharmacology Biochemistry and Behavior* **6**, 245–250.

Rolls, B. J., and Wood, R. J. (1977b). Excretion following drinking in the dog. *Journal of Physiology (London)* **272**, 73–74P.

Rolls, B. J., and Wood, R. J. (1979). Homeostatic control of drinking: A surviving concept. *Behavioral and Brain Sciences* **2**, 116–117.

Rolls, B. J., Jones, B. P., and Fallows, D. J. (1972). A comparison of the motivational properties of thirst induced by intracranial angiotensin and water deprivation. *Physiology and Behavior* **9**, 777–782.

Rolls, B. J., Wood, R. J., and Stevens, R. M. (1978). Effects of palatability on body fluid homeostasis. *Physiology and Behavior* **20**, 15–19.

Rolls, E. T. (1975). "The Brain and Reward." Pergamon, Oxford.

Rolls, E. T. (1978). The neurophysiology of feeding. *Trends in Neurosciences* **1**, 1–3.

Rolls, E. T. (1980). Activity of hypothalamic and related neurons in the alert animal. *In* "Handbook of the Hypothalamus" (P. J. Morgane and J. Panksepp eds.). Dekker, New York, in press.

Rolls, E. T., and Rolls, B. J. (1977). Activity of neurones in sensory, hypothalamic and motor areas during feeding in the monkey. *In* "Food Intake and Chemical Senses" (Y. Katsuki, M. Sato, S. Takagi, and Y. Oomura, eds.), pp. 525–549. University of Tokyo Press, Tokyo.

Rolls, E. T., Sanghera, M. K., and Roper-Hail, A. (1979). The latency of activation of neurones in the lateral hypothalamus and substantia innominata during feeding in the monkey. *Brain Research* **164**, 121–135.

Rowland, N. (1977). Regulatory drinking: Do physiological substrates have an ecological niche? *Biobehavioral Reviews* **1**, 261–272.

Schmitt, M. (1973). Influences of hepatic portal receptors on hypothalamic feeding and satiety centers. *American Journal of Physiology* **225**, 1089–1095.

Schwob, J. E., and Johnson, A. K. (1977). Angiotensin-induced dipso-genesis in domestic fowl *(Gallus gallus)*. *Journal of Comparative and Physiological Psychology* **91**, 182–188.

Simpson, J. B., and Routtenberg, A. (1973). Subfornical organ: Site of drinking elicitation by angiotensin II. *Science* **818**, 1172–1174.

Simpson, J. B., Epstein, A. N., and Camardo, J. S. (1977). The localization of receptors for the dipsogenic action of angiotensin II in the subfornical organ. *Journal of Comparative and Physiological Psychology* **91**, 1220–1231.

Simpson, J. B., Reid, I. A., Ramsay, D. J., and Kipen, H. (1978). Mechanism of the dipsogenic action of tetradecapeptide renin substrate. *Brain Research* **157**, 63–72.

Sobocińska, J. (1978). Gastric distension and thirst: Relevance to the osmotic thirst threshold and metering of water intake. *Physiology and Behavior* **20**, 497–501.

Stricker, E. M. (1973). Thirst, sodium appetite, and complementary physiological con-tributions to the regulation of intravascular fluid volume. *In* "The Neuropsychology of Thirst: New Findings and Advances in Concepts (A. N. Epstein, H. R. Kissileff, and E. Stellar, eds.), pp. 73–98. Wiley, New York.

Stricker, E. M. (1978). The renin-angiotensin system and thirst: Some unanswered questions. *Federation Proceedings* **37**, 2704–2710.

Stricker, E. M., Bradshaw, W. G., and McDonald, R. H., Jr. (1976). The renin-angiotensin system and thirst: A reevaluation. *Science* **194**, 1169–1171.

Swanson, L. W., Kucharczyk, J., and Mogenson, G. J. (1978). Autoradiographic evidence for pathways from the medial preoptic area to the midbrain involved in the drinking response to angiotensin II. *Journal of Comparative Neurology* **178**, 645–660.

Thrasher, T. N., Jones, R. G., and Ramsay, D. J. (1978). Effect of third ventricular infusions of hypertonic solutions on thirst in the dog. *Abstracts of the Society for Neuroscience,* Vol. 4.

Toates, F. M. (1979). Homeostasis and drinking. *Behavioral and Brain Sciences* **2**, 95–139.

Towbin, E. J. (1949). Gastric distension as a factor in the satiation of thirst in esophagostomized dogs. *American Journal of Physiology* **159**, 533–541.

Trippodo, N. C., McCaa, R. E., and Guyton, A. C. (1976). Effect of prolonged angiotensin II infusion on thirst. *American Journal of Physiology* **230**, 1063–1066.

Verney, E. G. (1947). The antidiuretic hormone and the factors which determine its release. *Proceedings of the Royal Society, London, Series B* **135**, 25–106.

Vincent, J. D., Arnauld, E., and Bioulac, B. (1972). Activity of osmosensitive single cells in the hypothalamus of the behaving monkey during drinking. *Brain Research* **44**, 371–384.

Weiss, C. S., and Almli, C. R. (1975). Lateral preoptic and lateral hypothalamic units: In search of the osmoreceptors for thirst. *Physiology and Behavior* **15**, 713–722.

Wolf, A. V. (1950). Osmometric analysis of thirst in man and dog. *American Journal of Physiology* **161**, 75–86.

Wood, R. J., Rolls, B. J., and Ramsay, D. J. (1977). Drinking following intracarotid infusions of hypertonic solutions in dogs. *American Journal of Physiology* **232**, R88–R92.

Zimmermann, M. B., Stricker, E. M., and Blaine, E. H. (1979). Water intake after volume depletion in sheep: Effects of crushing the left atrial appendage. *Society for Neuroscience Abstracts* **5**, 226.

PROGRESS IN PSYCHOBIOLOGY AND PHYSIOLOGICAL PSYCHOLOGY, VOL. 9

# The Pineal Gland:
# A Regulator of Regulators[1]

Russel J. Reiter

*Department of Anatomy*
*University of Texas*
*Health Science Center at San Antonio*
*San Antonio, Texas*

## I. Prefatory Remarks

If ubiquity of actions were synonymous with importance and if the alleged interactions of the pineal with other endocrine and nonendocrine organs are unequivocally substantiated, then surely the pineal gland, previously suspected of being vestigial, would now have to be considered one of the most influential glands in the mammalian organism. Indeed, although reluctantly admitted by some endocrine physiologists, the anterior pituitary gland often has an obsequious position relative to the pineal gland in the hierarchy of neuroendocrine regulation. As recently as 10 to 12 years ago such a statement would certainly have been considered paralogistic, whereas now it is practically axiomatic, if not among peripheral endocrinologists at least among informed neuroendocrinologists and pinealologists.

A veritable avalanche of new information has surfaced which puts the pineal gland into biological perspective (see, e.g., Quay, 1974; Reiter, 1977, 1978a; Nir *et al.*, 1978). Its position is now seen to be that of a regulator of other controlling processes, in effect, a "regulator of regulators," a phrase introduced a number of years ago to describe its actions (Reiter and Hester, 1966a). The pineal is now known to apprise the endocrine organs, presumably via the neuroendocrine axis, of the status of the environment, particularly of the photoperiod, and to adjust the activity of the hypothalamo-hypophyseal system accordingly. This

---

[1] Work by the author was supported by grants from the NSF and from the NIH.

323

Copyright © 1980 by Academic Press, Inc.
All rights of reproduction in any form reserved.
ISBN 0-12-542109-5

interaction is carried out by means of hormonal envoys produced and secreted by the pineal gland. Because of the importance of light and darkness to pineal biochemistry, the rigorous control of the artificial photoperiods used in most laboratory animal facilities has severely hindered research into the endocrine role of the pineal gland. The highly regulated long photoperiods used in most laboratory settings markedly quell its endocrine capabilities. Under such conditions surgical extirpation of the pineal, a method widely used in endocrine research to prove the organ of origin of a particular hormone, is virtually without effect. Indeed, in such experiments the pineal gland appears to be a functionless vestige. I have previously likened removal of the pineal gland from animals under controlled long photoperiods to removal of the ovaries from previously hypophysectomized animals (Reiter, 1973). In neither case are the consequences of the endocrinectomies, i.e., pinealectomy or ovariectomy, very dramatic. This, however, does not justify the conclusion that the organs are inconsequential.

The simpliest way to illustrate the endocrine capability of the pineal gland is to place a photosensitive species, e.g., the Syrian hamster, in a restricted photoperiodic environment and allow the pineal gland to achieve maximal activity; then the effects of its removal become conspicuous. A fact that is often overlooked, or simply ignored, by many scientists is that controlled long photoperiods impose an abnormal situation on animals that have evolved in their natural habitats under seasonally changing daylengths. Under the latter conditions the pineal becomes of paramount importance in adjusting the level of endocrine activity to suit the particular season of the year (Reiter, 1978b).

The objectives of the following review are 3-fold: to convince the skeptics who doubt the endocrine capability of the pineal gland of its importance as an organ of internal secretion; to present in an objective manner the data relating to the wide variety of potential pineal hormones; to put the pineal into biological perspective, i.e., to attempt to define its role in the normal economy of the organism.

## II. Anatomical Link between Eyes and Pineal Gland

Whereas in some reptilian and avian species the pineal gland, and possibly other parts of the central nervous system, responds directly to photic information which penetrates the scalp, in mammals photoreception has been relegated exclusively to the lateral eyes. Since the pineal gland in these animals still depends on environmental photoperiodic information they have had to evolve either a humoral or a neural connection between the eyes and the gland so the latter would be apprised of the light:dark situation. Mammals seemed to have opted for the neural route. This in itself is not surprising. What is of considerable interest, however, is the complicated and circuitous neuronal network involved in transferring the message, which originates in the retina, to its destination in the pineal gland. Despite its complexity, so far as is known, most mammals rely on basically the same neural pathways to connect the central structures to the gland. These involve peripheral sympathetic axons which form distinct nervi conarii that penetrate the apex of the gland (Kappers, 1960, 1965). Within the pineal gland the fibers terminate primarily in the perivascular spaces (Wartenberg, 1968; Matsushima and Reiter, 1977) and rarely in opposition to the pineal parenchymal elements (Matsushima and Reiter, 1978). The pineal in a few species may also be endowed with a parasympathetic innervation, e.g., the monkey (Kenny, 1961) and the rabbit (Romijn, 1975).

A great deal of effort has been expended in identifying the neural connections which relay information from the eyes to the preganglionic sympathetic neurons in the thoracic cord. It has been rewarded with the partial identification of at least a potential, and possibly an actual, chain of neurons which relate the eyes to the pineal. The eyes themselves must be present in order for the pineal to respond to ambient lighting providing evidence that the photoreceptor which eventually cues pineal activity resides in these structures. However, the classic photoreceptor elements in the retinas seem to be of little importance. For example, pineals of rats in which the rods have been totally or near totally destroyed by exposure of the animals to continuous light are still capable of responding to changes in the photoperiod in the normal manner (Reiter and Klein, 1971). Also, if the retinas are removed surgically but the remainder of the eye is left intact the pineal gland is no longer inhibited by light and the animals respond as if they are in darkness (Reiter and Johnson, 1974). In this case the retinas were removed by cutting the globes, everting the retinas, and removing them.

The neural impulses which arise in the retina and are destined for the pineal gland are carried to the brain via axons of the retinal ganglion cells which terminate in the suprachiasmatic nuclei (SCN) of the hypothalamus. These direct projections were identified in the early 1970s (Moore and Lenn, 1972; Hendrickson et al., 1972; Moore, 1973). The projection from a single retina is reportedly bilateral with the contralateral suprachiasmatic nucleus receiving roughly twice as many terminals as the ipsilateral. The ventral and lateral portions of the SCN receive the bulk of the terminals. This direct projection of axons from the retinas to the SCN seems to be a widespread component of the visual system of mammals (Moore, 1973). The neural pathways beyond the

SCN which project through the hypothalamus have been crudely mapped by lesion studies which indicate that fiber bundles descending or
ascending in the lateral hypothalamic area were critical for the normal
functioning of the pineal gland (Moore *et al.,* 1968; Reiter, 1972). The
most likely means whereby neural information from the SCN is eventually transferred to the upper thoracic spinal cord includes efferents
from the SCN which project caudally to the periventricular and tuberal
areas of the hypothalamus (Szentagothai *et al.,* 1968; Swanson and
Cowan, 1975). Axons from the ventral tuberal area project to the lateral
hypothalamus (Szentagothai *et al.,* 1968) and, finally, axons of neurons
in the lateral hypothalamic area project through the brain stem directly
to the intermediolateral cell column (preganglionic sympathetic neurons)
of the upper thoracic cord (Saper *et al.,* 1976). This sequence of
neurons, proposed by Moore (1978), is depicted in Fig. 1 and may explain the transferral of neural information from the SCN to the
peripheral sympathetic nervous system. The efferents of the preganglionic sympathetic parikarya in the intermediolateral cell column
exit the spinal cord and pass up the sympathetic trunk bilaterally to
synapse eventually in the superior cervical ganglia. Postganglionic

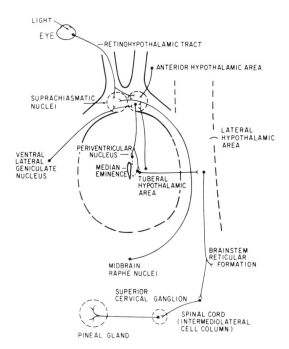

Fɪɢ. 1. Presumed neural pathways which connect the eyes to the pineal gland in mammals. From Moore (1978).

neurons carry the information to the pineal gland. The essential role of the superior cervical ganglia in influencing the synthesis of pineal indoleamines (Wurtman *et al.,* 1964) and the inhibitory reproductive effects of the gland (Reiter and Hester, 1966b) was demonstrated rather early and has been repeatedly confirmed in recent years.

In support of the anatomical findings, Nishino *et al.* (1976) provided electrophysiological evidence that the eyes and the SCN are capable of altering the propagation of action potentials through the superior cervical ganglia. Electrical stimulation of the SCN by means of stereotaxically implanted electrodes greatly decreased the frequency of action potentials in the cervical sympathetic trunk. Likewise, shining a light into the rat's eyes also diminished neural activity. When stimulated, other areas of the hypothalamus had very little influence on the electrical activity of the peripheral sympathetic nervous system. Nishino and co-workers (1976) interpreted their findings to mean that under normal situations photic stimulation of the eyes augments the electrical activity of the SCN which, in turn, suppresses the activity of the preganglionic sympathetic neurons resident in the intermediolateral cell column. The reduced activity in the sympathetic trunk causes a decreased release of norepinephrine within the gland (the neurotransmitter in the post-ganglionic sympathetic nerve endings) and, as a consequence, the organ remains in an inactive state. Conversely, during darkness the pineal gland is activated due to the augmented release of norepinephrine. The stimulatory effect of darkness on the melatonin-synthesizing enzymes (Quay, 1974; Nir *et al.,* 1978) and the physiologic (Reiter, 1973) aspects of the pineal is known.

The neuronal circuitry outlined in the previous paragraphs is reasonably well documented but it has been garnered primarily from studies in the rat. Other species may utilize slightly different central pathways to relay the neural signal from the SCN to the intermediolateral cell column. However, it seems safe to conclude that all mammals probably rely on the sympathetic nervous system to carry information about the photoperiod from the thoracic cord to the pineal gland. Within the gland the transduction of neural information into chemical factors is well documented (Axelrod, 1974). This involves a stimulation of adenylate cyclase activity by norepinephrine resulting in a rise in cyclic AMP levels and protein synthesis.

## III. Pineal Hormones

Hormones, by definition, are produced in a cell, are secreted and transferred to a distant target site via a bodily fluid, and there exert an action. Although various investigators have claimed hormonal status for many pineal constituents, few actually qualify for this role when the criteria previously mentioned are used. Nevertheless, it is the opinion of the present reviewer that not one, but several structurally diverse compounds will prove to be endocrine factors of the pineal gland. It has been conjectured that the pineal and pituitary gland may be functional mirror images, i.e., where one stimulates the other inhibits Wiener, 1968). Although this statement constituted rank speculation at the time it was rendered, it is now becoming increasingly apparent that this proposal may have validity. Certainly, considering the large number of processes which the pineal gland reportedly influences it would be scientifically naive to assume that all of the actions are propagated by a single hormone. The diversity of actions of the pineal gland practically requires that there be several endocrine factors produced within and discharged from it, possibly even as many as from its companion diencephalic structure the anterior pituitary gland. Like the pituitary, the pineal influences the function of the gonads, the adrenal cortex, the thyroid gland along with bodily growth, as well as several extrapituitary-regulated endocrine glands (Reiter, 1977, 1978a; Nir *et al.*, 1978).

Since the pineal gland is an outgrowth of the ectodermally derived central nervous system, one would anticipate that it may have some commonality with the neural tissue. Within the brain two major categories of constituents, amines and polypeptides, are liberated from cells and act on often adjacent, and sometimes distant, tissues. Investigations have revealed that the pineal is also concerned with the production of amines and polypeptides much in the same manner as the brain itself. Because of this it would seem worthwhile to duplicate many of the experiments originally carried out on neural tissue with the pineal; this is particularly true with regard to the studies which involved the amines. For the same reason, experimental paradigms used in testing for the secretion of polypeptides from the posterior pituitary gland (another ectodermal derivative) may prove to be informative when applied to the pineal gland.

A. INDOLEAMINES

The metabolism of indoleamines in the pineal gland has received a great deal of attention over the last decade. One substance in particular, $N$-acetyl-6-methoxytryptamine or melatonin, has attracted great interest. Its synthesis from tryptophan via serotonin has been carefully worked out (Axelrod, 1974; Klein, 1974; Quay, 1974). Serotonin is synthesized in the pinealocyte from tryptophan. This amino acid is taken up from the blood and is 5-hydroxylated in the presence of the enzyme tryptophan hydroxylase (Lovenberg *et al.*, 1967) and then decarboxylated by aromatic amino acid decarboxylase (Lovenberg *et al.*, 1962). The product, serotonin, is found in very high concentrations in the pineal gland. It is acted upon by *N*-acetyltransferase with the resultant formation of *N*-acetylserotonin (Klein and Weller, 1970) which is *O*-methylated by hydroxyindole-*O*-methyltransferase (HIOMT) resulting in the production of melatonin (Axelrod and Weissbach, 1960). The methyl group for this enzymatic step is provided by *S*-adenosylmethionine. Other indole derivatives are produced from serotonin within the pineal gland. The action of monoamine oxidase on serotonin causes the formation of an unstable metabolite, 5-hydroxyindole acetylaldehyde. This compound is either oxidized to 5-hydroxyindole acetic acid or reduced to 5-hydroxytryptophol (Quay, 1974). HIOMT methylates 5-hydroxytryptophol to form 5-methoxytryptophol (McIsaac *et al.*, 1965).

The step which regulates the amount of melatonin produced seems to be at the level of the acetylating enzyme (Klein, 1974). During times of peak performance, i.e., during the dark portion of the light:dark cycle, the activity of this enzyme increases, depending on the species, from several to many fold (Rudeen *et al.*, 1975). The enzyme HIOMT, initially thought to be rate limiting in melatonin synthesis, shows a much lower level of diurnal fluctuation (Lynch and Ralph, 1970).

## 1. Melatonin

Judging from its appearance in the blood and reduction after pinealectomy, this methoxyindole is believed to be released from the pineal gland. It is found in significant concentrations in several bodily fluids (Pang and Ralph, 1975; Ozaki and Lynch, 1976; Rollag and Niswender, 1976) and small amounts of unmetabolized melatonin are excreted in the urine (Lynch *et al.*, 1975). Its endocrine, particularly reproductive, influences have been extensively investigated.

*a. Antigonadotrophic Effects.* Shortly after its discovery, melatonin was tested for its ability to inhibit reproduction. Although these early studies (Wurtman and Axelrod, 1965) left investigators with the provisional impression that melatonin had a suppressive influence on reproductive physiology, the results were tantalizingly incomplete and did not convince scientists as a whole of its endocrine capabilities. The earliest papers reporting the antireproductive effects of melatonin appeared in the early 1960s. The following results are typical of these studies. Melatonin was injected (1 or 20 $\mu$g) either intraperitoneally or subcutaneously into maturing female rats for 28 consecutive days. At the conclusion of the experiment animals that received 20 $\mu$g melatonin daily possessed ovaries that were subnormal in weight. The 1 μg dosage produced a less dramatic change and was effective only when administered by means of the subcutaneous route. Additionally, rats that had smaller than normal ovaries exhibited a decreased incidence of vaginal "estrus." In this case the term "estrus" referred to smears that were classified, on the basis of cellular composition, as either being proestrous, estrous, or metestrous; this classification was later to be questioned by a number of scientists.

In subsequent years an incredible array of experimental paradigms was devised to test for the reproductive consequences of melatonin administration. Every conceivable route of administration was used and the dosages of melatonin employed varied widely among the experiments. Endpoints in these studies included gonadal and accessory organ weights, gonadotrophin levels in the pituitary and plasma, gonadal steroid concentrations in the blood, ovulation in females and spermatogenesis in males, and even mating behavior. The most common experimental animal in these studies was the rat while the mouse was used much less frequently. The findings of an overwhelming majority of these experiments indicated that melatonin's character was generally antigonadotrophic but scientists were uneasy with this assessment because of the marginal effects that were often produced by the compound. Moreover, on some occasions melatonin completely lacked significant antigonadotrophic capabilities. Variable results such as these encouraged investigators to continue examining the physiologic properties of the methoxyindole but also raised their suspicions about the hormonal nature of the compound. The findings of many of these studies have been dutifully tabulated in a review by Reiter et al. (1975c).

The use of the rat as an experimental subject in many of these experiments was unfortunate inasmuch as the neuroendocrine–reproductive axis in this species is relatively insensitive to darkness and to the antigonadotrophic influence of the pineal gland and, therefore, also to melatonin (Turek et al., 1976). Such species have been classified as nonphotoperiodic. Using certain experimental perturbations it is possible to sensitize the reproductive system of rats to the gonad-inhibiting ability of light restriction and the pineal gland. These manipulations are referred to as potentiating factors and include rendering the animals anosmic, the injection of gonadal steroids shortly after birth, and underfeeding (Reiter and Sorrentino, 1971). The mechanisms whereby these procedures change the reactivity of the neuroendocrine axis to the pineal remain unknown.

The reputation of melatonin as a pineal antigonadotrophic agent was greatly buoyed by the observation that the methoxyindole exerts a potent controlling influence on the genital apparatus of the Syrian hamster *(Mesocricetus auratus)*. This observation was noteworthy since the hamster is the species which has provided the most convincing evidence that the pineal is a legitimate functional organ of internal secretion (Reiter, 1978b). Even the most outspoken critics of the pineal cannot deny the unequivocal data which has surfaced inextricably linking the pineal and the reproductive system in the hamster. When adult male or female hamsters are placed in a photoperiodic environment which provides less than 12.5 hours of light per day their reproductive organs totally involute (Elliott, 1976). This collapse is associated with alterations in both pituitary and plasma gonadotrophin levels, gonadal morphology, steroid secretion, and in the size of the secondary sex organs (Reiter, 1978b; Reiter and Johnson, 1974). All of these changes are known to be a consequence of the activation of the pineal gland by photoperiods of reduced length. Unfortunately, virtually nothing has been done to determine whether the sexual behavior of these animals also is altered by photoperiod and the pineal gland.

The administration of melatonin, using a clearly defined scheme, can duplicate the reproductive effects of shortened photoperiods suggesting that it may be responsible for the gonadal involution seen in dark-exposed hamsters. It was only recently that this observation was made, however (Tamarkin *et al.,* 1975). In a 1974 review, I graphically illustrated the results of experiments that had been conducted in my laboratory and which showed that neither daily injections of melatonin nor the subcutaneous implantation of melatonin-beeswax pellets had significant effects on the sexual system of hamsters (Reiter, 1974a). The melatonin injections in this case had been made early in the light phase of the light:dark cycle, a point which was later shown to be a critical shortcoming of the experiments.

One year following the previously referred to review, Tamarkin *et al.* (1975) presented a paper at the annual Neuroscience meetings which convincingly demonstrated that daily subcutaneous injection of melatonin into male hamsters could induce total gonadal regression. This revolutionaly finding was attributed to the fact that the single daily injections of melatonin were made during a very restricted portion of the light phase of the light:dark cycle. The degree of atrophy of the reproductive system was equivalent to that which follows the exposure of hamsters to short daily photoperiods. What Tamarkin and colleagues had done was to compare the efficacy of morning versus afternoon injections of melatonin in influencing the status of the gonads. This treatment protocol uncovered a previously unrecognized rhythm in the sensitivity of the neuroendocrine–reproductive axis to melatonin. Only

when given late in the light period were single daily injections of the indoleamine capable of inducing gonadal atrophy. A later study revealed
that in hamsters kept in a light:dark cycle of 14:10 the period during
which the animals are sensitive falls between 6.5 and 13.75 hours after
lights on (Tamarkin *et al.,* 1976). Not only were the gonads regressed
but the anticipated changes in the gonadotrophins were apparent as well.
The effective daily dosages of melatonin in these studies ranged from 10
to 25 $\mu$g.

These findings were readily confirmed and, furthermore, it was shown
that daily single injections of melatonin could inhibit reproduction only
in hamsters in which the pineal gland was intact and sympathetically innervated (Reiter *et al.,* 1976a). Hence, in hamsters that were subjected to
either pinealectomy or superior cervical ganglionectomy prior to the
commencement of the melatonin injections the indole lacked the ability
to inhibit reproduction. This finding implied that the exogenous
melatonin given late in the afternoon was possibly synergizing with endogenously released melatonin (during darkness) to cause gonadal involution. This is supported by the later observation that three daily injections of melatonin into pinelectomized rats can cause the same degree
of gonodal involution as that experienced by intact hamsters treated
with single doses (Tamarkin *et al.,* 1977). Other pineal indoles including
5-methoxytryptophol, *N*-acetylserotonin, and 6-hydroxymelatonin do
not share melatonin's ability to suppress reproductive physiology in the
hamster when given by means of the same treatment protocol (Sackman
*et al.,* 1977).

Some of the antigonadotrophic interactions of acutely administered
melatonin with the reproductive system of the hamster are summarized
in Fig. 2. Under long photoperiodic conditions melatonin administered
at the appropriate time during the light period will inhibit the neuroendocrine–reproductive system. This culminates in alterations in pituitary
and plasma gonadotrophin and prolactin levels, atrophy of the end
organs, cessation of spermatogenesis in males and ovulation in females,
and reduction in steroid production by the gonads. The final result is
that the animals are rendered completely incapable of reproducing. This
is a state the animals normally experience under field conditions in the
fall of the year when they are preparing for hibernation. For melatonin
to induce total gonadal collapse, it must be administered for 6–8 weeks.
This is slightly less than the period of time required for short
photoperiods to induce sexual regression.

Based on the results of the studies summarized in the previous
paragraphs, even the most parsimonious scientist can no longer deny the
endocrine capabilities of melatonin. It could well be an important pineal

Photoperiod                    Treatment protocol              Gonadal status

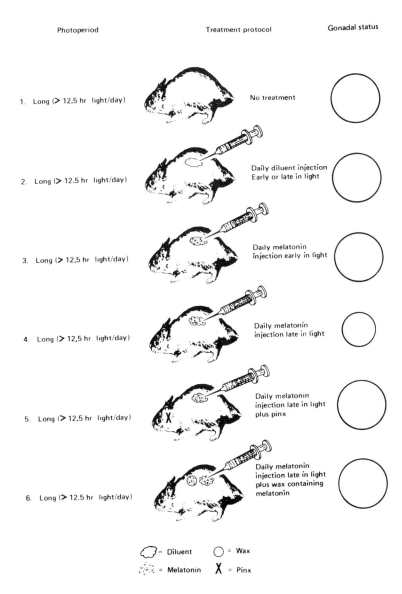

1. Long (> 12.5 hr light/day)                    No treatment

2. Long (> 12.5 hr light/day)          Daily diluent injection
                                       Early or late in light

3. Long (> 12.5 hr light/day)          Daily melatonin
                                       injection early in light

4. Long (> 12.5 hr light/day)          Daily melatonin
                                       injection late in light

5. Long (> 12.5 hr light/day)          Daily melatonin
                                       injection late in light
                                       plus pinx

6. Long (> 12.5 hr light/day)          Daily melatonin
                                       injection late in light
                                       plus wax containing
                                       melatonin

⟨⟩ = Diluent      ◯ = Wax

⋰ = Melatonin     X = Pinx

FIG. 2. Diagrammatic representation of the effects of single daily acute injections of melatonin and of subcutaneous beeswax-melatonin pellets on the gonadal status of intact or pinealectomized (pinx) hamsters maintained in long daily photoperiods. The large circles under "gonadal status" signify sexually mature gonads while small circles indicate anatomically and functionally atrophic reproductive organs.

antigonadotrophic factor in the hamster as well as in other species. This proposition was first put forth about 15 years ago on the basis of very fragmentary data (Wurtman and Axelrod, 1965). Now the findings are unequivocal. This does not mean that melatonin is the exclusive gonad-inhibiting factor of pineal origin. Indeed, in the subsequent sections of the present review a case will be made for similar function by other pineal-derived indoleamines and polypeptides.

    b. *Counter-antigonadotrophic Effects.* Having attempted to convince the reader that melatonin has a documented inhibitory effect on the sexual organs, the present section will review data showing that chronically available (as opposed to acutely administered) melatonin exerts a counter-antigonadotrophic (Reiter *et al.,* 1975a), or progonadal (Turek *et al.,* 1975) influence. Some of these findings actually accumulated prior to the demonstration that acutely injected melatonin possessed potent antigonadotrophic actions.

    In 1974, Hoffmann (1974) and Reiter *et al.* (1974) working independently and on different species observed that short daylengths acting on the pineal gland were unable to cause gonadal regression in hamsters if the animals contained a subcutaneous reservoir of releasable melatonin. Hoffmann (1974) utilized an experimentally rare species of rodent,. the dwarf hamster *(Phodopus sungorus),* in which to illustrate this action of melatonin. Normally, when male dwarf hamsters are placed under restricted photoperiodic conditions the animals experience involution of the sexual organs. However, if melatonin-beeswax pellets were implanted subcutaneously into animals kept in short light cycles, darkness, acting by way of the pineal gland, was incapable of suppressing reproductive physiology. Similar observations were made in the Syrian hamster by myself and colleagues (1974). In this case, adult male animals were placed in a light:dark cycle which provided 1 hour of light per 24-hour period. Subcutaneous deposits of melatonin (in beeswax), like surgical removal of the pineal gland, negated the effect of darkness on reproduction. Indeed, in reference to all sexual parameters that were investigated, chronically available melatonin was as effective as pinealectomy itself in preventing short photoperiods from exerting their inhibitory control over the sexual organs. In essence, the melatonin released from the subcutaneous depot caused a "functional pinealectomy."

    One potential explanation for the counter-antigonadotrophic actions of chronic melatonin administration which was initially considered was that the response was due to a pharmacological dosage of the indoleamine. In the aforementioned studies 1 mg of melatonin was implanted weekly. Assuming the bulk of the melatonin escaped from the beeswax pellet each week, the animals were possibly being exposed to rather substantial quantities of melatonin (about 143 μg/day). In an attempt to allay doubts concerning the massive dose hypothesis, in a subsequent study we changed the experimental paradigm to overcome this criticism (Reiter et al., 1975d). This was achieved in one of two ways, either by decreasing the frequency of pellet implantation or by decreasing the amount of melatonin per beeswax pellet. Hence, light-deprived male hamsters received 1 mg melatonin (in 24 mg beeswax) either once per week, or per 2, 3, 4, 6, and 12 weeks. Regardless of the frequency of pellet implantation, melatonin overcame the inhibitory effect of darkness on reproduction. When beeswax pellets containing either 1 mg, 500, 100, 50, or 1 μg melatonin were placed subcutaneously at 2-week intervals, all but the smallest dosage of melatonin prevented the gonads from regressing. Again, after making the assumption that the melatonin in the subcutaneous depots is totally dissolved from all of the implanted pellets the maximal daily dosage to which the animals were exposed was calculated. Such calculations revealed that as little as 3.6 μg melatonin daily was capable of preventing the antigonadotrophic capabilities of short daily photoperiods. The effectiveness of this rather small dose indicates that the massive dose probably does not explain the counter-antigonadotrophic actions of continuously available melatonin. Rather, an alternative explanation which relates to the reactivity of the receptors to melatonin will be considered later in this article.

When melatonin is administered by another mode, namely, by means of subcutaneously placed melatonin-filled silastic (polydimethylsiloxane) capsules, the responses to the indoleamine are similar to those following the implantation of melatonin-beeswax pellets (Turek et al., 1975). However, the responses to melatonin administered in this manner apparently vary widely. Thus, a dosage of only 50 μg/day (from a 100-mm melatonin-filled silastic capsule) was effective in reversing gonadal atrophy attendant on the exposure of Syrian male hamsters to short days. Conversely, dosages of 14, 26, 73, and 101, μg daily were ineffective. These results are difficult to explain and were not confirmed in later studies in which doses of melatonin (from silastic capsules) over a wide range prevented the gonadal regression which is a normal consequence of the exposure of male hamsters to natural photoperiods during the winter months (Reiter et al., 1978).

The counter-antigonadotrophic actions of subcutaneous reservoirs of melatonin which release the indoleamine continuously are summarized in Figs. 3 and 4. The first of these illustrates this action in hamsters maintained in the laboratory under artificially shortened days while the latter reviews this action in hamsters exposed to the naturally shortened

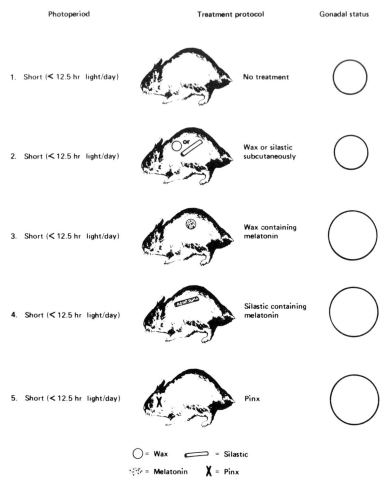

FIG. 3.  Diagrammatic representation of the effects of subcutaneously placed melatonin-beeswax pellets or melatonin-filled silastic capsules on the gonadal status of intact and pinealectomized (pinx) hamsters kept under short daily photoperiods. Large and small circles as in Fig. 2.

photoperiods which occur during the winter months. As noted in the figures and above, the effects of continuously available melatonin duplicate those of pinealectomy.

The ability of melatonin depots to prevent the reproductive inhibitory effects of darkness and the pineal gland are not confined to the hamster. In both blind-anosmic (Reiter *et al.*, 1975a) and in androgen-sterilized blind rats (Banks and Reiter, 1975), two treatment procedures which severely delay maturation of the reproductive systems, the pituitary-

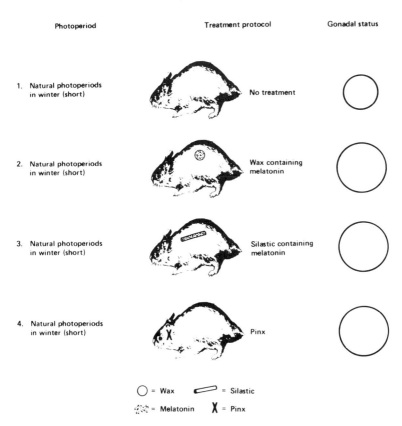

Photoperiod                              Treatment protocol                    Gonadal status

1. Natural photoperiods
   in winter (short)                                                No treatment

2. Natural photoperiods
   in winter (short)                                                Wax containing
                                                                    melatonin

3. Natural photoperiods
   in winter (short)                                                Silastic containing
                                                                    melatonin

4. Natural photoperiods
   in winter (short)                                                Pinx

○ = Wax        ⊏⊐ = Silastic

= Melatonin      X = Pinx

FIG. 4. Diagrammatic representation of the effects of subcutaneously placed melatonin-beeswax pellets or melatonin-filled silastic capsules on the gonadal status of intact and pinealectomized (pinx) hamsters kept under natural photoperiods during the winter months. Large and small circles as in Fig. 2.

gonadal axis flourishes if the animals possess subcutaneous deposits of melatonin.

It seems paradoxical that a single compound could possess both anti- and counter-antigonadotrophic effects. In one case the continual release of melatonin from a depot under the skin prevents the gonad-inhibiting effects of reduced daylengths. On the other hand, if the same daily dosage of melatonin is acutely administered as a bolus injection late in the light period to hamsters kept on long daily photoperiods it completely suppresses reproductive physiology. Hence, it is obvious that the mode and time of administration of melatonin are critical in determining whether the indoleamine acts as an inhibitory or stimulatory factor.

The overall problem is confounded by another perplexing observation concerning the action of melatonin. It has already been mentioned that both dark exposure and daily melatonin injections (late in the light period) induce sexual involution in hamsters. Likewise, it has been shown that pinealectomy prevents the gonad-inhibitory effect of acute daily melatonin injections. The question which obviously arises is whether chronic melatonin pellets would also prevent the inhibitory effects of acute melatonin injections, i.e., would melatonin prevent its own action? This possibility was tested in the following manner. Male hamsters maintained in light:dark cycles of 14:10 received 25 $\mu$g melatonin injections daily 1 hour before lights out. Half of the animals also were provided with a weekly subcutaneous melatonin (in beeswax) pellet. After 50 days of treatment various parameters of reproduction were examined. As anticipated, the regular melatonin injections markedly suppressed gonadal and accessory sex organ weights, spermatogenesis, and pituitary luteinizing hormone and prolactin levels unless the animals had additionally received a subcutaneous melatonin-beeswax pellet each week. This latter group of animals had reproductive organs and hormone levels indistinguishable from the highly functional sexual systems of untreated control hamsters (Reiter *et al.*, 1977) (Fig. 2, group 6). Indeed, chronically available melatonin had prevented the action of acute melatonin injections.

Such findings are difficult to accept. There is very little precedence in the scientific literature for a hormone restricting its own action. Although there are several possible and plausible explanations for this apparently paradoxical finding, the following hypothesis is the one currently receiving the greatest attention. Melatonin's effects presumably depend on interaction with a receptor. After it acts, the compound may render the receptor temporarily insensitive (increased threshold) to additional melatonin, i.e., the receptor may become transiently refractory. This would explain why melatonin injections given early in the light period are ineffective in inducing gonadal regression while identical amounts of the indoleamine given later in the light period possess gonad-inhibiting ability. Early in the light phase the receptors on which the melatonin acts are still in the refractory condition produced by the endogenous melatonin secreted by the pineal gland during the previous dark period. By late in the light phase the refractory state is lost (threshold is decreased). When melatonin is continuously available due to the presence of a subcutaneous pellet the receptors remain in a persistently refractory condition thus prohibiting either endogenously secreted (during periods of light restriction) or exogenously injected melatonin from acting to induce gonadal atrophy. This working hypothesis is amenable to experimentation.

## 2. Other Indoles

As noted earlier in this article, indole metabolism within the pineal gland is well defined. Several of these constituents have been tested for their endocrine capabilities but not nearly to the same extent as melatonin. Serotonin, the parent compound of many of the pineal indoles, is found in very high concentrations within the gland (Quay and Halevy, 1962) and, although it has been proposed as a pineal hormone (Albertazzi *et al.*, 1966), this idea is not currently widely accepted among scientists working in the field. It is difficult to envisage how a substance as widely distributed in the organism as serotonin could be a hormone of the pineal gland. Even though it is in high concentration in the gland the amount released, if indeed it escapes from the pineal, would be negligible in terms of the total amount of serotonin available in the body.

N-Acetylserotonin is a product of serotonin metabolism and the immediate precursor of melatonin (Quay, 1974). Its physiologic effects have been sparingly investigated and the compound has been essentially ignored as a pineal secretory product. When it was used, the results obtained were either inconsequential in terms of a significant effect on reproduction or the findings were contradictory. Although N-acetylserotonin was found to curtail the growth of the remaining ovary 9 days after unilateral ovariectomy in mice (Vaughan *et al.*, 1972), when administered by intraocular injection to immature rats it augmented the ovulatory response induced by the injection of pregnant mare's serum gonadotrophin (PMSG) (Pomerantz and Reiter, 1974). Similar divergent actions have been reported when the compound was injected intraventricularly into adult rats. Under these conditions, N-acetylserotonin either stimulated or inhibited circulating levels of luteinizing hormone (LH) (Kamberi *et al.*, 1970; Porter *et al.*, 1971/72). This discrepancy was presumably not due to technical variations in the experiments since both reports derived from the same laboratory. Unlike melatonin, late afternoon injections of N-acetylserotonin into hamsters have no measurable inhibitory effect on reproduction (Sackman *et al.*, 1977) and, likewise, its chronic administration by means of a subcutaneous pellet (in beeswax) does not counteract the antigonadotrophic effect of the pineal gland (Reiter and Vaughan, 1975). Although the proper experiment may not have been performed, the findings reported to date are generally consistent with the notion that the precursor of melatonin, N-acetylserotonin, is insignificant in terms of the endocrine capabilities of the pineal gland.

An early study with 5-hydroxytryptophol indicated that it was incapable of suppressing either the growth of the ovaries or the estrous cycles of rats (McIsaac *et al.*, 1964). However, a subsequent report claimed that it inhibited ovulation in young rats treated with PMSG (Pomerantz and Reiter, 1974). In mice, the indole reportedly restricted the growth of the remaining ovary after unilateral ovariectomy (Vaughan *et al.*, 1972). According to Fraschini *et al.* (1971), 5-hydroxytryptophol, like melatonin, curtails the synthesis of LH in the anterior pituitary gland when the indole is implanted into the brain. This observation has yet to be confirmed in another laboratory. The small amount of data available precludes an unequivocal judgment concerning the endocrine role of 5-hydroxytryptophol.

Although 5-methoxytryptophol was isolated from the pineal gland rather early (McIsaac *et al.*, 1965), interest in the reproductive consequences of this methoxyindole has never been very great. In 1964, it was reported to be at least as effective as melatonin in altering estrous cyclicity in rats (McIsaac *et al.*, 1974). According to Hipkin (1970) 5-methoxytryptophol also exhibits greater activity than melatonin in restricting the growth of uteri in mice treated exogenously with human chorionic gonadotrophin (HCG). Also in mice, the methoxyindole inhibits compensatory ovarian hypertrophy when it is given at the time of unilateral ovariectomy (Vaughan *et al.*, 1972).

One recent discovery may well stimulate interest in 5-methoxytryptophol as a hormonal constituent of the pineal gland. Using a highly specific gas chromatography–mass spectrometric method, Wilson *et al.* (1978) not only identified the methoxyindole in the peripheral circulation of the rat but also found a strong correlation between serum and pineal levels of this constituent. The pineal concentrations of 5-methoxytryptophol were found to be greater than those of melatonin and to exhibit a pronounced change over a 24-hour period. Highest concentrations were found during periods of darkness. In the sera, 5-methoxytryptophol exhibited a bimodal rhythm with elevated levels being detected at mid-light and mid-darkness. In view of these findings, 5-methoxytryptophol may well be considered a putative pineal hormone although physiologic evidence supporting this notion remains sparce.

## 3. Secretion of Indoleamines

For a substance to be classified as a hormone it must escape from the cell in which it is produced, travel to a distant site, and exert an action. From the data presented above it is apparent that melatonin (Rollag and Niswender, 1976), and possibly 5-methoxytryptophol (Wilson *et al.*, 1978), are discharged from the pineal gland into the systemic circulation. Classically, the peripheral circulation is considered to be the means whereby hormones are shunted throughout the body. However, if pineal constituents have their primary site of action within the brain then another potential route of transfer becomes apparent, namely, by way of the cerebrospinal fluid (CSF). The proximity of the pineal gland to the third ventricle in many vertebrate species has always made this idea enticing (Reiter *et al.*, 1975b). In the hamster where the pineal gland has migrated, during embryologic development, to a more superficial position there are modifications of the ventricular system which keep the pineal in close contact with the ventricular CSF (Sheridan *et al.*, 1969; Gregorek *et al.*, 1977).

With the advent of sensitive radioimmunoassays, melatonin has been routinely identified in the blood of submammals and mammals (Matthews *et al.*, 1976), however, it should be noted that melatonin in bodily fluids may not be entirely derived from the pineal gland (Kennaway *et al.*, 1977). In the blood, melatonin levels are higher at night than during the day (Pang and Ralph, 1975; Rollag and Niswender, 1976). The diurnal melatonin rhythms in the blood are paralleled by a similar pattern of urinary excretion (Lynch *et al.*, 1975).

The most thorough study concerned with the possible secretion of melatonin directly into the CSF is that of Hedlund *et al.* (1977). Plasma and ventricular CSF (collected via indwelling cannulae) concentrations of melatonin were estimated, by radioimmunoassay, in calves at various times of the day and night. In both fluids immunoreactive melatonin values were obviously higher during the period of darkness than during daylight hours. The rhythm in the CSF was more pronounced than in the plasma. One implication of these findings is that melatonin is normally released either directly or indirectly into the CSF. However, this assumption has yet to be proven. Rollag *et al.* (1978) also measured CSF and plasma levels of melatonin in sheep. They then calculated the rates of melatonin secretion into the two compartments. From this study they estimated that the quantity of melatonin discharged into the blood is more than $100\times$ that released into the CSF. Because of this, it is their opinion that the blood is the normal route of release of pineal melatonin. These observations require documentation in other species. Figure 5 summarizes possible routes of secretion and sites of action of pineal hormonal envoys.

There are obvious advantages to the release of melatonin, or other indoleamines, into the CSF. These include the fact that (*a*) release via this route would circumvent the problem of the rapid deactivation of these substances by the liver and other organs, and (*b*), the dilution factor would be much less in the CSF than in the blood and, as a result, smaller amounts would be required for secretion.

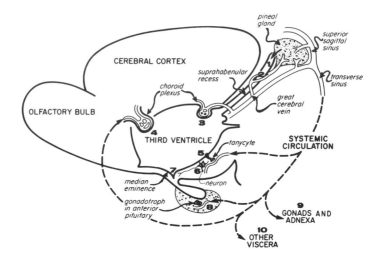

FIG. 5. Schematic representation of the possible routes of secretion of pineal hormones (1–5) and potential sites of action of pineal substances (6–10). Potential routes of secretion of pineal hormones include (1), release directly into the third ventricle; (2), release into pineal capillaries and secondarily into the ventricular system via a capillary plexus in the posterodorsal aspect of the third ventricle; (3), release into the sinuses surrounding the pineal followed by secretion through the choroid plexus in the posterodorsal area of the third ventricle (Quay, 1974); (4), release into the third ventricle after their systemic circulation; and (5), secretion into capillary beds in the pineal and eventual transferral to the third ventricle via the tanycytes lining the ventricular system. Possible sites of action of pineal hormones include (6), neurons or glia of the central nervous system; (7), hypothalamic-releasing hormone cells of the medial basal hypothalamus; (8), cells of the anterior pituitary gland; (9), the gonads; and (10), various visceral organs, e.g., the liver. From Reiter et al. (1975b).

## B. Polypeptides and Proteins

The discovery of potential peptidic hormones from the pineal gland preceded that of the indoleamines; however, research concerned with the specific identification of these factors has proceeded slowly with the exception of arginine vasotocin which is discussed in Section III, B, 1. On the other hand, scientists are now on the verge of characterizing pineal polypeptide hormones which appear to exert a marked controlling influence on reproductive physiology (Ebels, 1976; Benson, 1977). Although the bulk of these factors are antigonadotrophic when administered to experimental animals, some may also stimulate gonadal functions. The claim has been made that, on a weight basis, the polypeptides may be many times more potent than the indoleamines in suppressing reproduction (Benson et al., 1972).

The indoleamine-polypeptide controversy will not soon be resolved. An important fact to remember is that the two "schools" are not mutually exclusive. It is quite reasonable to assume that the pineal may secrete both categories of hormones. Indeed, considering the large number of endocrine functions governed by the pineal it seems unrealistic to imagine that the organ secretes only one active factor.

## 1. Arginine Vasotocin

Not until after it was biochemically synthesized was arginine vasotocin (AVT) actually discovered in nature. Milcu *et al.* (1963) extracted a polypeptide from bovine pineal tissue which has pressor and oxytocic activity and was biologically and chromatographically similar to AVT. AVT was definitively identified in the pineal in 1970 by Cheeman (1970) who utilized amino acid analysis and mass spectrometry. Confirmation of AVT in pineal tissue came from radioimmunoassay studies in 1974 (Rosenbloom and Fisher, 1974). There is some disagreement as to the actual localization of AVT within the epiphysis. Benson *et al.* (1976a) contend that the AVT which is present is confined to the stalk region (possibly to the ependymal cells of the pineal recess) of the bovine pineal while immunocytochemical evidence indicates its presence throughout the rat pineal gland (Bowie and Herbert, 1976). The simplest explanation for these apparently disparate reports would be species differences. Possibly further investigation will uncover other factors which contributed to the variability.

Although there are numerous reports concerned with indoleamine-reproductive interactions, studies that used AVT are much less frequent. This may be related to the greater commercial availability of melatonin and the other indoles. The treatment of prepuberal mice with 10 mU AVT for 2 weeks caused a highly significant reduction in the weights of the seminal vesicles and prostates without influencing the growth of the testes (Pavel, 1969). Likewise, daily injections over a shorter interval (3 days) into immature hamsters retarded the development of the accessory sex glands but spared the gonads (Vaughan *et al.,* 1974). Using several doses of AVT which they synthesized in their own laboratory, Benson *et al.* (1976b) were unable to confirm the inhibitory effect of the peptide in 7- and 10-week-old male mice. A number of studies have shown that laboratory rodents are most sensitive to the pineal polypeptides at or just prior to puberty and, hence, Benson and colleagues may have merely missed the sensitive period because the animals were too old. However, another explanation for the variable results can be suggested. As with melatonin, in order for AVT (or other peptides) to be antigonadotrophic it may have to be administered at a specific time each day, a factor the experimentalists working in this area have overlooked to date.

Possibly one of the most significant effects of AVT may be its ability to interfere with pregnancy in mice. When timed pregnant mice were injected with AVT (2 $\mu$g daily) the nonapeptide delayed parturition and resulted in a majority of stillborn pups (Vaughan *et al.*, 1976b). The mechanism involved in this outcome has not been investigated. Although the deliveries were not premature, the authors proposed that since AVT has significant oxytocic activity it may have initiated labor and delivery of the pups at a time which was not conducive to their survival. As an alternate explanation, the volume and flow of the amniotic fluid may have been affected as a result of the antidiuretic activity of AVT resulting in the death of the pups (Vaughan and Blask, 1978). These findings are sufficiently noteworthy to warrant further investigation. If AVT were shown to possess abortive properties when administered very early in pregnancy it could possibly have utility as an abortifacient.

The growth of the reproductive organs that is induced by exogenously administered hormones is also attenuated by concurrent treatment of the animals with AVT. In mice, ovarian and uterine growth which results from the injection of PMSG, a substance with primarily FSH-like activity, is less if the animals also receive AVT (Pavel and Petrescu, 1966). Ovulation which follows the treatment of immature rats with PMSG is also reduced by AVT although the associated surges in LH and FSH, rather than being reduced, are somewhat exaggerated (Johnson *et al.*, 1978). .The latter results contrast somewhat with the observation that spontaneous ovulations in adult rats are also inhibited by AVT but, in this case, the normal hormonal surges are suppressed (Cheesman *et al.*, 1977; Osland *et al.*, 1977. The finding of Johnson and colleagues (1978) in immature animals is consistent with the idea that AVT restricts the action of gonadotrophins at the ovarian level while the results of Cheesman *et al.* (1977) imply that the nonapeptide impedes the functioning of the hypothalamo-pituitary unit. The major difference between the two experiments was the age of the animals and although the end result was the same (inhibition of ovulation) the mechanisms were clearly different.

As with melatonin, the complexity and variability of the gonadotrophin responses to AVT is remarkable. It is thus imperative that investigators working in the field closely define the precise methods employed to check for the actions of AVT. As an example of the variable changes, results of work conducted in my own laboratory are cited. In 1975, we (Vaughan et al., 1975) reported that the addition of 5 μg AVT to culture media containing male rat pituitaries caused a 4- to 6-fold stimulation of LH released into the culture fluid. In similar in vitro experiments, AVT potentiated the stimulatory action of luteinizing hormone-releasing hormone (LH-RH) on LH released from cultured pituitary glands collected from castrated female rats primed with estrogen and progesterone (Vaughan et al., 1976c). More recently, Blask et al. (1978) tested the influence of AVT on the estrogen-induced surge of LH and FSH in adult ovariectomized rats. In this case, multiple 1 μg doses of AVT completely prevented the LH surge while failing to alter the pattern of FSH. An important factor which comes into play when comparing in vitro with in vivo experiments is the hormonal milieu to which the pituitary glands are exposed. The in vivo pituitary is under the influence of a gamut of hormones which may alter its response to AVT or, for that matter, any pineal envoy.

In addition to its effects on LH and FSH, AVT also influences prolactin secretion. Many of the studies of this issue were stimulated by the extraction of a nonmelatonin-related factor from bovine, human, and rat pineal glands which possessed prolactin-releasing activity (Blask et al., 1976). Whether this activity is specifically related to the presence of AVT in the extracts is unknown. However, there is no longer any doubt that AVT can cause the release of prolactin from the anterior pituitaty gland; in effect, it acts as a prolactin-releasing factor (Vaughan and Blask, 1978). In vitro, any dosage of AVT ranging from 100 ng to 10 μg promotes the release of prolactin from pituitaries bathed in culture medium (Vaughan et al., 1975). Likewise, the intravenous injection of the peptide into male rats primed with estrogen and progesterone is followed by a dose-related rise in plasma prolactin within 10 minutes (Vaughan et al., 1976a). The action of AVT on prolactin release may vary with the anesthesia employed to sedate the animals (L. Y. Johnson, M. K. Vaughan, and R. J. Reiter, unpublished observations). Thus the effects of AVT on prolactin are not unlike those on LH and FSH in that they vary with the experimental design.

At this time it is difficult to categorize AVT as a pineal antigonadotrophic factor. It has never been utilized over long periods of time to induce gonadal involution. The nonapeptide has been shown to both promote and inhibit the release of reproductively active hormones from the pituitary. Even its presence within the pineal gland has been questioned. Yet, Pavel (1978) is adamant about the physiological importance of AVT released from the pineal. The complex interactions of AVT with the neuroendocrine-reproductive axis have been the subject of two recent reviews (Pavel, 1978; Vaughan and Blask, 1978).

## 2. Other Pineal Peptides and Proteins

Benson (1977) and Ebels and Benson (1978) are convinced that the antigonadotrophic capabilities of the pineal gland cannot be attributed solely to melatonin or to other indoleamines. Furthermore, they doubt whether AVT is an important pineal factor. Rather, they feel that yet unidentified substances may at least be partially responsible for the ability of the pineal to restrain the growth and function of the reproductive organs. This factor (or group of factors) was initially referred to as PAG (pineal antigonadotrophin) (Benson et al., 1972). A partially purified melatonin-free extract from bovine pineals was found to be signigicantly more potent than melatonin in restricting compensatory ovarian hypertrophy after unilateral ovariectomy in mice. The bovine PAG is inactivated by treatment with trypsin or chymotrypsin (Matthews and Benson, 1973). Partially purified preparations of PAG have been characterized and it is now felt that it is a polypeptide or contains a peptidic moiety which is essential for its biological activity (Rosenblum et al., 1979). At this time sufficient quantities of the compound are not available to test for the effects of its chronic administration.

Two antigonadotrophic fractions, designated A1 and A3, have been isolated from bovine pineal extract by Bensinger et al. (1973). All tests indicate that these substances are peptidic in nature. Both factors have been shown to inhibit compensatory ovarian hypertrophy in laboratory mice. Furthermore, the A3 fraction at a dose of 100 mg Eq (mg pineal tissue equivalents) restrains the growth of the ventral prostate and testes of immature wild house mice (Vaughan et al., 1974). In vitro, both A1 and A3 promote the release of prolactin from the anterior pituitary gland (Blask et al., 1976). Thus, the effects of these compounds are not unlike those of another pineal polypeptide, AVT.

The urine of rats (Ota et al., 1970) and humans (Ota et al., 1968) contains a factor, gonadotrophin-inhibiting substance (GIS), which is believed to be derived from the pineal gland (Ota et al., 1971) and which, when injected into immature mice, significantly inhibits PMSG + HCG (human chorionic gonadotropin)-induced ovulation. The authors argue that GIS is a rather specific inhibitor of LH. The same group of workers (Ota et al., 1975) have isolated fractions with antigonadotrophic properties from bovine pineal tissue using extraction procedures very similar to those used to isolate GIS from urine. The factor(s) is distinct from melatonin and AVT and probably also differs from other water-soluble antigonadotrophic substances isolated from bovine and ovine pineal glands. Whether the pineal factor is identical to the one recovered from the urine is unknown.

Most recently, Orts et al. (1978) identified the structure of a pineal tripeptide (containing the amino acids threonine, serine, and lysine) which possesses the ability to inhibit compensatory hypertrophy of the remaining ovary in mice. In contrast to the compound recovered from the urine by Ota and colleagues (1970), the tripeptide is believed to specifically inhibit FSH.

## 3. Secretion of Polypeptides

Pavel (1978) is convinced that AVT is released either directly or indirectly into the CSF and only secondarily gains access to the systemic circulation. This idea originated in 1970 when he (Pavel, 1970) tentatively identified AVT in human CSF obtained by means of suboccipital puncture. Pavel (1973) also feels strongly that melatonin is the releasing factor for pineal AVT. This postulate has attracted our attention (Reiter et al., 1976b) since another group of amines, the monoamines, apparently serve to release an important category of polypeptides from the medial basal hypothalamus, namely, the hypothalamic-releasing hormones. Quay (1974) has also provisionally suggested that pineal indoleamines may function as intermediaries in the pineal gland to facilitate the release of factors such as AVT. Pavel (1978) has recently shown that the discharge of AVT from the pineal gland exhibits a diurnal sensitivity to melatonin. Thus, at so-called physiological concentrations (10 ng) melatonin was ineffective in releasing AVT during the day, however, during darkness the same dose of melatonin readily induced the release of the nonapeptide. This is the suggested reason why the concentration of AVT drops in the rat pineal gland at night (Calb et al., 1977). The same authors believe that they have another justification for the claim that AVT is normally secreted into the CSF. When 0.5 $\mu$U of synthetic AVT was administered into the third ventricle of mice it completely inhibited compensatory ovarian hypertrophy in the animals. The same dose injected either intravenously or intraperitoneally was ineffective in suppressing the induced ovarian growth. Only when the dose of AVT reached 25 (intravenously) or 50 (intraperitoneally) $\mu$U did it curtail enlargement of the remaining ovary. From these data Pavel et al. (1973) concluded that AVT is released into the CSF and that it acts centrally to control the neuroendocrine–reproductive axis.

The actual mechanisms of secretion of pineal polypeptides have not

been elucidated although one interesting theory has been presented
(Lukaszyk and Reiter, 1975). The theory relies heavily on what is known
about the posterior pituitary, another diencephalic outgrowth, which
secretes the hormones oxytocin and vasopressin that are structurally very
similar to AVT. Judging from what is known about the intracellular
transport and discharge of posterior pituitary hormones it seems likely
that the pineal polypeptides, be they AVT or as yet unidentified peptidic
factors, exist in the pineal cell in conjunction with carrier proteins. Both
Krass et al. (1971) and Reinharz et al. (1974) have extracted and purified
tissue proteins from bovine pineal which share biochemical and im-
munological properties with the neurophysins (the carrier proteins of oxytocin and vasopressin). As Lukaszyk and Reiter (1975) envision it, the
pineal polypeptide hormones exist in the pineal secretory cells in conjunction with a carrier protein provisionally referred to as a neuroepiphysin. The polypeptide-neuroepiphysin complex is believed to
be released from the intracellular compartment to the extracellular space
by an exocytotic process. Calcium, by a process very similar to that in
the posterior pituitary, is then exchanged for the polypeptide hormone
with the resultant secretion of the latter into the vascular system. The
calcium in the extracellular space then forms a complex with the carrier
protein which is deposited on cellular debris. The debris is believed to be
produced at the time of the exocytotic release of the polypeptide-
neuroepiphysin complex. The entire process, in addition to explain-
ing the discharge of polypeptides from the pineal gland, also accounts
for the formation of corpora arenacea (calcium deposits) which exist in
the pineal of some species. This theory is graphically depicted in Fig. 6.
Interestingly, procedures which prevent the synthesis and secretion of
active pineal factors also prevent the deposition of calcium within the
pineal gland (Reiter et al., 1976c). These theoretical mechanisms provide
a working basis for the studies on the release of pineal peptidic hormones.

## IV. Concluding Remarks

To recapitulate, it is obvious that the photoperiod is the single most
important factor in the control of the endocrine activity of the pineal
gland of mammals. Information about the photoperiod is transferred
from the eyes to the epithalamus over a complex and circuitous network
of neurons. Within the gland the neural information is transduced into a
humoral output. The exact nature of all of the hormonal products as
well as the mode of secretion of these envoys are under debate at this
time. In the previous discussion an attempt was made to objectively ap-

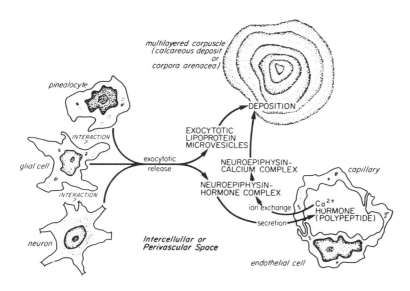

FIG. 6. Theoretical scheme for the secretion of polypeptides from and the formation of corpora arenacea (multilayered corpuscles) in the pineal gland. The cell of origin (pinealocyte, glia, or neuron) of the pineal polypeptides remains unknown. From Lukaszyk and Reiter (1975).

praise the published data, albeit in a rather concise manner. The allotment of verbiage to the various putative hormones should not be taken as an index of the presumed importance of these factors. Rather, it is merely an indication of the relative amounts of experimental data available for consideration.

The essence of pineal research, of course, is to identify the niche of this gland in the normal economy of the animal. Thus, the logical question that can be asked is, what advantage does the pineal gland afford? The strategy of the pineal seems to be the control of the annual cycle of reproduction in some mammals (Reiter, 1974b, 1978b). Most species which inhabit the temperate and polar regions of the earth are seasonal breeders in their natural habitat. The variable that keeps their reproductive behavior in synchrony with the environment is the length of the photoperiod. Although it is continually changing from day to day it does so in a very reproducible manner from year to year. Over eons of time animals have evolved an organ, the pineal gland, to take advantage of this information. Hence, the photoperiod acting by way of the pineal dictates the exact timing of sexual activity and, more importantly, delivery of the young which most often coincides with the spring of the year. This increases the chances of survival of the young and ensures perpetuation of the species. In the absence of a pineal gland animals (at least hamsters) breed continually irrespective of season and the young are often born during the winter months (Reiter, 1973/74). Because of the harsh environment and possibly the scarcity of food, many of the animals born under these conditions die shortly after birth. Losses such as this are more than any species can tolerate. A prolonged lack of synchronization between the time of delivery and the appropriate season for this event, i.e., the spring, could result in the disappearance of a species. Thus, whereas the pineal may not be essential for survival of the individual animal it is vital to the survival of the species.

## References

Albertazzi, E., Barbanti-Silva, C., Trentini, G.P., and Bottcelli, A. (1966). Influence de l'epiphysectomie et du treatment avec la 5-hydroxytryptamine sur le cycle oestral de la Ratte albinos. *Annales d'Endocrinologie* 27, 93-100.

Axelrod, J. (1974). The pineal gland: A neurochemical transducer. *Science* 184, 1341-1348.

Axelrod, J., and Weissbach, H. (1960). Enzymatic O-methylation of N-acetylserotonin to melatonin. *Science* 62, 554–559.

Banks, A. F., and Reiter, R. J. (1975)). Melatonin inhibition of pineal antigonadotrophic activity in male rats. *Hormone Research* 6, 351–356.

Bensinger, R., Vaughan, M. K., and Klein, D. C. (1973). Isolation of non-melatonin lipophylic antigonadotrophic factor from the bovine pineal gland. *Federation Proceedings* 32, 252.

Benson, B. (1977). Current status of pineal polypeptides. *Neuroendocrinology* 24, 241–258.

Benson, B., Matthews, M. J., and Rodin, A. E. (1972). Studies on a non-melatonin pineal antigonadotrophin. *Acta Endocrinologica* 69, 257–266.

Benson, B., Matthews, M. J., Hadley, M. E., Powers, S., and Hruby, V. J. (1976a). Differential localization of antigonadotrophic and vasotocin activities in bovine and rat pineal. *Life Sciences* 19, 747–754.

Benson, B., Matthews, M. J., and Hruby, V. J. (1976b). Characterization and effects of a bovine pineal antigonadotrophic peptide. *American Zoologist* 16, 17–24.

Blask, D. E., Vaughan, M. K., Reiter, R. J., Johnson, L. Y., and Vaughan G. M. (1976). Prolactin-releasing and release-inhibiting factor activities in the bovine, rat and human pineal gland: *In vitro* and *in vivo* studies. *Endocrinology* 99, 152–162.

Blask, D. E., Vaughan, M. K., Reiter, R. J., and Johnson, L. Y. (1978). Influence of arginine vasotocin on the estrogen-induced surge of LH and FSH in adult ovariectomized rats. *Life Sciences* 23, 1035-1040.

Bowie, E. P., and Herbert, D. C. (1976). Immunocytochemical evidence for the presence of arginine vasotocin in the rat pineal gland. *Nature (London)* 261, 5555.

Calb, M., Goldstein, R., and Pavel, S. (1977). Diurnal rhythm of vasotocin in the pineal gland. *Acta Endocrinologica* 84, 523–526.

Cheesman, D. W. (1970). Structural elucidation of a gonadotropin-inhibiting substance from the bovine pineal gland. *Biochemica et Biophysica Acta* 207, 247–253.

Cheesman, D. W., Osland, R. B., and Forsham, P. H. (1977). Suppression of the preovulatory surge of luteinizing hormone and subsequent ovulation in the rat by arginine vasotocin. *Endocrinology* **101**, 1194-1202.

Ebels, I. (1976). Isolation of avian and mammalian pineal indoles and anti-gonadotrophic factors. *American Zoologist* **16**, 5-15.

Ebels, I., and Benson, B. (1978). A survey of the evidence that unidentified pineal substances affect the reproductive system in mammals. In "The Pineal and Reproduction" (R. J. Reiter, ed.), pp. 51-89. Karger, Basal.

Elliott, J. (1976). Circadian rhythms and photoperiodic time measurements in mammals. *Federation Proceedings* **35**, 2339-2346.

Fraschini, F., Collu, R., and Martini, L. (1971). Mechanisms of inhibitory action of pineal principles on gonadotrophin secretion. In "The Pineal Gland"(G. E. W. Wolstenholme and J. Knight, eds.), pp. 259-278. Churchill Livingstone, London.

Gregorek, J. C., Seibel, H. R., and Reiter, R. J. (1977). The pineal complex and its relationship to other epithalamic structures. *Acta Anatomica* **99**, 425-434.

Hedlund, L., Lischki, M. M., Rollag, M. D., and Niswender, G. D. (1977). Melatonin: Daily cycle in plasma and cerebrospinal fluid of calves. *Science* **195**, 686-687.

Hendrickson, A. E., Wagoner, N., and Cowan, W. M. (1972). An autoradiographic and electron microscopic study of retino-hypothalamic connections. *Zeitschrift für Zellforschung und Mikroskopic Anatomie* **135**, 1-26.

Hipkin, L. J. (1970). Effect of 5-methoxytryptophol and melatonin on uterine weight responses to human chorionic gonadotrophin. *Journal of Endocrinology* **48**, 287-288.

Hoffmann, K. (1974). Testicular involution in short photoperiods inhibited by melatonin. *Naturwissenschaften* **61**, 364-365.

Johnson, L. Y., Vaughan, M. K., Reiter, R. J., Blask, D. E., and Rudeen, P. K. (1978). The effects of arginine vasotocin on pregnant mare's serum-induced ovulation in the immature female rat. *Acta Endocrinologica* **87**, 367-376.

Kamberi, I., Mical, R. S., and Porter, J. C. (1970). Effect of anterior pituitary perfusion and intraventricular injection of catecholamines and indoleamines on LH release. *Endocrinology* **87**, 1-12.

Kappers, J. A. (1960). The development, topographical relations and innervation of the epiphysis cerebri in the albino rat. *Zetschrift Für Zellforschung und Mikroskopic Anatomie* **52**, 163-215.

Kappers, J. A. (1965). Survey of the innervation of the epiphysis cerebri and the accessory pineal organ of vertebrates. In "Structure and Function of the Epiphysis Cerebri" (J. A. Kappers and J. P. Schade, eds.), pp. 87-153. Elsevier, Amsterdam.

Kennaway, D. J., Frith, R. G., Phillipou, G., Matthews, C. D., and Seamark, R. F. (1977). A specific radioimmunoassay for melatonin in biological tissue and fluid and its validation by gas chromatography-mass spectrometry. *Endocrinology* **101**, 119-129.

Kenny, G. C. J. (1961). The "nervus conarii" of the monkey. *Journal of Neuropathology and Experimental Neurology* **20**, 563-570.

Klein, D. C. (1974). Circadian rhythms in indole metabolism in the rat pineal gland. In "The Neurosciences Third Study Programme"(F. O. Schmidt, ed.), pp. 509-515. MIT Press, Cambridge.

Klein, D. C., and Weller, J. L. (1970). Indole metabolism in the pineal gland: A circadian rhythm in *N*-acetyltransferase. *Science* **169**, 1093-1095.

Krass, M. E., LaBella, F. S. Shin, S. H., and Minnich, J. (1971). Biochemical features of the pineal compared with other endocrine and nervous structures. In "Subcellular Organization and Function in Endocrine Tissues" (H. Heller and K. Lederis, eds.), pp. 49-76. Cambridge Univ. Press, Cambridge.

Lovenberg, W., Weissbach, H., and Udenfrined, S. (1962). Aromatic L-amino acid decarboxylase. *Journal of Biological Chemistry* **237**, 89-92.

Lovenberg, W., Jequier, E., and Sjoerdsma, A. (1967). Tryptophan hydroxylation: Measurements in pineal gland, brain stem, and carcinoid tumor. *Science* **155**, 217–218.

Lukaszyk, A., and Reiter, R. J. (1975). Histophysiological evidence for the secretion of polypeptides by the pineal gland. *American Journal of Anatomy* **143**, 451–464.

Lynch, H. J., and Ralph, C. L. (1970). Diurnal variation in pineal melatonin and its non-relationship to HIOMT activity. *American Zoologist* **10**, 300.

Lynch, H. J., Ozaki, Y., Shakal, D., and Wurtman, R. J. (1975). Melatonin excretion of man and rats: Effect of time of day, sleep, pinealectomy and food consumption. *International Journal of Biometeorology* **19**, 267–279.

McIsaac, W. M., Taborsky, R. G., and Farrell, G. (1964). 5-Methoxytryptophol: Effect on estrus and ovarian weight. *Science* **145**, 63–64.

McIsaac, W. M., Farrell, G., Taborsky, R. G., and Taylor, A. N. (1965). Indole compounds: Isolation from pineal tissue. *Science* **148**, 102–103.

Matsushima, S., and Reiter, R. J. (1977). Fine structural features of adrenergic nerve fibers and endings in the pineal gland of the rat, ground squirrel and chinchilla. *American Journal of Anatomy* **148**, 463–478.

Matsushima, S., and Reiter, R. J. (1978). Electron microscopic observations on neuron like cells in the ground squirrel pineal gland. *Journal of Neural Transmission* **42**, 223–237.

Matthews, C. D., Kennaway, D. J., Frith, R. G., Phillipou, G., LeCornu, A., and Seamark, R. F. (1976). Plasma melatonin values in man and some domestic animals: Initial observation on the effects of pregnancy in man and pinealectomy in sheep. *Journal of Endocrinology* **73**, 41P–42P.

Matthews, M. J., and Benson, B. (1973). Inactivation of pineal antigonadotropin by proteolytic enzymes. *Journal of Endocrinology* **56**, 339–340.

Milcu, S. M., Pavel, S., and Neascu, C. (1963). Biological and chromatographic evidence of a polypeptide with pressor and oxytocic activities isolated from bovine pineal gland. *Endocrinology* **72**, 563–566.

Moore, R. Y. (1973). Retinohypothalamic projection in mammals: A comparative study. *Brain Research* **49**, 403–409.

Moore, R. Y. (1978). Central neural control of circadian rhythms. *In* "Frontiers in Neuroendocrinology" (W. F. Ganong and L. Martini, eds.), Vol. 5, pp. 185–206. Raven, New York.

Moore, R. Y., and Lenn, N. J. (1972). A retinohypothalamic projection in the rat. *Journal of Comparative Neurology* **146**, 1–14.

Moore, R. Y., Heller, A., Bhatnager, R. K., Wurtman, R. J., and Axelrod, J. Central control of the pineal gland: Visual pathways. (1968). *Archives of Neurology* **18**, 208–218.

Nir, I., Reiter, R. J., and Wurtman, R. J. (eds.). (1978) The pineal gland. *Journal of Neural Transmission,* Supplement 13.

Nishino, H., Koizumi, K., and Brooks, C. McC. (1976). The role of suprachiasmatic nuclei of the hypothalamus in the production of circadian rhythm. *Brain Research* **112**, 45–59.

Orts, R. J., Liao, T.-H., Sartin, J. L., and Bruet, B. (1978). Purification of a tripeptide with anti-reproductive properties isolated from bovine pineal gland. *The Physiologist* **21**, 87.

Osland, R. B., Cheesman, D. W., and Forsham, P. H. (1977). Studies on the mechanism of the suppression of the preovulatory surge of luteinizing hormone in the rat by arginine vasotocin. *Endocrinology* **101**, 1203–1209.

Ota, M., Dronkert, A., and Gates, A. H. (1968). The presence of a gonadotrophin-inhibiting substance in human urine. *Fertility and Sterility* **19**, 100–109.

Ota, M., Hsieh, K. S., and Obara, K. (1970). Presence of a gonadotropin-inhibiting substance in the urine of albino rats. *Endocrinology Japonica* **17**, 333–337.

Ota, M., Hsieh, K. S., and Obara, K. (1971). Absence of gonadotrophin-inhibiting substance in the urine of pinealectomied rats. *Endocrinology* **88**, 816–820.

Ota, M., Horiuchi, S., and Obara, K. (1975). Inhibition of ovulation induced with PMS and HCG by a melatonin-free extract of bovine pineal powder. *Neuroendocrinology* **18**, 311–321.

Ozaki, Y., and Lynch, H. J. (1976). Presence of melatonin in plasma and urine of pinealectomized rats. *Endocrinology* **99**, 641–644.

Pang, S. F., and Ralph, C. L. (1975). Pineal and serum melatonin at midday and midnight following pinealectomy or castration in male rats. *Journal of Experimental Zoology* **193**, 275–280.

Pavel, S. (1969). Effects of pineal and synthetic arginine vasotocin on the gonads of prepuberal male mice. *Fifth Conference of European Comparative Endocrinologists*, Utrecht, Abstract 129.

Pavel, S. (1970). Tentative identification of arginine vasotocin in human cerebrospinal fluid. *Journal of Clinical Endocrinology* **31**, 369–371.

Pavel, S. (1973). Arginine vasotocin release into cerebrospinal fluid of cats induced by melatonin. *Nature (London)* **246**, 183–184.

Pavel, S. (1978). Arginine vasotocin as a pineal hormone. *Journal of Neural Transmission, Supplement* **13**, 135–155.

Pavel, S., and Petrescu, S. (1966). Inhibition of gonadotrophin by a highly purified pineal peptide and by synthetic arginine vasotocin. *Nature (London)* **212**, 1054.

Pavel, S., Petrescu, M., and Vicoleanu, N. (1973). Evidence of central gonadotropin inhibiting activity of arginine vasotocin in the female mouse. *Neuroendocrinology* **11**, 370–374.

Pomerantz G, and Reiter, R. J. (1974). Influence of intraocularly-injected pineal indoles on PMS-induced ovulation in immature rats. *International Journal of Fertility* **19**, 117–120.

Porter, J. C., Mical, R. S., and Cramer, O. M. (1971/72). Effect of serotonin and other indoles on the release of LH, FSH, and prolactin. *Gynecologic Investigation* **2**, 13–21.

Quay, W. B. (1974). "Pineal Chemistry in Cellular and Physiological Mechanisms." Thomas, Springfield, Ill.

Quay, W. B. and Halevy, A. (1962). Experimental modification of the rat pineal's content of serotonin and related indole amines. *Physiological Zoology* **35**, 1–7.

Reinharz, A. C., Czernichow, P., and Vallotton, M. B. (1974). Neurophysin-like protein in bovine pineal gland. *Journal of Endocrinology* **62**, 35–44.

Reiter, R. J. (1972). Surgical procedures involving the pineal gland which prevent gonadal degeneration in adult male hamsters. *Annales d'Endocrinologie* **33**, 571–581.

Reiter, R. J. (1973). Comparative physiology: Pineal gland. *Annual Reviews of Physiology* **35**, 305–328.

Reiter, R. J. (1973/74). Influence of pinealectomy on the breeding capability of hamsters maintained under natural photoperiodic and temperature conditions. *Neuroendocrinology* **13**, 366–370.

Reiter, R. J. (1974a). Pineal regulation of the hypothalamo-pituitary axis: Gonadotrophins. *In* "Handbook of Physiology, Endocrinology IV, Part 2" (E. Knobil and W. H. Sawyer, eds.), pp. 519–550. American Physiological Society, Washington.

Reiter, R. J. (1974b). Circannual reproductive rhythms in mammals related to photoperiod and pineal function: A review. *Chronobiologia* **1**, 365–395.

Reiter, R. J. (1977). *"The Pineal—1977."* Eden, Montreal.

Reiter, R. J. (1978a). *"The Pineal—1978."* Eden, Montreal.

Reiter, R. J. (1978b). Interaction of photoperiod, pineal and seasonal reproduction as exemplified by findings in the hamster. *In* "The Pineal and Reproduction" (R. J. Reiter, ed.), pp. 169–190. Karger, Basel.

Reiter, R. J., and Hester, R. J. (1966a). Neuroendocrinological interrelationships. In "Metabolic Regulation of Physiological Activity" (B. Sacktor, R. J. Reiter, J. E. Wilson, H. J. Smith, C. G. Tiekert, and R. J. Hester, eds.), pp. 13–18. Research Laboratories US Army, Edgewood Arsenal, Md.

Reiter, R. J., and Hester, R. J. (1966b). Interrelationships of the pineal gland, the superior cervical ganglia, and the photoperiod in the regulation of the endocrine system of hamsters. *Endocrinology* **79,** 1168–1170.

Reiter, R. J., and Johnson, L. Y. Depressant action of the pineal gland on pituitary luteinizing hormone and prolactin in male hamsters. *Hormone Research* **5,** 311–320.

Reiter, R. J., and Klein, D. C. (1971). Observations on the pineal gland, the Harderian glands, the retina, and the reproductive organs of adult female rats exposed to continuous light. *Journal of Endocrinology* **51,** 117–125.

Reiter, R. J., and Sorrentino, S., Jr. (1971). Factors influential in determining the gonad-inhibiting activity of the pineal gland. *In* "The Pineal Gland" (G. E. W. Wolstenholme and J. Knight, eds.), pp. 329–340. Churchill Livingstone, London.

Reiter, R. J., and Vaughan, M. K. (1975). A study of indoles which inhibit pineal antigonadotrophic activity in male hamsters. *Endocrine Research Communications* **2,** 299–308.

Reiter, R. J., Vaughan, M. K., Blask, D. E., and Johnson, L. Y. (1974). Melatonin: Its inhibition of pineal antigonadotrophic activity in male hamsters. *Science* **185,** 1169–1171.

Reiter, R. J., Blask, D. E., and Vaughan, M. K. (1975a). A counter antigonadotrophic effect of melatonin in male rats. *Neuroendocrinology* **19,** 72–80.

Reiter, R. J., Vaughan, M. K., and Blask, D. E. (1975b). Possible role of the cerebrospinal fluid in the transport of pineal hormones in mammals. *In* "Brain-Endocrine Interaction II" (K. M. Knigge, D. E. Scott, H. Kobayashi, and S. Ishii, eds.), pp. 337–354. Karger, Basel.

Reiter, R. J., Vaughan, M. K., Vaughan, G. M., Sorrentino, S., Jr., and Donofrio, R. J. (1975c). The pineal gland as an organ of internal secretion. *In* "Frontiers of Pineal Physiology" (M. D. Altschule, ed.), pp. 54–174. MIT, Cambridge.

Reiter, R. J., Vaughan, M. K., and Waring, P. J. (1975d). Studies on the minimal dosage of melatonin required to inhibit pineal antigonadotrophic activity in male golden hamsters. *Hormone Research* **6,** 258–267.

Reiter, R. J., Blask, D. E., Johnson, L. Y., Rudeen, P. K., Vaughan, M. K., and Waring, P. K. (1976a). Melatonin inhibition of reproduction in the male hamster: Its dependency on time of day of administration and on an intact and sympathetically innervated pineal gland. *Neuroendocrinology* **22,** 107–116.

Reiter, R. J., Lukaszyk, A. J., Vaughan, M. K., and Blask, D. E. (1976b). New horizons of pineal research. *American Zoologist* **16,** 93–101.

Reiter, R. J., Welsh, M. G., and Vaughan, M. K. (1976c). Age related changes in the intact and sympathetically denervated gerbil pineal gland. *American Journal of Anatomy* **146,** 427–432.

Reiter, R. J., Rudeen, P. K., Sackman, J. W., Vaughan, M. K., Johnson, L. Y., and Little, J. C. (1977). Subcutaneous melatonin implants inhibit reproductive atrophy in male hamsters induced by daily melatonin injections. *Endocrine Research Communications* **4,** 35–44.

Reiter, R. J., Rudeen, P. K., and Philo, R. C. (1978). Influence of chronic melatonin availability on the reproductive quiescent period in male hamsters exposed to natural photoperiods during the winter months. *In* "Current Studies of Hypothalamic Function, 1978, Vol, 2, Metabolism and Behavior'' (W. L. Veale and K. Lederis, eds), pp. 175-182. Karger, Basel.

Rollag, M. D., and Niswender, G. D. (1976). Radioimmunoassay of serum concentrations of melatonin in sheep exposed to different lighting regimes. *Endocrinology* **98**, 482-489.

Rollag, M. D., Morgan, R. J., and Niswender, G. D. (1978). Utilization of the convoluted integral to calculate rates of melatonin secretion into blood CSF of sheep. *ISA Transactions* **16**, 91-96.

Romijn, H. J. (1975). The ultrastructure of the rabbit pineal gland after sympathectomy, parasympathectomy, continuous illumination, and continuous darkness. *Journal of Neural Transmission* **36**, 183-194.

Rosenbloom, A. A., and Fisher, D. A. (1974). Radioimmunoassay of arginine vasotocin: Studies of bovine pineal. *Endorcrinology* **94**, A-296.

Rosemblum, I. Y., Benson, B., Bria, C. F., McDonnell, D., and Hruby, V. J. (1979). Localization and chemical characterization of a partially purified bovine pineal antigonadotropin. *Journal of Neural Transmission* **44**, 197-220.

Rudeen, P. K., Reiter, R. J., and Vaughan, M. K. (1975). Pineal serotonin-*N*-acetyltransferase activity in four mammalian species. *Neuroscience Letters* **1**, 225-229.

Sackman, J. W., Little, J. C., Rudeen, P. K., Waring, P. J., and Reiter, R. J. (1977). The effects of pineal indoles given late in the light period on reproductive organs and pituitary prolactin levels in male golden hamsters. *Hormone Research* **8**, 84-92.

Saper, C. B., Loewy, A. D., Swanson, L. W., and Cowan, W. M. (1976). Direct hypothalamo-autonomic connections. *Brain Research* **117**, 305-312.

Sheridan, M. N., Reiter, R. J., and Jacobs, J. J. (1969). An interesting anatomical relationship between the hamster pineal gland and the ventricular system of the brain. *Journal of Endocrinology* **45**, 131-132.

Swanson, L. W., and Cowan, W. M. (1975). The efferent connections of the suprachiasmatic nucleus of the hypothalamus. *Journal of Comparative Neurology* **160**, 1-12.

Szentagothai, J., Flerko, B., Mess, B., and Halasz, B. (1968).''Hypothalamic Control of the Anterior Pituitary.'' Akademiai Kiado, Budapest.

Tamarkin, L., Brown, S., and Goldman, B. (1975). Neuroendocrine regulation of seasonal reproductive cycles in the hamster. *Abstracts of the 5th Annual Meeting of the Society of Neuroscience,* New York, p. 458.

Tamarkin, L., Westrom, W. K., Hamill, A. I., and Goldman, B. D. (1976). Effect of melatonin on the reproductive systems of male and female Syrian hamsters: A diurnal rhythm in sensitivity to melatonin. *Endocrinology* **99**, 1534-1541.

Tamarkin, L., Hollister, C. W., Lefebvre, N. G., and Goldman, B. D. (1977). Melatonin induction of gonadal quiescence in pinealectomized Syrian hamsters. *Science* **198**, 953-955.

Turek, F. W., Desjardins, C., and Menaker, M. (1975). Melatonin: Antigonadal and progonadal effects in male golden hamsters. *Science* **190**, 280-282.

Turek, F., Desjardins, C., and Menaker, M. (1976). Differential effects of melatonin on the testes of photoperiodic and nonphotoperiodic rodents. *Biology of Reproduction* **15**, 94-97.

Vaughan, M. K., and Blask, D. E. (1978). Arginine vasotocin—A search for its function in mammals. *In* "The Pineal and Reproduction" (R. J. Reiter, ed.), pp. 90-115. Karger, Basel.

Vaughan, M. K., Reiter, R. J., Vaughan, G. M., Bigelow, L., and Altschule, M. D. (1972). Inhibition of compensatory ovarian hypertrophy in the mouse and vole: A comparison of Altschule's pineal extract, pineal indoles, vasopressin, and oxytocin. *General and Comparative Endocrinology* **18**, 372-377.

Vaughan, M. K., Reiter, R. J., McKinney T., and Vaughan, G. M. (1974). Inhibition of growth of gonadal dependent structures by arginine vasotocin and purified bovine pineal fractions in immature mice and hamsters. *International Journal of Fertility* **19**, 103-106.

Vaughan, M. K., Blask, D. E., Johnson, L. Y., and Reiter, R. J. (1975). Prolactin-releasing activity of arginine vasotocin *in vitro*. *Hormone Research* **6**, 342-350.

Vaughan, M. K., Blask, D. E., Vaughan, G. M., and Reiter, R. J. (1976a). Dose-dependent prolactin releasing activity of arginine vasotocin in intact and pinealectomized estrogen-progesterone treated adult male rats. *Endocrinology* **99**, 1319-1322.

Vaughan, M. K., Reiter, R. J., and Vaughan, G. M. (1976b). Fertility patterns in female mice following treatment with arginine vasotocin. *International Journal of Fertility* **21**, 65-68.

Vaughan, M. K., Vaughan, G. M., Blask, D. E., Barnett, M. P., and Reiter, R. J. (1976c). Arginine vasotocin: Structure-activity relationships and influence on gonadal growth and function. *American Zoologist* **16**, 25-34.

Wartenburg, H. (1968). The mammalian pineal organ: Electron microscopic studies on the fine structure of the pinealocytes, glial cells, and on the perivascular compartment. *Zeitschrift fur Zellforschung und Mikroskopic Anatomie* **86**, 74-97.

Wiener, H. (1968). External chemical messengers. IV., Pineal gland. *New York State Journal of Medicine* **68**, 912-938.

Wilson, B. W., Lynch, H. J., and Ozaki, Y. (1978). 5-Methoxytryptophol in rat serum and pineal: Detection, quantitation, and evidence for daily rhythmicity. *Life Sciences* **23**, 1019-1024.

Wurtman, R. J., and Axelrod, J. (1965). The formation, metabolism, and physiologic effects of melatonin in mammals. *In* "Structure and Function of the Epiphysis Cerebri" (J. A. Kappers and J. P. Schade, eds.), pp. 520-529. Elsevier, Amsterdam.

Wurtman, R. J., Axelrod, J., and Fischer, J. E. (1964). Melatonin synthesis in the pineal gland: Effect of light mediated by the sympathetic nervous system. *Science* **143**, 1329-1330.

# Author Index

Numbers in italics refer to the pages on which the complete references are listed.

## A

Abeles, M., 5, *38*
Abdelaal, A. E., 287, *315*
Abraham, S. F., 285, *315*
Acuna, C., 9, *40,* 64, 66, 67, *81*
Adachi, A., 270, *315*
Adams, R. D., 126, *223, 230*
Adamuk, E., 45, *77*
Adolph, E. F., 282, 290, 298, 299, 302, *315*
Aghajanian, G. K., 249, *255, 261*
Akert, K., *80,* 272, *317*
Albano, J. E., *83*
Albeitazzi, E., 339, *350*
Aleksandrov, Yu. I., 135, *229*
Alexander, M., 74, *81*
Alger, B., 188, *223*
Alger, B. E., 241, *255*
Allman, J. M., 7, 8, 23, 25, 30, *36*
Almli, C. R., 269, *321*
Altman, J., 126, 127, 189, 194, *223*
Altschule, M. D., 339, 340, *355*
Amit, Z., 244, 250, *255*
Andersen, R. A., 14, 21, 22, 24, 39, 30, *37*
Anderson, B., 265, *315, 316*
Andrews, R. J., 97, *120, 121*
Angelergues, R., 126, 158, *223*
Antem, A., 236, *256*
Antin, J., 297, *316*
Apter, J. T., 45, *77*
Arduini, A., 127, 180, *225*
Arnauld, E., 269, 294, *316, 321*
Arnold, A. P., 101, 111, *120, 123*
Arthur, J. B., 253, *255*
Ashe, J. H., 236, 237, 243, 251, 252, 253, *259, 260*
Assaf, S. Y., 273, *318*
Astruc, J., 76, *77*
Atkin, L. M., 22, *40*
Axelrod, J., 326, 327, 328, 329, 334, *350, 352, 356*

## B

Baizer, J. S., 61, 63, 74, *77, 82*
Baker, J. F., 30, *40*

Baker, L. J., 240, *255*
Baker, T. B., 240, *255*
Baldwin, F. M., 111, *120*
Baleydier, C., 52, 53, *77*
Bambridge, R., 251, *256*
Banks, A. F., 336, *350*
Barbanti-Silva, C., 339, *350*
Barbizet, J., 126, *223*
Barchfiel, J. L., 9, *37*
Bard, P., 9, *41, 42*
Baril, L. L., 246, *261*
Barker, D. J., 126, 127, 160, *230*
Barker, J. P., 282, *315*
Barker, L. M., 234, 239, *256*
Barlett, J. R., 61, 70, *77, 78*
Barnett, M. P., 345, *356*
Barnett, S. A., 240, *256*
Baum, M., 244, *255*
Bayer, S. A., 126, 127, 189, 194, *223*
Beaton, R., 76, *77*
Beecher, M. D., 95, *124*
Bellows, R. T., 300, *316*
Bender, D. B., 5, *38*
Bennett, C. T., 283, 300, *317*
Bennett, T. L., 127, 181, 202, *223, 228*
Bensinger, R., 346, *350*
Benson, B., 342, 343, 346, *350, 351, 352, 355*
Benson, D. A., 76, *79*
Benevento, L. A., *37,* 63, *77*
Berger, B. D., 243, 248, 252, *256*
Berger, R., 274, *318*
Berger, T. W., 128, 132, *223*
Berlyne, D. E., *77*
Berman, N., 46, 47, *78*
Berman, R. F., 253, *258*
Bernard, C., 290, *316*
Best, M. R., 234, *256*
Best, P. J., 252, *256*
Bhatnager, R. K., 326, *352*
Bigelow, L., 339, 340, *355*
Bioulac, B., 269, 294, *321*
Bishop, G. H., *37*
Bizzi, E., 64, *77*
Black, A., 189, *227*
Black, A. H., 128, 204, 207, 213, *223, 231*

357

Luria, A. R., 31, *39*
Lynch, G., 241, *257*
Lynch, G. S., 132, *223*
Lynch, H. J., 329, 340, 341, *352, 353, 356*
Lynch, J. C., 9, *40,* 64, 66, 67, *80, 81*

**M**

McCaa, R. E., 287, *320*
McCleary, R. A., 126, 127, 159, 160, 194, *227, 230*
McDonald, R. H., Jr., 285, *320*
McDonnell, D., *355*
McEwen, B. S., 112, 115, *122*
McFarland, D. J., 272, *318, 319*
McGaugh, J. L., 251, *258, 259*
McGowan, B. K., 239, 240, 249, 252, *259*
McIntosh, H., 243, *256*
McIntosh, J., 5, *38*
McIsaac, W. M., 329, 340, *352*
McKinney, T., 343, 346, *355, 356*
Mackintosh, N. J., 157, 172, *227, 229*
McNeely, D. A., 215, *228*
Madarasz, I., 127, 181, 194, *225*
Maddison, S., 291, 302, 303, *318*
Magnin, M., 52, 53, *77*
Magoun, H. W., 69, *80, 81*
Makous, W., 236, *259*
Malamud, M., 126, *227*
Malmo, R. B., 269, *318*
Malpeli, J. G., 17, 63, *40, 82*
Malvin, R. L., 286, *318*
Manning, E., 93, 94, *124*
Margules, D. L., 249, *259*
Marler, P., 110, 118, 119, *122, 124*
Marrocco, R. T., *80*
Marshall, W. H., 9, *41, 42,* 296, *319*
Martin, J. R., 247, *259*
Martini, L., 340, *351*
Mathers, L. H., 63, *80*
Matsunami, K., *82*
Matsushima, S., 325, *352*
Matthews, C. D., 341, *351, 352*
Matthews, M. J., 342, 343, 346, *350, 352*
Means, L. W., 127, 199, *227*
Mehta, V. H., 249, *258*
Meibach, R. C., 179, *227*
Meizer, F. M., 30, *40*

Menaker, M., 110, *122,* 330, 334, 335, *355*
Mercer, P. F., 287, *315*
Merzenich, M. M., 9, 10, 11, 13, 14, 16, 18, 21, 22, 26, 27, 28, 29, 30, *37, 39, 40*
Mess, B., 326, *355*
Mesulam, M. M., 74, *80*
Metfessel, M., 111, 118, *120, 123*
Mical, R. S., 339, *351, 353*
Micco, D. J., 211, *227*
Michael, C. R., 61, *81*
Middlebrooks, J. C., 28, *39*
Milcu, S. M., 343, *352*
Miller, C. R., 190, 239, 252, *259*
Miller, J. D., 128, 131, 132, 134, 190, *225*
Miller, J. M., 76, *77*
Miller, R. F., 44, *81*
Milner, B., 126, 127, 128, *227, 228, 229*
Milner, T. A., 132, *223*
Minnich, J., 348, *351*
Miselis, R. R., 274, *318*
Mishkin, M., 63, *80,* 127, 164, *227*
Mogenson, G. J., 202, *231,* 264, 273, 274, 287, 308, *315, 318, 320*
Mohler, C. W., 46, 48, 49, 51, 52, 53, 54, 55, 56, 57, 58, 59, 60, 61, 62, 64, 65, 76, *81, 83*
Moody, D. B., 95, *124*
Mook, D. G., 290, *319*
Moore, J. W., 127, 202, 203, 207, 211, 212, *227, 229*
Moore, R. Y., 161, *227,* 325, 326, *352*
Moray, N., 72, *81*
Morest, D. K., 22, *39,* 236, 247, 249, *259*
Morgan, M. J., 95, *121*
Morgan, R. J., 341, *355*
Morrell, J. I, 112, *123*
Moruzzi, G., 69, *81*
Mott, F. W., 2, *39*
Mountcastle, V. B., 9, 17, 18, *39, 40,* 64, 66, 67, *80, 81, 83*
Mouw, D., 286, *318*
Mulligan, J. A., 118, *123*
Mundl, W. J., 269, *318*
Murphy, L. R., 252, *259*
Murton, R. K., 110, *122*
Myers, R. E., 63, *81*
Myerson, F. M., 30, *40*

# Subject Index

COLORADO COLLEGE LIBRARY
COLORADO SPRINGS,
COLORADO